T0198271

COVID-19 Infection

Editors

RACHEL A. BENDER IGNACIO
RAJESH T. GANDHI

INFECTIOUS DISEASE CLINICS
OF NORTH AMERICA

www.id.theclinics.com

Consulting Editor
HELEN W. BOUCHER

June 2022 • Volume 36 • Number 2

ELSEVIER

1600 John F. Kennedy Boulevard • Suite 1800 • Philadelphia, Pennsylvania, 19103-2899.
http://www.theclinics.com

INFECTIOUS DISEASE CLINICS OF NORTH AMERICA Volume 36, Number 2
June 2022 ISSN 0891–5520, ISBN-13: 978-0-323-91979-1

Editor: Kerry Holland
Developmental Editor: Hannah Almira Lopez

Infectious Disease Clinics of North America (ISSN 0891–5520) is published in March, June, September, and December by Elsevier Inc., 360 Park Avenue South, New York, NY 10010-1710. Periodicals postage paid at New York, NY and additional mailing offices. Subscription prices are $357.00 per year for US individuals, $950.00 per year for US institutions, $100.00 per year for US students, $408.00 per year for Canadian individuals, $979.00 per year for Canadian institutions, $445.00 per year for international individuals, $979.00 per year for international institutions, $100.00 per year for Canadian students, and $200.00 per year for international students. To receive student rate, orders must be accompained by name of affiliated institution, date of term, and the *signature* of program/residency coordinator on institution letterhead. Orders will be billed at individual rate until proof of status is received. Foreign air speed delivery is included in all *Clinics* subscription prices. All prices are subject to change without notice. **POSTMASTER:** Send address changes to *Infectious Disease Clinics of North America*, Elsevier Health Sciences Division, Subcription Customer Service, 3251 Riverport Lane, Maryland Heights, MO 63043. **Customer Service: 1-800-654-2452 (US). From outside of the US and Canada, call 1-314-447-8871. Fax: 1-314-447-8029. E-mail: JournalsCustomerService-usa@elsevier.com (print support) or JournalsOnlineSupport-usa@elsevier.com (online support).**

Infectious Disease Clinics of North America is also published in Spanish by Editorial Inter-Médica, Junin 917, 1er A 1113, Buenos Aires, Argentina.

Reprints. For copies of 100 or more, of articles in this publication, please contact the Commercial Reprints Department, Elsevier Inc., 360 Park Avenue South, New York, New York 10010-1710. Tel. 212-633-3874, Fax: 212-633-3820, E-mail: reprints@elsevier.com.

Infectious Disease Clinics of North America is covered in *MEDLINE/PubMed (Index Medicus), Current Contents/ Clinical Medicine, Science Citation Alert, SCISEARCH,* and *Research Alert.*

Contributors

CONSULTING EDITOR

HELEN W. BOUCHER, MD, FIDSA, FACP
Director, Infectious Diseases Fellowship Program, Division of Geographic Medicine and Infectious Diseases, Tufts Medical Center, Associate Professor of Medicine, Tufts University School of Medicine, Boston, Massachusetts

EDITORS

RACHEL A. BENDER IGNACIO, MD, MPH
Assistant Professor, Division of Allergy and Infectious Diseases, University of Washington, Medical Director, COVID-19 Clinical Research Clinic, Assistant Professor, Vaccine and Infectious Diseases Division, Fred Hutchinson Cancer Research Center, Seattle, Washington

RAJESH T. GANDHI, MD
Director of HIV Clinical Services and Education, Massachusetts General Hospital, Co-Director, Harvard University Center for AIDS Research, Professor of Medicine, Harvard Medical School, Boston, Massachusetts

AUTHORS

MICHELE P. ANDRASIK, EDM, PhD
Senior Staff Scientist, Vaccine and Infectious Disease Division, Fred Hutchinson, Seattle, Washington

MARWAN M. AZAR, MD, FAST, FIDSA
Assistant Professor, Department of Infectious Diseases, Yale School of Medicine, New Haven, Connecticut

TAISON D. BELL, MD, MBA
Assistant Professor, Internal Medicine, Divisions of Pulmonary/Critical Care and Infectious Diseases and International Health, University of Virginia School of Medicine, Charlottesville, Virginia

ADARSH BHIMRAJ, MD
Department of Infectious Diseases, Cleveland Clinic, Cleveland, Ohio

ERIC J. CHOW, MD, MS, MPH
Division of Allergy and Infectious Diseases, Department of Medicine, University of Washington, Seattle, Washington

BIANCA B. CHRISTENSEN, MD, MPH
Medical Microbiology Fellow, Department of Pathology, Massachusetts General Hospital, Boston, Massachusetts

JANET A. ENGLUND, MD
Division of Pediatric Infectious Diseases, Department of Pediatrics, University of Washington, Seattle Children's Research Institute, Seattle, Washington

ZERELDA ESQUER GARRIGOS, MD
Division of Infectious Diseases, University of Mississippi Medical Center, Jackson, Mississippi

TERESA H. EVERING, MD, MS
Assistant Professor, Department of Medicine, Division of Infectious Diseases, Weill Cornell Medicine, New York, New York

WILLIAM O. HAHN, MD
Division of Infectious Diseases, Department of Medicine, University of Washington, Seattle, Washington

R. ALFONSO HERNANDEZ ACOSTA, MD
Department of Internal Medicine, John H. Stroger Jr. Hospital of Cook County, Chicago, Illinois

DAVID C. HOOPER, MD
Chief, Infection Control Unit, Professor of Medicine, Associate Chief, Division of Infectious Diseases, Massachusetts General Hospital, Harvard Medical School, Boston, Massachusetts

ALUKO A. HOPE, MD, MSCE
Associate Professor of Medicine, Division of Pulmonary, Allergy, and Critical Care Medicine, School of Medicine, Oregon Health & Science University

NIYATI JAKHARIA, MD
Infectious Diseases Fellow, Department of Medicine, Division of Infectious Diseases, Stanford University School of Medicine, Stanford, California

DENISE J. JAMIESON, MD, MPH
James Robert McCord Professor and Chair, Emory University School of Medicine, Department of Gynecology and Obstetrics, Atlanta, Georgia

JONATHAN Z. LI, MD, MMSc
Brigham and Women's Hospital, Harvard Medical School, Boston, Massachusetts

YIJIA LI, MD
Brigham and Women's Hospital, Massachusetts General Hospital, Harvard Medical School, Boston, Massachusetts

JASMINE R. MARCELIN, MD
Division of Infectious Diseases, University of Nebraska Medical Center, Omaha, Nebraska

ALIKA K. MAUNAKEA, PhD
Associate Professor, Department of Anatomy, Biochemistry, and Physiology, John A. Burns School of Medicine, University of Hawaii, Honolulu, Hawaii

ERIC A. MEYEROWITZ, MD
Montefiore Medical Center, Bronx, New York

LINDA OSESO, MPH
Project Manager, Vaccine and Infectious Disease Division, Fred Hutchinson, Seattle, Washington

SONJA A. RASMUSSEN, MD, MS
Professor, Department of Pediatrics, Department of Obstetrics and Gynecology, University of Florida College of Medicine, University of Florida, Department of Epidemiology, University of Florida College of Public Health and Health Professions and College of Medicine, Gainesville, Florida

AARON RICHTERMAN, MD, MPH
Hospital of the University of Pennsylvania, Philadelphia, Pennsylvania

CARLOS E. RODRIGUEZ-DIAZ, PhD, MPH
Associate Professor, Department of Prevention and Community Health, Milken Institute School of Public Health, The George Washington University, Washington, DC

ADRIENNE E. SHAPIRO, MD, PhD
Acting Assistant Professor, Department of Global Health, Department of Medicine, Division of Allergy and Infectious Diseases, University of Washington, Seattle, Washington

ERICA S. SHENOY, MD, PhD
Associate Chief, Infection Control Unit, Associate Professor of Medicine, Division of Infectious Diseases, Massachusetts General Hospital, Harvard Medical School, Boston, Massachusetts

AMY HIRSCH SHUMAKER, PharmD, BCPS, AAHIVP
Clinical Pharmacy Specialist, Infectious Disease, Cleveland, Ohio; Department of Pharmacy, VA Northeast Ohio Healthcare System, School of Medicine, Case Western Reserve University

ARUNA K. SUBRAMANIAN, MD
Clinical Professor, Department of Medicine, Division of Infectious Diseases, Stanford University School of Medicine, Stanford, California

SARAH E. TURBETT, MD
Instructor, Departments of Medicine and Pathology, Massachusetts General Hospital, Boston, Massachusetts

PRAKHAR VIJAYVARGIYA, MBBS
Division of Infectious Diseases, University of Mississippi Medical Center, Jackson, Mississippi

STEPHAUN WALLACE, PhD
Staff Scientist, Vaccine and Infectious Disease Division, Fred Hutchinson, Seattle, Washington

KARINA WALTERS, PhD
Co-Director/Full Professor, Indigenous Wellness Research Institute, University of Washington, Seattle, Washington

ZANTHIA WILEY, MD
Division of Infectious Diseases, Department of Medicine, Emory University, Infectious Diseases Clinic, Atlanta, Georgia

MARISA L. WINKLER, MD, PhD
Infectious Disease Fellow, Infection Control Unit, Division of Infectious Diseases, Massachusetts General Hospital, Harvard Medical School, Boston, Massachusetts

MICHI YUKAWA, MD, MPH
Clinical Professor, Division of Geriatrics, University of California, San Francisco, Geriatric Palliative and Extended Care, San Francisco VA Medical Center, San Francisco, California

Contents

Preface: COVID-19: Where We Are, Where We Need to Be   xiii

Rachel A. Bender Ignacio and Rajesh T. Gandhi

COVID-19 Pathogenesis and Clinical Manifestations   231

R. Alfonso Hernandez Acosta, Zerelda Esquer Garrigos, Jasmine R. Marcelin, and Prakhar Vijayvargiya

> In this review, we summarize the current knowledge about the virology, the host-pathogen interactions and pathogenesis of coronavirus disease 2019 in humans. We also describe the various clinical presentations of the disease including respiratory system and extrapulmonary manifestations.

SARS-Cov-2 Virology   251

Yijia Li and Jonathan Z. Li

> Severe acute respiratory syndrome coronavirus 2 (SARS-Cov-2) was first identified in 2020 and has led to an unprecedented global pandemic. Understanding the virology behind SARS-Cov-2 infection has provided key insights into our efforts to develop antiviral agents and control the COVID-19 pandemic. In this review, the authors focus on the genomic features of SARS-Cov-2, its intrahost and interhost evolution, viral dynamics in respiratory tract, and systemic dissemination.

SARS-Cov-2 Transmission and Prevention in the Era of the Delta Variant   267

Eric A. Meyerowitz and Aaron Richterman

> The severe acute respiratory syndrome coronavirus 2 (SARS-Cov-2) delta variant transmits much more rapidly than prior SARS-Cov-2 viruses. The primary mode of transmission is via short range aerosols that are emitted from the respiratory tract of an index case. There is marked heterogeneity in the spread of this virus, with 10% to 20% of index cases contributing to 80% of secondary cases, while most index cases have no subsequent transmissions. Vaccination, ventilation, masking, eye protection, and rapid case identification with contact tracing and isolation can all decrease the transmission of this virus.

Awakening: The Unveiling of Historically Unaddressed Social Inequities During the COVID-19 Pandemic in the United States   295

Michele P. Andrasik, Alika K. Maunakea, Linda Oseso, Carlos E. Rodriguez-Diaz, Stephaun Wallace, Karina Walters, and Michi Yukawa

> The violence and victimization brought by colonization and slavery and justified for over a century by race-based science have resulted in enduring inequities for black, Indigenous and people of color (BIPOC) across the United States. This is particularly true if BIPOC individuals have other intersecting devalued identities. We highlight how such longstanding inequities paved the way for the disproportionate burdens of

coronavirus disease 2019 (COVID-19) among the BIPOC populations across the country and provide recommendations on how to improve COVID-19 mitigation strategies with the goal of eliminating disparities.

Infection Prevention and Control of Severe Acute Respiratory Syndrome Coronavirus 2 in Health Care Settings   309

Marisa L. Winkler, David C. Hooper, and Erica S. Shenoy

The authors describe infection prevention and control approaches to severe acute respiratory syndrome coronavirus 2 in the health care setting, including a review of the chain of transmission and the hierarchy of controls, which are cornerstones of infection control and prevention. The authors also discuss lessons learned from nosocomial transmission events.

Laboratory Diagnosis for SARS-CoV-2 Infection   327

Bianca B. Christensen, Marwan M. Azar, and Sarah E. Turbett

The optimal diagnostic test for SARS-CoV-2 infection should be selected based on a patient's clinical syndrome and presentation in relation to symptom onset. Molecular testing, most often reverse-transcriptase polymerase chain reaction, offers the highest sensitivity and specificity during acute infection, whereas antigen testing can also be useful for acute diagnosis when rapid turnaround of results is necessary or if molecular testing is unavailable. Serologic testing is often reserved for identifying individuals with prior or late COVID-19 infection.

Pharmacologic Treatment and Management of Coronavirus Disease 2019   349

Amy Hirsch Shumaker and Adarsh Bhimraj

Over the last 2 years, there has been gradual and sustained progress toward our understanding of pharmacotherapy for coronavirus disease 2019 (COVID-19) as a result of large- and small-scale randomized controlled trials. Numerous new and repurposed treatments have been evaluated; some have demonstrated benefit in clinically important outcomes like mortality and hospitalization, and optimism for oral antiviral treatments is growing. Given the rapidly evolving landscape of COVID-19 treatments, frontline clinicians should use treatment and management guidelines to guide their approach to each patient, with the individual's severity and location of illness in mind to appreciate the nuances in clinical evidence.

COVID-19 in the Critically Ill Patient   365

Taison D. Bell

The COVID-19 pandemic has led to significant mortality in the United States with more than 800,000 deaths in 2020 and 2021. The proportion of patients with COVID-19 who develop severe disease varies but is decreasing over time with growing population immunity and improved therapeutic options. Patients who are 65 years and older represent the largest proportion of deaths from COVID-19. Additional risk factors include immunosuppression and chronic medical conditions. Vaccination dramatically reduces the risk of severe COVID-19. Although critical illness from

COVID-19 is mostly driven by respiratory disease, critical illness can manifest in several ways and affect several organ systems.

Postacute Sequelae of Severe Acute Respiratory Syndrome Coronavirus 2 Infection   379

Aluko A. Hope and Teresa H. Evering

Postacute sequelae of severe acute respiratory syndrome coronavirus 2 (SARS-CoV-2) or long coronavirus disease (COVID) is an emerging syndrome characterized by multiple persisting or newly emergent symptoms following the acute phase of SARS-CoV-2 infection. For affected patients, these prolonged symptoms can have a relapsing and remitting course and may be associated with disability and frequent health care utilization. Although many symptom-driven treatments are available, management remains challenging and often requires a multidisciplinary approach. This article summarizes the emerging consensus on definitions, epidemiology, and pathophysiology of long COVID and discusses what is understood about prevention, evaluation, and treatment of this syndrome.

COVID-19 in the Immunocompromised Host, Including People with Human Immunodeficiency Virus   397

Niyati Jakharia, Aruna K. Subramanian, and Adrienne E. Shapiro

This review describes the incidence, epidemiology, and risk factors for mortality of COVID-19 in immunocompromised patients, including persons with human immunodeficiency virus. It describes various preventive measures, including vaccines and their effectiveness and the role of monoclonal antibodies for pre-exposure prophylaxis. It also reviews the different treatment options for immunocompromised individuals, including antivirals, monoclonal antibodies, and immunomodulators. Lastly, it describes the impact of COVID-19 on transplantation and continuity care of this population.

COVID-19 and Pregnancy   423

Sonja A. Rasmussen and Denise J. Jamieson

Pregnancy seems to be a risk factor for severe disease with COVID-19. Although SARS-CoV-2 intrauterine transmission seems to be rare, most studies show COVID-19 during pregnancy increases the risk for pregnancy complications, with higher risk among those with severe disease compared with those mildly affected. Studies suggest that COVID-19 vaccination during pregnancy is safe and effective. Antibodies to SARS-CoV-2 have been found in umbilical cord blood and breast milk following maternal vaccination, which might provide protection to the infant. However, vaccination rates during pregnancy remain low. Studies are needed to understand ways to address SARS-CoV-2 vaccine hesitancy among pregnant persons.

Severe Acute Respiratory Syndrome Coronavirus 2 Infections in Children   435

Eric J. Chow and Janet A. Englund

Severe acute respiratory syndrome coronavirus 2 (SARS-CoV-2) infections in children generally have milder presentations, but severe disease can occur in all ages. MIS-C and persistent post-acute COVID-19 symptoms can be experienced by children with previous infection and emphasize the need for infection prevention. Optimal treatment for COVID-19 is not known, and clinical trials should include children to guide therapy. Vaccines are the best tool at preventing infection and severe outcomes of COVID-19. Children suffered disproportionately during the pandemic not only from SARS-CoV-2 infection but because of disruptions to daily life, access to primary care, and worsening income inequalities.

COVID-19 Vaccines   481

William O. Hahn and Zanthia Wiley

This article is a narrative review of the rapidly moving coronavirus disease 2019 vaccine field with an emphasis on clinical efficacy established in both randomized trials and postmarketing surveillance of clinically available vaccines. We review the major clinical trials that supported authorization for general use of the Janssen (Ad.26.CoV2), Pfizer-BioNTech (BNT162b2), and Moderna (mRNA-1273) vaccines and the publicly available postmarketing information with the goal of providing a broad, clinically relevant comparison of efficacy and safety. This review is primarily focused on the US market.

INFECTIOUS DISEASE CLINICS OF NORTH AMERICA

FORTHCOMING ISSUES

September 2022
Lyme Disease and the Expanded Spectrum
of Blacklegged Tick-Borne Infections
Robert P. Smith, *Editor*

December 2022
Complex Infectious Disease Issues in the
Intensive Care Unit
Sameer Kadri and Naomi P. O'Grady,
Editors

RECENT ISSUES

March 2022
Pediatric Infections
Rebecca G. Same and Jason G. Newland,
Editors

December 2021
Infection Prevention and Control in
Healthcare, Part II: Clinical Management of
Infections
Keith S. Kaye and Sorabh Dhar, *Editors*

September 2021
Infection Prevention and Control in
Healthcare, Part I: Facility Planning
Keith S. Kaye and Sorabh Dhar, *Editors*

Preface

COVID-19: Where We Are, Where We Need to Be

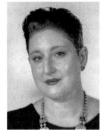 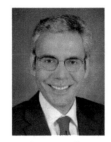

Rachel A. Bender Ignacio,   Rajesh T. Gandhi, MD
MD, MPH

Editors

The COVID-19 pandemic has drastically changed life across the globe. The severe acute respiratory syndrome coronavirus 2 (SARS-CoV-2) has directly caused hundreds of millions of cases and millions of deaths and has indirectly had far-reaching impacts on health and society. Many of the direct and indirect impacts of the COVID-19 pandemic disproportionately impact marginalized and less-resourced persons and communities around the world, and the disparate impacts, including wide-ranging differences in public health and political responses, have meant that we are all living through the same pandemic, but having vastly different experiences of its risks and hardships. In particular, the COVID-19 pandemic, and the response to it, has highlighted long-standing gaps in pathogen surveillance, public health infrastructure, access to care and social services, as well as the global inequities that cause worse health outcomes. At the same time, the scientific community has had remarkable achievements in two short (or very long) years. Within 4 months of the first detected case of the novel coronavirus infection in December 2019, there were many vaccines in human clinical trials, and several safe and effective vaccines were authorized for use less than a year from when the SARS-CoV-2 genome was sequenced. Now, those vaccines must be deployed around the world. We have novel and repurposed treatments for COVID-19, although there is much more that must be done to develop and equitably distribute safe and effective treatments that retain activity in the face of new variants of concern. We understand much more about SARS-CoV-2 transmission and how to prevent COVID-19 through a variety of nonpharmacologic measures; now we must overcome lingering distrust and societal divisions to implement the tools that we have.

Because nearly as much has been published on COVID-19 as has been published on HIV since the beginning of that pandemic, it is a dizzying task to stay current on

Infect Dis Clin N Am 36 (2022) xiii–xv
https://doi.org/10.1016/j.idc.2022.02.003
0891-5520/22/© 2022 Published by Elsevier Inc.

id.theclinics.com

both the scientific and the clinical advances in COVID-19. We hope that this *Infectious Disease Clinics of North America* issue provides a thorough primer on virology, pathogenesis, transmission, clinical manifestations, treatments, and vaccines, with important information pertaining to specific risk populations, such as pregnant persons, children, individuals with different types of immune compromise, and the risks disproportionately born by those with societally marginalized identities. We also know that new and ever-changing information will make some of what is included here outdated within a short period of time. This is inevitable given the record-breaking pace at which new knowledge is being generated and new interventions that are being developed to respond to this novel pathogen and its new variants. Our goal is to have provided foundational understanding for each of these topics, written by established and emerging leaders in their respective fields, such that as new information emerges, these summaries can continue to form a solid knowledge base and stepping-off point.

In addition to summarizing where we are in our understanding of COVID-19, we also define several areas where more progress is needed to bring us to where we need to be. First, we need to know more about the pathophysiology and treatment of various phenotypes of "long-COVID" or postacute sequelae of COVID-19. Second, we need more direct-acting antivirals that do not have some of the shortcomings of our current treatments. Third, we need vaccines that provide durable protection against a broader array of variants, a universal coronavirus vaccine. Fourth, outside the clinical sphere, we are in urgent need of a better understanding of how to improve indoor ventilation for the nonmedical spaces in which the world works, goes to school, and lives. Finally, we need to achieve a more equitable distribution of diagnostics, vaccines, and therapeutics around the globe. The lesson of COVID-19, and of HIV before it, is that a global pandemic requires a coordinated and equitable global response.

It is our privilege to have the opportunity to work with colleagues with wide-ranging expertise to create a comprehensive anthology for clinicians summarizing the current knowledge about COVID-19 just a few years since its first impact in the human population. We hope that this first COVID-19 issue of *Infectious Disease Clinics of North America* provides a succinct and accessible review of the current knowledge in early

2022, and, through these insights, sets the stage for how we might more effectively respond to COVID-19 and new pandemics in the future.

Rachel A. Bender Ignacio, MD, MPH
Division of Allergy and Infectious Diseases
University of Washington

Medical Director
COVID-19 Clinical Research Clinic
Vaccine and Infectious Diseases Division
Fred Hutchinson Cancer Research Center
Seattle, WA 98109, USA

Rajesh T. Gandhi, MD
Director, HIV Clinical Services and Education
Massachusetts General Hospital
Co-Director, Harvard University Center for AIDS Research
Professor of Medicine
Harvard Medical School
Boston, MA, USA

E-mail addresses:
rbi13@uw.edu (R.A. Bender Ignacio)
rgandhi@mgh.harvard.edu (R.T. Gandhi)

COVID-19 Pathogenesis and Clinical Manifestations

R. Alfonso Hernandez Acosta, MD[a], Zerelda Esquer Garrigos, MD[b],
Jasmine R. Marcelin, MD[c], Prakhar Vijayvargiya, MBBS[b],*

KEYWORDS

- COVID-19 • Severe acute respiratory syndrome coronavirus 2 • Pathogenesis
- Clinical manifestations • SARS-CoV-2

KEY POINTS

- SARS-CoV-2 can cause widespread damage in different organ systems mediated by the host's immune response. Severity of illness can range from asymptomatic infection to severe multiorgan failure.
- While SARS-CoV-2 is a respiratory virus, COVID-19 affects many organs and has a variety of clinical presentations. In this review, we cover various clinical manifestations of COVID-19 infection.
- Postacute sequelae of COVID-19 (also known as long COVID) is an area of developing knowledge that will require ongoing surveillance to fully characterize. It is generally defined as persistent symptoms for more than 3 months after initial infection.

INTRODUCTION

Severe acute respiratory syndrome coronavirus 2 (SARS-CoV-2) is a member of the *Betacoronavirus* genus (which also includes SARS 1 and Middle East respiratory syndrome–related coronavirus [MERS]), which are large positive-sense single-stranded RNA viruses (estimated size 70–200 nm) with zoonotic origins and transmissible from person to person. Coronaviruses are named after the projections from their membrane (*Corona*, Latin, "crown").[1] When it was first described, the virus had been named 2019-novel coronavirus, but was renamed SARS-CoV-2 owing to a greater similarity with SARS-CoV than initially thought. Since its emergence in late 2019 with the first cases described in Wuhan, China, its human-to-human transmission is clear, with uncounted active infections and millions of deaths worldwide. Furthermore, airborne spread[2] and transmission by asymptomatic individuals[3] further add to its potential for infection.

[a] Department of Internal Medicine, John H. Stroger Jr. Hospital of Cook County, Chicago, IL, USA; [b] Division of Infectious Diseases, University of Mississippi Medical Center, Jackson, MS, USA; [c] Division of Infectious Diseases, University of Nebraska Medical Center, Omaha, NE, USA
* Corresponding author. Division of Infectious Diseases, University of Mississippi Medical Center, 2500 N State Street, Jackson, MS 39216.
E-mail address: pvijayvargiya@umc.edu

Infect Dis Clin N Am 36 (2022) 231–249
https://doi.org/10.1016/j.idc.2022.01.003   id.theclinics.com
0891-5520/22/© 2022 Elsevier Inc. All rights reserved.

Global collaboration and sequencing technologies have helped to uncover the pathogenic mechanisms behind SARS-Cov-2 infection and its associated clinical manifestations, collectively called coronavirus disease 2019 (COVID-19). Nevertheless, COVID-19 remains a novel disease and its complete pathogenesis is yet to be elucidated. Several studies have been conducted to better understand the host–virus interactions and pathogenesis to develop strategies for prevention and treatment. Insight from previous infections caused by coronaviruses such as SARS and MERS has also been useful to understand the pathogenesis of this new virus. Even though several promising new (and repurposed) treatments are being studied, there is yet to be a clear and effective treatment modality. The development of effective vaccines as part of preventive strategies has also played a significant role in controlling this pandemic.[4] In this article, we review clinical and experimental evidence available for pathogenesis of COVID-19 and highlight various clinical presentations in human infection.

PATHOGENESIS
Structure of SARS-CoV-2

Coronaviruses have the largest RNA viral genomes, ranging from 26,000 to 32,000 bases,[5] and the genome is made up almost entirely of protein coding sequences.[6] SARS-CoV-2 is the seventh known coronavirus capable of causing human infection.[7] Whole genome sequencing revealed that SARS-CoV-2 has genomic similarities to be placed in the same *Betacoronavirus* clade like SARS-CoV, MERS-CoV, and SARS-like bat CoV; however, phylogenetic analysis and amino acid sequences have revealed enough differences in SARS-CoV-2 to confer structural and functional difference from other coronaviruses.[8] The genome of SARS-CoV-2 is about 29.9 kB[9] in length (in contrast, SARS-CoV is about 29.7 kB long[10]) of which about 79% to 82% includes a sequence[11] homology to SARS-CoV and 50% to MERS-CoV.[8] Unlike SARS-CoV, SARS-CoV-2 possesses a distinguishing polybasic cleavage site (RRAR) that is cleaved by furin and other proteases. The presence of this furin cleavage site has been suggested to confer SARS-CoV-2 with greater transmissibility than SARS-CoV and enhances its virulence.[12] Like SARS-CoV and other coronaviruses, SARS-CoV-2 codes for four structural proteins: spike (S), membrane (M), envelope (E), and nucleocapsid (N). The viral envelope is created by S, E, and M proteins together, whereas the N protein binds to the viral RNA.[13]

Origin and Transmission

Coronaviruses are diverse and pathogenic to a variety of animals, including pigs, cows, dogs, cats, and chickens. Bats act as a reservoir for coronaviruses, including SARS-CoV-2.[6] When the first cases of pneumonia were described in the Hubei province in China in late 2019, genome sequencing and phylogenetic analysis identified the pathogen as a novel coronavirus with bat and pangolin genetic sequences, further adding evidence to a zoonotic origin of the virus.[14]

Viral Entry and Initial Infection

Infection occurs when the viral particles are inhaled, enter the airways, and bind to the receptors on host cell surface. Like other coronaviruses, the S protein of SARS-CoV-2 binds to the angiotensin-converting enzyme 2 (ACE2), a metalloproteinase found in large amounts in airway epithelial and endothelial cells that undergoes a conformational change to permit the fusion of viral and host cell membranes.[15] Although this mechanism is shared by SARS-CoV, a recent study using biophysical assays found that the S protein of SARS-CoV-2 binds 10 to 20 times more strongly to ACE2.[16] The higher binding affinity to ACE2 has been proposed to be responsible for increased viral transmissibility and severity of disease compared with SARS-CoV.

The S protein is composed of 2 subunits: S1 and S2.[17] When the S1 subunit attaches to the ACE2 receptor on the host cell, a transmembrane protease, serine 2 (TMPRSS2) cleaves the S protein to reveal S2 subunit, and ACE2. The S protein undergoes dramatic conformational changes, leading to the fusion of the viral membrane with the host cell. The viral particle is then engulfed in an endosome. The virion escapes the endosome when it is cleaved by a host cell protease, cathepsin, or by a decrease in the pH (acidification).[18] Cathepsin has been proposed as a therapeutic target to prevent infection with SARS-CoV-2.[19]

High expression of ACE2 on the surface of lung alveolar epithelium and enterocytes of the small intestine was proposed to contribute to the viral entry of SARS-CoV, a mechanism that SARS-CoV-2 likely mirrors.[20] Besides these locations, ACE2 is widely expressed in various human tissues, including the heart, kidneys, and arterial and venous endothelial cells. The presence of ACE2 in these tissues likely contributes to extrapulmonary manifestations, such as diarrhea, acute renal injury, cardiac injury, and vascular endothelial damage with multisystem organ failure.[21] Children have lower ACE2 expression, which might explain lower early COVID-19 acquisition rates in children but higher rate of multisystem inflammatory syndrome in older children. The tissues expressing ACE2 do not participate equally in the pathogenesis of COVID-19, suggesting that other factors are involved in contributing to tissue damage.[22]

PHASES OF INFECTION

Early after the discovery of SARS-CoV-2, COVID-19 infection was described in 2 phases: a viral response phase and a host inflammatory response phase (also referred to as the cytokine storm phase) (**Fig. 1**). This general principle has remained relevant over time, but the relative contribution of each phase to the illness remains to be characterized. Viral loads of SARS-CoV-2 are high in the initial days of infection and decrease steadily over time in immunocompetent hosts (**Fig. 2**). In these first few days, SARS-CoV-2 infection can range from asymptomatic to mildly symptomatic in most patients, and generally includes upper respiratory symptoms and/or a systemic influenza-like illness. Severe COVID-19 usually develops at least after 1 week of illness onset, which could imply a greater role for a dysregulated immune response rather than a direct viral cytopathic effect. An evaluation of the timeline of events suggests that median time from onset of symptoms to hospital admission, dyspnea, acute respiratory distress syndrome (ARDS), mechanical ventilation, and intensive care unit (ICU) admission were 7.0, 8.0, 9.0, 10.5, and 10.5 days, respectively,[23] for the original virus, although the timelines differ slightly depending on the responsible variant, further supporting the hypothesis of dysregulated immune response driving severe COVID-19.

HOST IMMUNE RESPONSES
Innate Immune Response

The innate immune response is activated when pathogen-associated molecular patterns (PAMPs) are recognized by host receptors.[24] PAMPs are small molecules, such as lipopolysaccharides, peptidoglycan, lipoteichoic acid, and nucleic acids, that are present in different patterns and trigger immune cascades when recognized by the host. The protein receptors in the host responsible for detecting PAMPs are called pattern recognition receptors. These pattern recognition receptors include Toll-like receptors, C-type lectin receptors, NOD-like receptors, and RIG-I-like

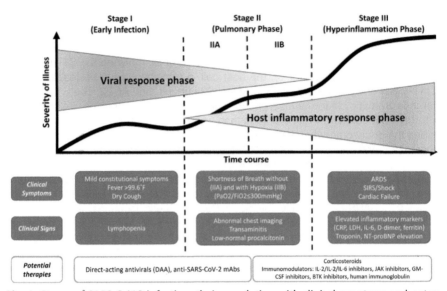

Fig. 1. Stages of SARS-CoV-2 infection, their correlation with clinical symptoms and potential therapies that have been identified. (*Adapted from*: Siddiqi HK, Mehra MR. COVID-19 illness in native and immunosuppressed states: A clinical-therapeutic staging proposal. *J Heart Lung Transplant*. 2020 May;39(5):405–407. https://doi.org/10.1016/j.healun.2020.03.012 with permission from Elsevier)

receptors. Once activated, these receptors initiate downstream signaling pathways leading to secretion of type I and type III interferons, and the assembly and activation of the NOD-like receptor P3 inflammasome and other inflammasome complexes that promote secretion of proinflammatory cytokines including IL-1β and IL-18.[25] The activation of antigen-presenting cells by proinflammatory cytokines also recruits the adaptive immunity to enhance viral clearance by antibody-mediated neutralization and T-cell–mediated cytotoxicity.[24] The inflammasome pathway triggers the coagulation cascade, contributing to coagulopathy and the thrombotic events seen in severe COVID-19.[26]

Like PAMPs, host cells are also activated by damaged or stressed cells in the setting of inflammation,[24] necrosis, or hypoxia even if no microbial PAMPs are present. These are called damage-associated molecular patterns. Although the activated PAMP and damage-associated molecular pattern pathways contribute to viral clearance, an overactivated response leads to a dysregulated immune system and exacerbates inflammation and damage through a cytokine storm[26] (**Fig. 3**). These pathways have been described for viral infections in the past, but corresponding pathways specific to SARS-CoV-2 remain to be identified.

One proinflammatory cytokine, IL-6, garnered attention after reports of ARDS became common in patients with severe COVID-19. IL-6 is a mediator of both innate and adaptive immune responses and acts as both a proinflammatory cytokine and an anti-inflammatory myokine. IL-6 is secreted by macrophages when PAMPs bind to pattern recognition receptors. An elevated IL-6 was reported to be associated with a poor prognosis and, consequently, much emphasis was placed on the treatment of severe COVID-19 with IL-6 receptor antagonists.[4] Clinical trials have suggested there is some benefit to limiting hyperactive immune responses through blocking IL-6 in severe COVID-19.[27]

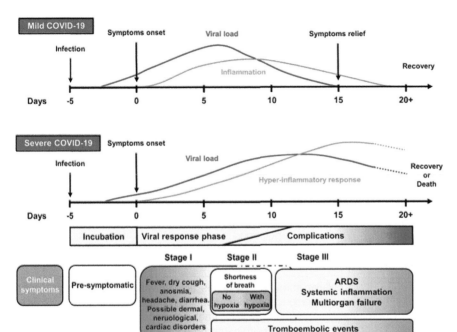

Fig. 2. Timeline of mild and severe COVID-19 and its correlation with viral activity and clinical manifestations. (*From* Lariccia and colleagues Challenges and Opportunities from Targeting Inflammatory Responses to SARS-CoV-2 Infection: A Narrative Review, *Journal of Clinical Medicine.* 2020; 9(12):4021. https://doi.org/10.3390/jcm9124021. © 2020 by the authors. Licensee MDPI, Basel, Switzerland. Under Creative Commons (CC BY 4.0) license)

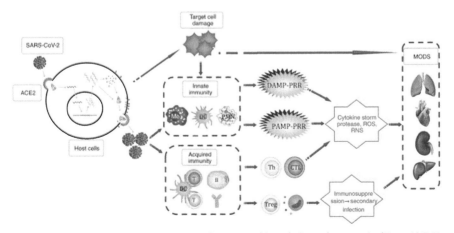

Fig. 3. Immune response to SARS-CoV-2 infection and its role in pathogenesis. (*From* Li C, He Q, Qian H, Liu J. Overview of the pathogenesis of COVID-19 (Review). *Exp Ther Med.* 2021;22(3):1011. https://doi.org/10.3892/etm.2021.10444. © Li and colleagues Under Creative Commons Attribution License)

An early innate immune response is critical in activating the T- and B-cell immune systems and terminating the infection at asymptomatic or mild to moderate stage.[28] A delayed or absent innate immune response, either by immune evasion by the virus or defective host immunity (or both), fails to prime the adaptive immune system and contributes to a high risk of severe or fatal COVID- 19.

Antigen Presentation

Antigen-presenting cells are the initial component of antiviral response by the host. The specific mechanism of antigen presentation of SARS-CoV-2 is not well-understood; however, some of it can be extrapolated based on data from other betacoronaviruses, which mainly depends on major histocompatibility complex 1 molecules. Several HLA types have been associated with increased susceptibility or protection against SARS-CoV.[29] It is highly likely there exist HLA alleles that predict increased susceptibility to SARS-CoV-2 and correlate with more severe outcomes, although research in diverse populations is ongoing.

Adaptive Immunity

Both humoral and cellular immune responses are activated by antigen-presenting cells as suggested by presence of virus-specific B and T cells in convalescent cases.[30] Coordinated humoral and cellular immune responses have been hypothesized to be protective, and an uncoordinated response has been blamed for uncontrolled disease[31] (Fig. 4.) Moreover, a delayed activation of adaptive immunity has been correlated with a higher viral burden and severe or fatal COVID-19. It has been hypothesized that the innate immune response attempts to fill the gap left by the absence of a functional adaptive immune system response, leading to an overactivated innate cytokine and chemokine responses and exacerbated neutrophil-driven lung damage, as evidenced by the presence of a substantial number of neutrophils in end-stage COVID-19.[28,32]

It has been demonstrated that neutralizing antibody titers and quantity of virus-specific T cells are positively correlated.[30] As with other acute viral infections, IgG and IgM subtype antibodies are produced, primarily against the S and N proteins.[33] IgM antibodies persist for 4 to 6 weeks after the onset of symptoms, whereas IgG persists for approximately 6 months after symptom onset in most cases. Persons who experienced asymptomatic infection have been shown to have lower seropositivity and delayed seroconversion when compared with persons who developed symptomatic COVID-19. Furthermore, antibodies in people who have recovered from COVID-19 may persist for well over 6 months.[30]

The T-cell response to SARS-CoV-2 includes both CD4+ and CD8+ T cells. It has been suggested that CD4+ T cells are more abundant and effective against SARS-CoV-2 infection than CD8+ T cells.[31] A predominantly CD4+ T-cell response is seen against S, M, and N proteins, although CD4+ cells respond against almost all SARS-CoV- 2 proteins. After symptom onset, a CD4+ T-cell response can be detected within 2 to 4 days, whereas a CD8+ T-cell response can be detected as early as 1 day after symptoms develop.[28]

A study found that although the overall number of CD4 and CD8 T cells in patients with COVID-19 is decreased, cells are excessively activated, with increased expression of proinflammatory HLAs and coreceptors. CD8 T cells were found to have an increased density of cytotoxic granules.[34] This factor likely contributes to the cytokine storm causing ARDS and systemic inflammation, through the release of proinflammatory cytokines (including interferon, IL-6, and tumor necrosis factor-α) and

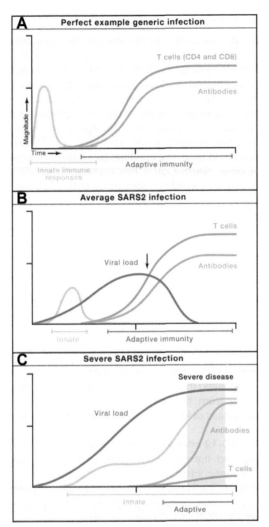

Fig. 4. Timeline of immune response and viral load in SARS-CoV-2 infection. (*A*) Perfect example generic infection. (*B*) Average SARS-CoV-2 infection. (*C*) Severe SARS-CoV-2 infection. (*From* Sette A, Crotty S. Adaptive immunity to SARS-CoV-2 and COVID-19. *Cell.* 184(4), 861–880. Copyright 2021 with permission from Elsevier; with permission)

chemokines (CCL5, CXCL8, etc). This exaggerated immune response is what leads to the multiorgan involvement and high mortality seen in COVID-19.

Although long-term memory immunity is not yet clarified for SARS-CoV-2, it is known that CD4 and CD8 memory T cells persist for years after recovery from SARS-CoV infection and can respond to SARS-CoV antigens even after 6 years. In contrast, it seems that memory B-cell response is almost absent after 6 years after recovery from SARS.[35] In follow-up of early SARS-CoV-2 infections and after vaccination, it also seems clear that T-cell responses are longer than antibody responses. Longer term follow-up will be required to fully elucidate the duration of postinfection responses.

Immune Evasion and Variants

It is believed that SARS-CoV-2 uses similar mechanisms to evade the host's immune response as other coronaviruses. Viral proteins interfere with the function and maturation of antigen-presenting cells and activate pathways that decrease the transcription and transport of antiviral proteins (such as interferons). Antigenic variation, particularly in the M protein, also decreases the production of interferons.[36]

Another mechanism of immune evasion of particular concern is S protein mutations, which alter the ultrastructure and function of the epitope domain, impairing the function of antibodies against the immunodominant protein.[37] These mutations in structural proteins have caused (and will continue to cause) the emergence of different variants of SARS-CoV-2. SARS-CoV-2 has undergone significant mutations, with some lineages emerging as variants of concern as defined by the World Health Organization. These variants are so named because of their potential for higher transmissibility, more severe disease, or high risk of immune escape. See William O. Hahn and Zanthia Wiley's article, "COVID-19 Vaccines," in this issue.

CLINICAL FEATURES

Several medical comorbidities have been identified as risk factors for severe COVID-19, including cardiovascular disease,[38] chronic kidney disease, immunocompromising conditions, and metabolic diseases.[39] It should be noted that the rates of infection, hospitalization, and death from COVID-19 in Black,[40] Hispanic,[41] and American Indian/Alaska Native communities[42] have been disproportionately higher than other racial or ethnic groups. The role of biology and the disproportionate prevalence of medical comorbidities has not been enough to explain these inequities, in addition to a wealth of data suggesting that these differences are driven by social and structural vulnerabilities resulting from the impacts of structural racism in these communities.[43,44] Additional details of inequities seen with COVID-19 will be presented elsewhere in this collection.

The severity of COVID-19 infection varies depending on both the virulence of the SARS-CoV-2 variant and the host immune response, with clinical manifestations ranging from asymptomatic infection to severe inflammatory syndrome and multiorgan dysfunction. As such, the National Institutes of Health established a classification system for COVID-19 disease, delineating the criteria for asymptomatic, mild, moderate, severe, and critical COVID-19. These categories are not mutually exclusive, and many patients progress from 1 category to another during the course of the disease.[45]

The incubation period following exposure to SARS-CoV-2 has been estimated anywhere between 2 and 14 days, and varies by variants of concern. In a pooled analysis of 181 confirmed COVID-19 cases from China the median incubation period was estimated to be 5.1 days (95% confidence interval, 4.5–5.8 days).[46] Noteworthy, compared with earlier variants of concern, shorter incubation periods have been documented in infections with Delta and Omicron variants, with a median incubation period of 4 days.[47]

Asymptomatic Infection

Asymptomatic infections involve individuals who test positive for SARS-CoV-2 but have no symptoms. It is estimated that 50% of persons who test positive for SARS-CoV-2 are asymptomatic at the time of diagnosis.[3] The overall proportion of asymptomatic infections was estimated at approximately 25% in one meta-analysis, but the proportion of asymptomatic infections is generally higher in persons with pre-existing immunity.[48]

Asymptomatic infections are more common in young and middle-aged patients (<50 years of age), women, and individuals without underlying comorbid conditions.[49] In an early study including 55 cases of asymptomatic infection,[50] the median age at the time of diagnosis was 49 years. Despite absence of symptoms, more than half patients (37/55) in this study had evidence of pneumonia on computed tomography scans.

Importantly, a small proportion of patients initially classified as asymptomatic may eventually develop symptoms of infection, generally within 48 hours of SARS-CoV-2 RNA being detectable in the nasopharynx and are referred to as presymptomatic. However, many patients remain asymptomatic at follow-up.[49]

Mild Disease

Mild COVID-19 cases include individuals with symptoms of fever, sore throat, myalgia, and/or malaise, but without shortness of breath, dyspnea, or abnormal chest imaging indicating the presence of lower respiratory tract disease. The majority of symptomatic infections result in mild COVID-19 (81%).[51] Gastrointestinal symptoms such as diarrhea, nausea, and emesis have also been reported, but with lower frequencies (<20%) than in SARS or MERS infections.[52] The incidence of symptoms such as loss of smell or taste varies significantly among studies, with frequencies between 10% and 40%.[23] Loss of taste or smell (anosmia and ageusia, respectively), however, are often recognized by patients as a hallmark, or pathognomonic feature, of COVID-19, and frequently precede the onset of other flu-like symptoms. This peculiar manifestation has been studied, with one of the proposed theories being that the specialized cells in the olfactory bulb and olfactory epithelium have the ACE2 receptors for viral entry and subsequent infection, although there are detectable changes in brain imaging in some persons with anosmia.[53,54] Most patients recover over the course of a few weeks; however, persistent anosmia and ageusia are also frequently described and remain under study.

Moderate, Severe, and Critical Disease

Patients with moderate disease have evidence of lower respiratory disease on physical examination or chest imaging, but maintain an oxygen saturation of equal or greater than 94% on room air at sea level.[45] Individuals with severe disease have an oxygen saturation on room air of less than 94% at sea level, a ratio of arterial partial pressure of oxygen to fraction of inspired oxygen of less than 300 mm Hg, or a respiratory rate of greater than 30 breaths/min, or lung infiltrates greater than 50%.[45] Critical disease is defined as respiratory failure, septic shock and/or multiorgan failure.[45]

During the initial phase of the pandemic, severe disease accounted for up to 14% of cases and critical illness was seen in about 5% of cases according to the Chinese Center for Disease Control and Prevention.[55] The rate of severe disease, however, varies depending on several factors, including history of prior infection, vaccination status, variant causing the infection and available health care resources. For example, the Omicron variant seems to be associated with milder disease compared with Delta variant.[56] The risk of progression to severe and critical disease is markedly decreased in persons with prior immunity, especially after vaccination.

The hallmark of COVID-19 is respiratory disease, which is the consequence of severe inflammation and damage of lung tissue. The pathogenesis of COVID-19 is still being extensively studied. The replication of the virus inside the respiratory epithelium causes a proinflammatory state through the production of chemokines and cytokines, including IL-1, IL-6, and tumor necrosis factor-α, among many others.[57] The main mechanism of lung injury in COVID-19 is diffuse alveolar damage.[56] The damage to the endothelium mediated by fibrin and inflammation causes edema and thrombosis of lung vessels. This process can cause extensive injury and edema of the alveoli with formation of protein deposits and hyaline membranes. This inflammation in the lung parenchyma manifests as mucus production, cough, and dyspnea. On imaging, patchy opacities can be seen on radiograph or ground glass opacities on computed tomography scans. These opacities are usually of peripheral or subpleural distribution bilaterally. Pneumonia can be significant enough to cause hypoxemic respiratory failure and, in some cases, may progress to ARDS, and ultimately, death. Risk factors for progression to ARDS have been identified: age greater than 65 years, diabetes mellitus, hypertension, and obesity, and nonreceipt of SARS-CoV-2 vaccination, among other factors.[58]

Acute Respiratory Distress Syndrome

ARDS is a clinical entity that presents with bilateral pulmonary infiltrates and severe hypoxemia, which results from extensive damage and edema of the alveolar system owing to infiltration by inflammatory cells and mediators. Inflammatory cells, lytic enzymes, and cytokines produce thickening and fibrosis of the alveolar-blood barrier, destruction of alveoli, formation of proteinaceous hyaline membranes and severe edema of the interstitium. It is characterized by noncardiac pulmonary edema and severe hypoxemia with a ratio of arterial partial pressure of oxygen to fraction of inspired oxygen of less than 300. The severity of disease is classified according to the ratio of arterial partial pressure of oxygen to fraction of inspired oxygen.[59]

ARDS develops in approximately 30% to 50% of patients presenting with COVID-19 pneumonia and hypoxemia, although this number could change with the implementation of steroid therapy, vaccination, and outpatient therapeutics. In a study of 13 patients admitted to the ICU,[60] 30% developed ARDS at a median time of 9 days and 10% required mechanical ventilation. The mortality rate of ARDS in patients with COVID-19 seems to be higher than that of other causes of ARDS.[60] This could be due to multiple factors, including the added damage from the virus to the lung parenchyma and the thrombotic microangiopathy and thrombosis that develops in severe COVID-19.

COVID-19–Associated Pulmonary Aspergillosis

Like influenza, pulmonary epithelial damage resulting from COVID-19 increases risk of invasive pulmonary aspergillosis. A systematic review described 85 cases of invasive pulmonary aspergillosis in patients with critical COVID-19, with an estimated prevalence of 5% to 30%, although this high estimate has been questioned.[61] Risk factors for death from CAPA were age, male sex, and pre-existing lung disease. Importantly, not all patients had a predisposing immunosuppressive state for invasive disease, although many received corticosteroids.[61] It is important to note that not all cases of COVID-19–associated pulmonary aspergillosis clearly represent an infection versus colonization, and this clinical entity is an area of developing study, especially as cross-sectional imaging, bronchoalveolar lavage, and definitive diagnostics are often deferred in patients with COVID-19 to reduce transmission potential and procedures. Owing to the degree of lung damage and long duration of ventilation and extracorporeal life support required for some with critical COVID-19, it is important to keep vigilance for COVID-19–associated pulmonary aspergillosis and treat with appropriate antifungals if suspicion is high.

Extrapulmonary Manifestations of COVID-19

Cutaneous manifestations

Cutaneous manifestations are rare with reported rates of less than 2% and usually nonspecific.[62] However, certain features accompanying cutaneous manifestations have been reported in the literature. Urticarial rash is commonly associated with moderate to severe COVID-19.[62] A maculopapular rash can be observed after the onset of systemic symptoms whereas papulovesicular exanthems frequently occur before the onset of symptoms. Livedo racemosa-like pattern lesions are often associated with severe coagulopathy and acral ischemia with cyanosis of toes (so-called COVID toes), skin blisters, and dry gangrene have been reported in patients with severe COVID-19.[63]

Neurologic Manifestations

Dizziness and headache are among the most common neurologic symptoms reported in the literature, although the prevalence.[64] A minority of patients with severe COVID-19 can present with acute encephalopathy, cerebrovascular accidents, changes in vision, seizures and radiculopathy.[65] So-called brain fog has also been described, particularly as a sequela of COVID, referring to a nonspecific and subjective inability to concentrate or to perform certain tasks. One of the proposed mechanisms is direct viral interference in mitochondrial function in neurons, although studies are ongoing.[66]

The prevalence of ischemic stroke in patients with COVID-19 has been estimated to be approximately 5%, and it carries a high mortality rate of 30% to 40%.[67] It is most commonly seen in patients older than 70 years of age, but it has also been reported in younger, previously healthy patients.[68] Risk factors include prior cerebrovascular events, hypertension, diabetes, chronic kidney disease, and chronic liver disease, among others. Depending on the vascular territory affected, patients may present with facial droop, aphasia, dysarthria, or unilateral weakness. The management for stroke in the setting of COVID-19 is the same as for other patients: the use of the tissue plasminogen activator alteplase or mechanical thrombectomy if patients meet criteria for either.[67] It is not yet clear if patients have a higher risk of hemorrhagic complications with the use of alteplase.

Cardiac Injury

Cardiac injury by COVID-19 has been reported in the literature mainly in patients with underlying cardiovascular conditions and carries a poor prognosis.[69] The range of manifestations can go from asymptomatic troponin elevation to severe myocarditis and heart failure.

The proposed pathogenic mechanisms include direct viral infection, cytokine storm, pulmonary emboli, coronary thrombosis, hypercoagulability, and an imbalance between demand and supply.[69] A study of 40 patients who died with cardiac-related COVID-19 complications revealed that microthrombi were the most common pathologic cause of myocyte necrosis.[70] Of note, the composition of these microthrombi was different from that of patients without COVID-19. Myocarditis associated with COVID-19 has also been described. The risk of myocarditis in people with COVID-19 is approximately 16 times that of people without COVID-19, and the highest risk is found in children aged less than 16 years and elderly patients ages more than 75 years.[71] Although there has been concern about infrequent cases of myocarditis associated with SARS-CoV-2 vaccination, the risk of myocarditis owing to COVID-19 itself is 4- to 40-fold higher than from vaccination with one of the mRNA vaccines.[71,72]

Thrombotic Episodes

Significant thrombotic events have been described in persons with both symptomatic and asymptomatic SARS-CoV-2 infection, ranging from an increased risk of deep venous thrombosis (DVT) and pulmonary embolism (PE), to stroke, thrombotic micro-angiopathy and disseminated intravascular coagulation, all of which further increase the morbidity and mortality of the disease.[73]

SARS-CoV-2 infects host cells via ACE2, which is present in high concentrations in the endothelial cells. Proinflammatory pathways are triggered in endothelial cells, with indirect activation of the kallikrein-kinin system and increased levels of bradykinin, which increase vascular permeability. Activation of the complement and subsequent direct endothelial injury and death causes denudation of the endothelium.[74] Procoagulant pathways are activated in response to exposure of the basement membrane, which triggers microvascular thrombosis and hemorrhage.[75] This proposed cascade of events is consistent with what is seen macroscopically in autopsy studies, where platelet and fibrin rich thrombi have been found in the lungs of patients who have died of COVID-19.[76] Tissue factor expression induces coagulation pathways, and anticoagulants like protein C and tissue factor pathway inhibitor are inhibited by the overwhelming procoagulant activation. The damaged endothelium expresses adherence molecules and cytokines that not only stimulate the production of platelets, but also their adhesion to the endothelium and formation of clots.[74]

Venous Thromboembolism

Venous thromboembolism, consisting of DVT and PE, is a common complication of hospitalized patients with COVID-19, and less frequently in persons whose COVID-19 respiratory infection is not severe enough to merit hospitalization. The prevalence has been identified to be particularly high in patients admitted to the ICU (from 50% to 80% depending on the series[77,78]), even when the clinical suspicion may be low.[73] However, patients that are admitted to acute care units also have an increased risk of DVT (20%–30% of patients).[79] These thrombotic events can happen despite pharmacologic prophylactic doses of anticoagulant.[79] PE is another potentially life-threatening complication that is more prevalent in patients with COVID-19, particularly those admitted to the ICU (20%–30%). Persons admitted to acute care for COVID-19 have PE rates of 10% to 20%.[79,80] DVT can be seen both in lower and upper extremities, and presents identically to non-COVID–associated VTE, subclinical, and asymptomatic presentations. The diagnosis of PE in patients who are mechanically ventilated may be challenging, especially given the many reasons for physiologic shunt present owing to microthrombi, airspace disease from COVID-19 pneumonia, and superimposed bacterial or fungal infection, and ARDS. The preferred diagnostic modality is computed tomography angiography.

Arterial Thrombosis

Thrombotic complications in arterial vessels have also been described. Acute limb ischemia has been observed in patients with COVID-19, regardless of pre-existing peripheral arterial disease.[73] Arterial thrombosis manifests as severe pain and discoloration of an extremity, cold and clammy extremities, and decreased pulses. Thrombosis of the thoracic or abdominal aorta has also been reported, manifesting as unilateral limb ischemia, bilateral loss of pulses in the lower extremities, bilateral loss of sensation, or acute periumbilical/epigastric pain.[81] Mesenteric ischemia can present with diarrhea and severe abdominal pain.[82] Arterial thrombotic complications often cause a marked elevation of D-dimer as well as inflammatory markers such as

C-reactive protein, although these markers are often drastically elevated in persons with severe or critical COVID-19, and the difficulty in making these diagnoses can result in delays in detection, and further increase their morbidity and mortality.

COVID-19 IN CHILDREN

COVID-19 is a disease that has been proven to affect children of all ages, especially as the incidence of pediatric COVID-19 increased during infection waves attributable to the delta and omicron variants. The most common clinical presentation in children is fever with cough, similar to adult infections. Many infections are asymptomatic, and in the majority, disease is mild or moderate. Children younger than 1 year old may have a higher incidence of critical disease and gastrointestinal symptoms.[83]

In May 2020, the US Centers for Disease Control and Prevention reported a severe inflammatory syndrome that presented in otherwise healthy children that had features similar to Kawasaki disease, with persistent fever, rash, and other various neurologic, gastrointestinal, dermatologic, cardiac, and renal manifestations.[84] This syndrome had been linked to COVID-19 infection and was named multisystem inflammatory syndrome in children. Further description of manifestations of COVID-19 in pediatric populations is discussed in Andrasik and colleagues' article, "Awakening: The Unveiling of Historically Unaddressed Social Inequities During the COVID-19 Pandemic in the United States," in this issue.

POSTACUTE SEQUELAE OF COVID-19

Postacute sequelae of COVID-19, also colloquially termed long COVID or long-haul COVID-19, is a clinical entity that has gained recognition as the pandemic continued into its second year in 2021. Although there is no consensus for a single definition, in general, postacute sequelae of COVID-19 refers to the persistence of symptoms for more than 3 months after the onset of symptoms.[85] The most common reported symptoms are shortness of breath and fatigue; however, an extensive list of symptoms involving multiple systems has been described. These symptoms include cognitive dysfunction (brain fog), mental disorders (depression, anxiety), headache, musculoskeletal complaints (myalgia, joint pain, chest wall pain), taste and smell disorders, chronic cough, alopecia, and insomnia, among many others.[86] Further details on pathophysiology, manifestations, and proposed treatments for postacute sequelae of COVID-19 are discussed in Eric A. Meyerowitz and Aaron Richterman's article, "SARS-CoV-2 Transmission and Prevention in the Era of the Delta Variant," in this issue.

SUMMARY

COVID-19 is a disease that affects multiple organ systems, and the prevailing theory is that most symptoms outside of the upper respiratory tract are predominately triggered by an exaggerated inflammatory response in the host. This inflammatory process results in a wide variety of clinical presentations, ranging from asymptomatic to severe multiorgan dysfunction. COVID-19 affects people of all age groups, including children, who also suffer from severe disease. Groups of people with poor access to health care such as Black and Hispanic/Latino communities have been disproportionately impacted by COVID-19, fueling increased awareness of health care disparities. Furthermore, the persistence of symptoms in people who recover from COVID-19 adds to its morbidity and impact on the workforce, mental health, and economic impacts in the long term. The complete pathogenesis of SARS-CoV-2 is slowly being unraveled through knowledge from similar respiratory viruses, as well as a rapid proliferation of research on this novel pathogen. Fully understanding the pathogenesis, especially of extrapulmonary manifestations of COVID-19 disease, will likely remain an area of developing knowledge for years to come.

CLINICS CARE POINTS

- COVID-19 can range from asymptomatic infection to severe multiorgan failure. The hallmark of the disease is exaggerated inflammation in the lung tissue that can progress to ARDS, although it also causes significant endothelial damage and thrombosis in other systems.
- COVID-19 affects different organs and systems, and the presentation depends on the organ systems affected. Not all patients present with respiratory symptoms.
- Although venous thrombosis is widely reported in COVID-19, arterial thrombosis can also be encountered as mesenteric or aortic thrombosis, as well as acute limb ischemia. These often cause significant elevations of D-dimer and C-reactive protein.
- Although COVID-19 is generally less severe in children than in adults, it can present with persistent fever, rash and multiorgan dysfunction (multisystem inflammatory syndrome in children) that often requires an ICU level of care.
- Postacute sequelae of COVID-19 (also known as long COVID) is generally defined as persistent symptoms for more than 3 months after the initial onset of symptoms of COVID-19.

DISCLOSURES

J.R. Marcelin Co-chairs the NIH/NIAID/CoVPN vaccine study CoVPN 3006/Prevent COVID U and receives salary support for this activity, not related to this article. All other authors have no potential conflicts of interest to disclose.

REFERENCES

1. Sawicki SG, Sawicki DL. Coronavirus transcription: a perspective. Coronavirus Replication Reverse Genet 2005;287:31–55.
2. Tabatabaeizadeh SA. Airborne transmission of COVID-19 and the role of face mask to prevent it: a systematic review and meta-analysis. Eur J Med Res 2021;26(1):1.
3. Prevalence of asymptomatic SARS-CoV-2 infection: a narrative review. Annals of Internal Medicine: vol 173, No 5. Available at: https://www.acpjournals.org/doi/10.7326/M20-3012. Accessed November 8, 2021.
4. Vijayvargiya P, Esquer Garrigos Z, Castillo Almeida NE, et al. Treatment considerations for COVID-19: a critical review of the evidence (or Lack Thereof). Mayo Clin Proc 2020;95(7):1454–66.
5. Frampton D, Rampling T, Cross A, et al. Genomic characteristics and clinical effect of the emergent SARS-CoV-2 B.1.1.7 lineage in London, UK: a whole-genome sequencing and hospital-based cohort study. Lancet Infect Dis 2021; 21(9):1246–56.
6. Singh D, Yi SV. On the origin and evolution of SARS-CoV-2. Exp Mol Med 2021; 53(4):537–47.
7. Zhu N, Zhang D, Wang W, et al. A novel coronavirus from patients with pneumonia in China, 2019. N Engl J Med 2020;382(8):727–33.

8. Lu R, Zhao X, Li J, et al. Genomic characterisation and epidemiology of 2019 novel coronavirus: implications for virus origins and receptor binding. Lancet 2020;395(10224):565–74.

9. Severe acute respiratory syndrome coronavirus 2 isolate Wuhan-Hu-1, complete genome. 2020. Accessed. http://www.ncbi.nlm.nih.gov/nuccore/NC_045512.2. [Accessed 7 November 2021]. Available at:.

10. The Genome Sequence of the SARS-Associated Coronavirus. Accessed. https://www.science.org/doi/10.1126/science.1085953. [Accessed 7 November 2021]. Available at:.

11. Chan JFW, Kok KH, Zhu Z, et al. Genomic characterization of the 2019 novel human-pathogenic coronavirus isolated from a patient with atypical pneumonia after visiting Wuhan. Emerg Microbes Infect 2020;9(1):221–36.

12. Hu B, Guo H, Zhou P, et al. Characteristics of SARS-CoV-2 and COVID-19. Nat Rev Microbiol 2020;1–14. https://doi.org/10.1038/s41579-020-00459-7.

13. Walls AC, Park YJ, Tortorici MA, et al. Structure, function, and antigenicity of the SARS-CoV-2 spike glycoprotein. Cell 2020;181(2):281–92.e6.

14. Lau SKP, Luk HKH, Wong ACP, et al. Possible Bat origin of severe acute respiratory syndrome coronavirus 2. Emerg Infect Dis 2020;26(7):1542–7.

15. Li W, Moore MJ, Vasilieva N, et al. Angiotensin-converting enzyme 2 is a functional receptor for the SARS coronavirus. Nature 2003;426(6965):450–4.

16. Wrapp D, Wang N, Corbett KS, et al. Cryo-EM structure of the 2019-nCoV spike in the prefusion conformation. Science 2020;367(6483):1260–3.

17. Huang Y, Yang C, Xin-Feng X, et al. Structural and functional properties of SARS-CoV-2 spike protein: potential antivirus drug development for COVID-19. Acta Pharmacol Sin 2020;41(9):1141–9.

18. Coronaviruses - a general introduction - CEBM. Available at: https://web.archive.org/web/20200522053938/https:/www.cebm.net/covid-19/coronaviruses-a-general-introduction/. Accessed November 8, 2021.

19. Zhao MM, Yang WL, Yang FY, et al. Cathepsin L plays a key role in SARS-CoV-2 infection in humans and humanized mice and is a promising target for new drug development. Signal Transduct Target Ther 2021;6(1):1–12.

20. Hamming I, Timens W, Bulthuis M, et al. Tissue distribution of ACE2 protein, the functional receptor for SARS coronavirus. A first step in understanding SARS pathogenesis. J Pathol 2004;203(2):631–7.

21. Nadim MK, Forni LG, Mehta RL, et al. COVID-19-associated acute kidney injury: consensus report of the 25th Acute Disease Quality Initiative (ADQI) Workgroup. Nat Rev Nephrol 2020;16(12):747–64.

22. Eun LY. Is multisystem inflammatory syndrome related with coronavirus disease 2019, Kawasaki disease, and angiotensin-converting enzyme 2 in children? Clin Exp Pediatr 2021;64(5):225–6.

23. Huang C, Wang Y, Li X, et al. Clinical features of patients infected with 2019 novel coronavirus in Wuhan, China. The Lancet 2020;395(10223):497–506.

24. Carty M, Guy C, Bowie AG. Detection of viral infections by innate immunity. Biochem Pharmacol 2021;183:114316.

25. Rodrigues TS, de Sá KSG, Ishimoto AY, et al. Inflammasomes are activated in response to SARS-CoV-2 infection and are associated with COVID-19 severity in patients. J Exp Med 2020;218(3):e20201707.

26. Inflammasome activation triggers blood clotting and host death through pyroptosis. Accessed. https://www.ncbi.nlm.nih.gov/pmc/articles/PMC6791531/. [Accessed 8 November 2021]. Available at:.

27. Interleukin-6 receptor antagonists in critically ill patients with Covid-19. N Engl J Med 2021;384(16):1491–502.
28. Sette A, Crotty S. Adaptive immunity to SARS-CoV-2 and COVID-19. Cell 2021; 184(4):861–80.
29. Chen YMA, Liang SY, Shih YP, et al. Epidemiological and genetic correlates of severe acute respiratory syndrome coronavirus infection in the hospital with the highest nosocomial infection rate in Taiwan in 2003. J Clin Microbiol 2006; 44(2):359–65.
30. Ni L, Ye F, Cheng ML, et al. Detection of SARS-CoV-2-specific humoral and cellular immunity in COVID-19 convalescent individuals. Immunity 2020;52(6): 971–7.e3.
31. Rydyznski Moderbacher C, Ramirez SI, Dan JM, et al. Antigen-specific adaptive immunity to SARS-CoV-2 in acute COVID-19 and associations with age and disease severity. Cell 2020;183(4):996–1012.e19.
32. Kuri-Cervantes L, Pampena MB, Meng W, et al. Comprehensive mapping of immune perturbations associated with severe COVID-19. Sci Immunol 2020;5(49): eabd7114.
33. Zhang X, Lu S, Li H, et al. Viral and antibody kinetics of COVID-19 patients with different disease severities in acute and convalescent phases: a 6-month follow-up study. Virol Sin 2020;35(6):820–9.
34. Xu Z, Shi L, Wang Y, et al. Pathological findings of COVID-19 associated with acute respiratory distress syndrome. Lancet Respir Med 2020;8(4):420–2.
35. Tang F, Quan Y, Xin ZT, et al. Lack of peripheral memory B cell responses in recovered patients with severe acute respiratory syndrome: a six-year follow-up study. J Immunol 2011;186(12):7264–8.
36. Bouayad A. Innate immune evasion by SARS-CoV-2: comparison with SARS-CoV. Rev Med Virol 2020;30(6):e2135.
37. Harvey WT, Carabelli AM, Jackson B, et al. SARS-CoV-2 variants, spike mutations and immune escape. Nat Rev Microbiol 2021;19(7):409–24.
38. Ssentongo P, Ssentongo AE, Heilbrunn ES, et al. Association of cardiovascular disease and 10 other pre-existing comorbidities with COVID-19 mortality: a systematic review and meta-analysis. PLoS One 2020;15(8):e0238215.
39. Zhou Y, Yang Q, Chi J, et al. Comorbidities and the risk of severe or fatal outcomes associated with coronavirus disease 2019: a systematic review and meta-analysis. Int J Infect Dis 2020;99:47–56.
40. Kullar R, Marcelin JR, Swartz TH, et al. Racial disparity of Coronavirus disease 2019 in African American communities. J Infect Dis 2020;222(6):890–3.
41. Macias Gil R, Marcelin JR, Zuniga-Blanco B, et al. COVID-19 pandemic: disparate health impact on the Hispanic/Latinx population in the United States. J Infect Dis 2020;222(10):1592–5.
42. Arrazola J, Masiello MM, Joshi S, et al. COVID-19 mortality among American Indian and Alaska Native persons — 14 States, January–June 2020. Morb Mortal Wkly Rep 2020;69(49):1853–6.
43. Khazanchi R, Evans CT, Marcelin JR. Racism, not race, drives inequity across the COVID-19 continuum. JAMA Netw Open 2020;3(9):e2019933.
44. Marcelin JR, Swartz TH, Bernice F, et al. Addressing and inspiring vaccine confidence in black, indigenous, and people of color during the Coronavirus disease 2019 pandemic. Open Forum Infect Dis 2021;8(9):ofab417.
45. Clinical Spectrum. COVID-19 treatment guidelines. Available at: https://www.covid19treatmentguidelines.nih.gov/overview/clinical-spectrum/.   Accessed October 24, 2021.

46. Lauer SA, Grantz KH, Bi Q, et al. The incubation period of Coronavirus disease 2019 (COVID-19) from publicly reported confirmed cases: estimation and application. Ann Intern Med 2020;172(9):577–82.

47. Wang Y, Chen R, Hu F, et al. Transmission, viral kinetics and clinical characteristics of the emergent SARS-CoV-2 delta VOC in Guangzhou, China. EClinicalMedicine 2021;40:101129.

48. Syangtan G, Bista S, Dawadi P, et al. Asymptomatic SARS-CoV-2 carriers: a systematic review and meta-analysis. Front Public Health 2021;8:587374.

49. Meng H, Xiong R, He R, et al. CT imaging and clinical course of asymptomatic cases with COVID-19 pneumonia at admission in Wuhan, China. J Infect 2020; 81(1):e33–9.

50. Wang Y, Liu Y, Liu L, et al. Clinical outcomes in 55 patients with severe acute respiratory syndrome Coronavirus 2 who were asymptomatic at hospital admission in Shenzhen, China. J Infect Dis 2020;221(11):1770–4.

51. Stokes EK, Zambrano LD, Anderson KN, et al. Coronavirus disease 2019 case surveillance - United States, January 22-May 30, 2020. MMWR Morb Mortal Wkly Rep 2020;69(24):759–65.

52. Bleibtreu A, Bertine M, Bertin C, et al. Focus on middle east respiratory syndrome coronavirus (MERS-CoV). Med Mal Infect 2020;50(3):243–51.

53. Brann DH, Tsukahara T, Weinreb C, et al. Non-neuronal expression of SARS-CoV-2 entry genes in the olfactory system suggests mechanisms underlying COVID-19-associated anosmia. Sci Adv 2020;6(31):eabc5801.

54. Kandemirli SG, Altundag A, Yildirim D, et al. Olfactory bulb MRI and paranasal sinus CT findings in persistent COVID-19 anosmia. Acad Radiol 2021;28(1): 28–35.

55. Wu Z, McGoogan JM. Characteristics of and important lessons from the Coronavirus disease 2019 (COVID-19) outbreak in China: summary of a report of 72 314 cases from the Chinese Center for Disease Control and Prevention. JAMA 2020; 323(13):1239–42.

56. Wang L, Berger NA, Kaelber DC, et al. Comparison of outcomes from COVID infection in pediatric and adult patients before and after the emergence of Omicron. medRxiv 2022. https://doi.org/10.1101/2021.12.30.21268495.

57. Azkur AK, Akdis M, Azkur D, et al. Immune response to SARS-CoV-2 and mechanisms of immunopathological changes in COVID-19. Allergy 2020. https://doi.org/10.1111/all.14364.

58. Wu C, Chen X, Cai Y, et al. Risk factors associated with acute respiratory distress syndrome and death in patients with Coronavirus disease 2019 pneumonia in Wuhan, China. JAMA Intern Med 2020;180(7):934–43.

59. Thompson BT, Chambers RC, Liu KD. Acute respiratory distress syndrome. In: Drazen JM, editor. N Engl J Med 2017;377(6):562–72.

60. Gibson PG, Qin L, Puah SH. COVID-19 acute respiratory distress syndrome (ARDS): clinical features and differences from typical pre-COVID-19 ARDS. Med J Aust 2020. https://doi.org/10.5694/mja2.50674.

61. Apostolopoulou A, Esquer Garrigos Z, Vijayvargiya P, et al. Invasive pulmonary aspergillosis in patients with SARS-CoV-2 infection: a systematic review of the literature. Diagnostics (Basel) 2020;10(10):E807.

62. Genovese G, Moltrasio C, Berti E, et al. Skin manifestations associated with COVID-19: current knowledge and future perspectives. Dermatology 2021; 237(1):1–12.

63. Zhang Y, Cao W, Xiao M, et al. [Clinical and coagulation characteristics of 7 patients with critical COVID-2019 pneumonia and acro-ischemia]. Zhonghua Xue Ye Xue Za Zhi 2020;41(0):E006.

64. Hassett CE, Gedansky A, Migdady I, et al. Neurologic complications of COVID-19. Cleve Clin J Med 2020;87(12):729–34.

65. Ye M, Ren Y, Lv T. Encephalitis as a clinical manifestation of COVID-19. Brain Behav Immun 2020;88:945–6.

66. Stefano GB, Ptacek R, Ptackova H, et al. Selective neuronal mitochondrial targeting in SARS-CoV-2 infection affects cognitive processes to induce "brain fog" and results in behavioral changes that favor viral survival. Med Sci Monit 2021;27: e930886.

67. Qureshi AI, Abd-Allah F, Al-Senani F, et al. Management of acute ischemic stroke in patients with COVID-19 infection: report of an international panel. Int J Stroke 2020;15(5):540–54.

68. Oxley TJ, Mocco J, Majidi S, et al. Large-vessel stroke as a presenting feature of Covid-19 in the young. N Engl J Med 2020;382(20):e60.

69. Tajbakhsh A, Gheibi Hayat SM, Taghizadeh H, et al. COVID-19 and cardiac injury: clinical manifestations, biomarkers, mechanisms, diagnosis, treatment, and follow up. Expert Rev Anti Infect Ther 2021;19(3):345–57.

70. Pellegrini D, Kawakami R, Guagliumi G, et al. Microthrombi as a major cause of cardiac injury in COVID-19: a pathologic study. Circulation 2021;143(10): 1031–42.

71. Boehmer TK. Association between COVID-19 and myocarditis using hospital-based administrative data — United States, March 2020–January 2021. MMWR Morb Mortal Wkly Rep 2021;70(35):1228–32.

72. Patone M, Mei XW, Handunnetthi L, et al. Risks of myocarditis, pericarditis, and cardiac arrhythmias associated with COVID-19 vaccination or SARS-CoV-2 infection. Nat Med 2021;14:1–13.

73. Avila J, Long B, Holladay D, et al. Thrombotic complications of COVID-19. Am J Emerg Med 2021;39:213–8.

74. Branchford BR, Carpenter SL. The role of inflammation in venous thromboembolism. Front Pediatr 2018;6:142.

75. Perico L, Benigni A, Casiraghi F, et al. Immunity, endothelial injury and complement-induced coagulopathy in COVID-19. Nat Rev Nephrol 2020;1–19.

76. Fox SE, Akmatbekov A, Harbert JL, et al. Pulmonary and cardiac pathology in African American patients with COVID-19: an autopsy series from New Orleans. Lancet Respir Med 2020;8(7):681–6.

77. Bo H, Li Y, Liu G, et al. Assessing the risk for development of deep vein thrombosis among Chinese patients using the 2010 Caprini risk assessment model: a prospective multicenter study. J Atheroscler Thromb 2020;27(8):801–8.

78. Nahum J, Morichau-Beauchant T, Daviaud F, et al. Venous thrombosis among critically ill patients with Coronavirus disease 2019 (COVID-19). JAMA Netw Open 2020;3(5):e2010478.

79. Artifoni M, Danic G, Gautier G, et al. Systematic assessment of venous thromboembolism in COVID-19 patients receiving thromboprophylaxis: incidence and role of D-dimer as predictive factors. J Thromb Thrombolysis 2020;50(1):211–6.

80. Grillet F, Behr J, Calame P, et al. Acute pulmonary embolism associated with COVID-19 pneumonia detected with pulmonary CT angiography. Radiology 2020;296(3):E186–8.

81. Kashi M, Jacquin A, Dakhil B, et al. Severe arterial thrombosis associated with Covid-19 infection. Thromb Res 2020;192:75–7.

82. Lia A B, Pacioni C, Ponton S, et al. Arterial mesenteric thrombosis as a complication of SARS-CoV-2 infection. Eur J Case Rep Intern Med 2020;7(5):001690.

83. Cui X, Zhao Z, Zhang T, et al. A systematic review and meta-analysis of children with Coronavirus disease 2019 (COVID-19). J Med Virol 2020. https://doi.org/10.1002/jmv.26398.

84. CDC. Multisystem inflammatory syndrome (MIS). Centers Dis Control Prev. 2020. Available at: https://www.cdc.gov/mis/mis-c.html. Accessed November 8, 2021.

85. Yomogida K. Post-acute sequelae of SARS-CoV-2 infection among adults aged ≥18 years — Long Beach, California, April 1–December 10, 2020. MMWR Morb Mortal Wkly Rep 2021;70(37):1274–7.

86. Yong SJ. Long COVID or post-COVID-19 syndrome: putative pathophysiology, risk factors, and treatments. Infect Dis (Lond) Engl.:1-18. doi:10.1080/23744235.2021.1924397

SARS-CoV-2 Virology

Yijia Li, MD[a,b], Jonathan Z. Li, MD, MMSc[a,*]

KEYWORDS

- SARS-CoV-2 • COVID-19 • Viremia • Receptor-binding domain
- Monoclonal antibody

KEY POINTS

- Severe acute respiratory syndrome coronavirus 2 (SARS-CoV-2) genome is homologous to several Sarbecoviruses, but its proteins have unique features.
- SARS-CoV-2 viral evolution is more prominent in immunocompromised hosts.
- There are several variants of concern and variants of interest, with Omicron, followed by Delta variants, being the most dominant variant currently.
- Upper and lower respiratory tract SARS-CoV-2 infection follows different viral dynamics.
- Systemic dissemination serves as a marker and mechanism for COVID-19 disease severity.

INTRODUCTION

Severe acute respiratory syndrome coronavirus 2 (SARS-CoV-2) has not ceased to wreak havoc since its identification in early 2020.[1,2] Despite its homology with several Betacoronavirus strains including SARS-CoV-1 and bat-derived SARS-related coronaviruses (SARSr-CoVs),[1] SARS-CoV-2 owns several unique features accounting for its pathogenesis and transmission. Clinically, coronavirus disease 2019 (COVID-19) demonstrates the full spectrum of symptomatology, ranging from asymptomatic, to mild/moderately symptomatic, to critical illness with acute respiratory distress syndrome (ARDS) and death.[3] In addition, presymptomatic transmission has greatly contributed to SARS-CoV-2 community spread.[4] Asymptomatic, paucisymptomatic, and presymptomatic transmission has made it difficult to trace and contain its transmission, leading to this global pandemic that has lasted more than 2 years, with more than 330 million confirmed cases and 5.5 million reported deaths, although the attributable mortality to the COVID-19 pandemic has been estimated to be 12 to 22 million by January 2022.[5] In this review, the authors discuss key aspects of SARS-CoV-2 virology that contribute to its variable clinical manifestations, evolution, replication dynamics in the respiratory tract, and systemic dissemination.

[a] Brigham and Women's Hospital, Harvard Medical School, Boston, MA, USA; [b] Massachusetts General Hospital, Harvard Medical School, Boston, MA, USA
* Corresponding author. 65 Landsdowne Street, Room 421 Cambridge, MA 02139.
E-mail address: jli@bwh.harvard.edu

Infect Dis Clin N Am 36 (2022) 251–265
https://doi.org/10.1016/j.idc.2022.01.004
0891-5520/22/© 2022 Elsevier Inc. All rights reserved.

id.theclinics.com

Genome Structure and Viral Proteins

SARS-CoV-2 is part of the Betacoronavirus genus and Sarbecovirus subgenus. It is a single-stranded, positive-sense, 29.9-kilobase (kb) RNA virus.[1] This virus shares 96.2% identity with a bat SarSr-CoV strain RaTG13 and 79.6% with SARS-CoV-1.[6] SarSr-CoV have also recently been recovered from pangolins (Manis javanica)[7] and different species of bats (eg, RpYN06 from Rhinolophus pusillus[8] in southern China and RshSTT182/RshSTT200 from Rhinolophus shameli in Cambodia[9]) with variable degrees of recombination detected in different regions of genome.

The SARS-CoV-2 genome consists of the following genes: open reading frame (ORF) 1a/1b, S, 3a/3b, E, M, 6, 7a/7b, 8, 9b, N, 10, with overlaps in certain regions[1,8] (Fig. 1). The S (Spike), E (Envelope), M (Membrane), and N (Nucleocapsid) genes encode essential structural proteins, whereas the rest of the genes encode nonstructural proteins (Nsps) from ORF1a/1b and accessory factors (ORFs 3–10). Of note, ORF1a/1b encode polyproteins that are subject to viral protease-mediated cleavage into Nsp1-Nsp16.[10] Nsps serve a variety of functions. For example, Nsp1 interacts with the ribosome subunit 40S and interrupts host protein translation,[11] whereas Nsps 7 to 10, 13 to 16 coordinate with Nsp12 to complete the replication cycle, RNA capping, and proofreads.[12] In addition, accessory factors carry additional functions necessary for immune evasion and viral replication. For example, ORF3b, 6, 7a, 8, 9b proteins have been reported to interfere with innate immune responses by antagonizing the interferon (IFN) signaling pathway.[13] In an in vitro cell model, Lei and colleagues[14] demonstrated that ORF6 protein inhibits both upstream type I IFN promotor activation and downstream IFN-stimulated gene expression. In another in vitro cell model, Xia and colleagues[15] further noted that the ORF6 protein could inhibit interferon regulatory factor 3 nuclear translocation, thus blocking its binding to IFN-α/β gene promotor. In addition, ORF7a/7b and ORF3a proteins in conjunction with nsp6, nsp1, and nsp13 inhibit signal transducer and activator of transcription 1 (STAT1)/STAT2 phosphorylation or nuclear translocation, thus further blocking the type I IFN downstream signal. SARS-CoV-2 accessory proteins are also capable of antagonizing other aspects of the home immune response. For example, the ORF8 protein is capable of downregulating human leukocyte antigen-I (HLA-I) by enhancing autophagy-related HLA-I degradation,[16] which may enhance escape from T-cell–mediated immunity in SARS-CoV-2 infection. Finally, many of the Nsps, accessory proteins, and structural proteins are polyfunctional. In an affinity-purification–mass spectrometry–based proteomics study, Gordan and colleagues[17] reported that almost 40% of SARS-CoV-2-interacting host proteins are associated with endomembrane and vesicle trafficking/rearrangement, in addition to their previously identified functions. For example, Nsp8 participates in forming primase for RNA-dependent RNA polymerization, interaction with signal recognition particle to hijack protein translocation pathway, glycosylation, and extracellular matrix regulation; N protein, as a structural protein, also participates in RNA processing and stress granule regulation.[17]

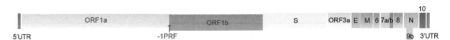

Fig. 1. SARS-CoV-2 genome structure. In SARS-CoV-2 genome, ORF1a/1b encodes polypeptides that undergo viral protease–mediated cleavage to nonstructural proteins 1 to 16. Spike (S), Envelope (E), Membrane (M), and N (nucleocapsid) genes encode corresponding structural proteins. Accessory factors including ORF3a, 6, 7a, 8, and 9b contribute to viral pathogenesis and immune evasion. ORF, open reading frame; UTR, untranslated region; −1PRF, −1 programmed ribosomal frameshifting.

Of all the Nsps, Nsp12 and Nsp5 have been the primary focus of therapeutic development. Nsp12 is the RNA-dependent RNA polymerase (RdRp) that is crucial for viral replication.[18] Remdesivir, an adenosine analogue inhibitor of RdRp, has been shown to shorten recovery time for hospitalized COVID-19 patients[19] and has been approved by the Food and Drug Administration (FDA). Accumulating evidence has also demonstrated its efficacy in decreasing hospitalization and death in the outpatient setting.[20] Nsp5 is the main protease of SARS-CoV-2 (3C-like protease) and is responsible for viral polypeptide cleavage and viral maturation.[21] Nirmatrelvir/PF-07321332[22] (boosted by ritonavir), a protease inhibitor targeting 3C-like protease, has been reported to decrease the risk of hospitalization and death and has been granted Emergency Use Authorization in the outpatient setting.[23]

Of all the structural proteins, Spike protein has been the center of research and therapeutic development. Spike protein consists of 2 subunits: S1 and S2. The S1 subunit contains the N-terminal domain and the receptor-binding domain (RBD) that mediate host cell binding, whereas the S2 domain is responsible for cell membrane fusion.[1] Host proteases are required to prime the Spike protein by cleavage at the boundary between S1 and S2 and the S2' site in S2 domain.[24] Similar to SARS-CoV-1 and SARSr-CoVs, SARS-CoV-2 binds to human angiotensin-converting enzyme 2 (ACE2) through interaction with the RBD.[6,25] However, SARS-CoV-2 Spike protein contains a unique polybasic cleavage site at S1/s2 boundary that is recognized by Furin, an ubiquitous host protease,[25] which contributes to SARS-CoV-2 pathogenesis and host adaptation.[24,26] Furin cleavage allows for the S2 subunit to mediate host cell fusion, promoting viral entry into target cells. The Spike protein is further cleaved at target cell surface by TMPRSS2 and on endocytosis, by Cathepsin L in the endosome.[27] Given its key role in SARS-CoV-2 lifecycle and cell entry, the Spike protein has been targeted by several monoclonal antibodies that can neutralize the virus, especially by targeting the RBD.[28,29]

Evolution and Variants

Similar to other RNA viruses, the SARS-CoV-2 RNA-dependent RNA polymerase has a relatively high error rate, although the error rate is mitigated in part by the presence of a proofreading mechanism mediated by the nsp14-encoded exonuclease.[12,30] There was initial optimism about the lack of genetic diversity seen in the early stages of the pandemic,[31] including relatively limited intrahost viral diversity in next-generation sequencing studies. Lythgoe and colleagues[32] demonstrate that average intrahost single-nucleotide variant (iSNV) count is 1.4 iSNVs per sample (0.47 base substitution per 10kb), and this observation was only seen at high viral loads, sampled a median of 6 days apart. In addition, the bottleneck size for intrahost variants is very small, indicating the difficulty of transmitting intrahost mutant variants to others.[32] However, in immunocompromised hosts, the situation seems different. In patients with cancer infected with SARS-CoV-2, intrahost diversity is far higher than in the immunocompetent control group (iSNV 0.77 vs 0.45 base substitution per 10kb),[33] and immunocompromised individuals are at risk of persistent COVID-19 infections.[34] One of the most extreme cases that has been reported is an individual with antiphospholipid antibody syndrome, who was receiving a broad spectrum of immunosuppressants targeting T cells, B cells, complement system, and innate immunity. This patient suffered from persistent COVID-19 over a 5-month period and harbored constantly evolving virus and eventually succumbed to COVID-19, despite Remdesivir and monoclonal antibody administration.[35] Viral genome sequencing at different time points demonstrated a dynamic pattern of mutations, with an overall accumulation of mutations. When comparing sequences from approximately 5 months after the initial diagnosis, there was an average of 4.67 base substitutions per 10kb (excluding the deletions in Spike protein region; compared with 0.45–0.47 in the aforementioned immunocompetent hosts), with mutations overrepresented in the Spike protein gene that highlights the Spike protein as the site of intense immune pressure.[35–37] In addition, the mutations that emerged in this patient were subsequently identified as key mutations in several variants of concern, suggesting that immunosuppressed individuals may be a source for the emergence of new variants. Similar cases in immunocompromised patients infected with SARS-CoV-2 further support the negative correlation between host immunity and accelerated intrahost evolution.[38–40]

From the population level, interhost mutations and evolution have certainly complicated this pandemic by multiple folds. D614G mutation on Spike protein was the first major mutation discovered since the beginning of this pandemic. D614G was rare before March 2020 but rapidly became the globally dominant mutation since May 2020.[41] This mutation is associated with enhanced infectivity and replication compared with the original strain with D614.[41,42] This enhanced infectivity is mediated by an increase in Furin cleavage efficiency and more frequent RBD "up" state[43] that characterizes a conformation facilitating ACE2 accessibility.[44] However, G614 and D614 strains have similar level of susceptibility to neutralization from convalescent plasma/serum.[45] With further global spread and replication, SARS-CoV-2 continues to diversify and has developed into multiple circulating variants. By the beginning of 2022, there have been 5 major variants of concern (VOC) and 6 variants of interest (VOI) documented on the GISAID database.[46,47] The VOCs and certain VOIs are summarized in **Table 1**.

Among all these VOC and VOI strains, the Delta variant merits further discussion. This variant was first detected in India in December 2020 and caused a disastrous surge in COVID-19 cases and death in early 2021. By July 2021 it has already supplanted the then-dominant strains (Alpha, Beta, and Gamma) to become the dominant strain in most countries of the world.[47,48] The Delta variant has several features that seem to enhance transmission. First, it contains several antibody evasion mutations.[49] Several neutralization studies have demonstrated that the Delta variant is associated with decreased sensitivity to convalescent sera, vaccinated sera, or bamlanivimab (a monoclonal antibody targeting the Spike protein), compared with the wild-type strains or the Alpha variant.[50,51] In addition, real-world data demonstrate that certain adenovirus-vector–based vaccine (ChAdOx1 nCoV-19) and mRNA-based vaccine (BNT162b2) have a modestly decreased vaccine efficacy against symptomatic disease.[48] Second, the Delta variant contains certain mutations that may escape preexisting cellular immunity from prior infection or vaccination. Two groups have demonstrated that L452R, the signature mutation in the Delta variant, is associated with decrease in HLA-A24– or HLA-A02–restricted CD8+ T-cell response to the T-cell epitope containing this mutation.[52,53] Third, the Delta variant is associated with more efficient membrane fusion independent of better ACE2 binding. Zhang and colleagues[54] demonstrated that Delta strain had higher fusion activity toward target cells in an in vitro system without having higher affinity to ACE2 compared with other variants. Last but not the least, Syed Abdullah and colleagues[55] used an SARS-CoV-2 virus-like particle model and demonstrated that key nucleocapsid mutations found in Delta variant, including R203M, are associated with enhanced viral RNA packaging and replication. Although the Beta and Gamma variants mediate a greater degree of escape against vaccine or natural immunity–mediated immune responses, the greater transmissibility of Delta allowed it to supplant these variants. Together, the features discussed earlier enable Delta variant to transmit efficiently and evade preexisting adaptive immunity, leading to higher viral shedding in the upper respiratory

Table 1
Summary of variants of concern and certain variants of interest per World Health Organization definition

Variants	First Identified	Key Spike Mutations	Impact on Antibody Neutralization	Impact on Viral Entry and Transmission
VOC				
Alpha[a]	United Kingdom	69–70del, **144del**, N501Y, A570D, D614G, P681H, T716I, S982A, D1118H	+/–	++
Beta[a]	South Africa	D80A, D215G, **241–243del**, K417N, **E484K**, N501Y, D614G, A701V	++	++
Gamma[a]	Japan/Brazil	**L18F, T20N, P26S**, D138Y, R190S, **K417T, E484K**, N501Y, <u>D614G, **H655Y**</u>, T1027I, V1176F	++	++
Delta	India	**T19R**, G142D, E156G, **157–158del, L452R, T478K**, D614G, **P681R**, D950N	++	+++
Omicron	South Africa	A67V, del69–70, T95I, G142D, **del143–145**, , del212, G339D, S371L, S373P, S375F, **K417N**, N440K, **G446S**, S477N, T478K, **E484A, Q493R**, G496S, **Q498R**, N501Y, Y505H, T547K, <u>D614G, **H655Y**</u>, N679K, **P681H**, N764K, D796Y, N856K, Q954H, N969K, L981F	++++	++++
VOI				
Lambda[a]	Peru	G75V, T76I, R246N, **del247–253, L452Q, F490S**, D614G, T859N	++	++
Iota[a]	United States	L5F, T95I, **D253G, E484K**, D614G	++	+
Mu[a]	Colombia	**T95I**, Y144S, Y145N, R346K, **E484K**, N501Y, D614G, P681H, D950N	+++	++
Kappa[a]	India	**L452R, E484Q**, <u>D614G, P681R</u>, Q1071H	+++	++

Bold font, adaptive immunity escape mutations. Underline, increase in ACE2 binding affinity and transmission.
[a] Currently listed as Variant Being Monitored (VBM) by US CDC.
Data from Refs[50,51,54,61,78,117–123]

tract,[56,57] more rapid transmission,[58] and vaccine "breakthrough" infection[59] compared with ancestral strains. Fortunately, vaccination is still associated with more rapid viral clearance in those Delta breakthrough cases compared with unvaccinated cases.[60]

The Omicron variant, first reported in South Africa in November 2021, has further led this pandemic into an uncharted water. The rate that the Omicron variant has spread world-wide has been unprecedented, and it has become the dominant strain worldwide.[61] The Omicron variant has developed an extensive set of mutations in the Spike protein[62–66]; this unfortunately leads to escape from multiple FDA-authorized monoclonal antibody treatments[62,63] and leads to substantial reductions in vaccine-induced neutralizing titers.[64,67,68] Somewhat reassuringly, CD4 and CD8 T cells from vaccinated and/or previously infected people retain activity against the Omicron strain,[69] although as many as 21% of the participants in one study has shown significant reduction in Omicron spike recognition by the CD8 T cells.[70] In addition, Omicron is not as efficiently antagonizing IFN signaling pathway as other variants and remain susceptible to most of the available antiviral small molecules authorized by the FDA.[71] Last but not the least, several in vitro and animal studies have demonstrated that the Omicron strain preferably replicate in the upper respiratory epithelium and does not replicate well in the lungs, causing less severe inflammation in the lung tissue in animal models.[72–74] These findings could potentially indicate differences in its clinical phenotypes and outcomes, as reported in a recent study from South Africa suggesting milder disease and lower morbidity/mortality,[75] but more evidence is needed.

Animal Reservoirs

SARS-CoV-2 seems to have broad tropism across species, and infection has been observed in a wide range of animals besides the bats.[76] Gu and colleagues[77] demonstrated that SARS-CoV-2 developed a de novo mutation in the Spike protein gene after 6 passages of a viral strain from clinical isolate in early 2020 (BetaCov/human/CHN/Beijing_IME-BJ05/2020), when VOCs/VOIs had not yet arisen. This mutation N501Y confers higher affinity to mice ACE2 and is associated with adaptation to mice[77] and is subsequently found in 4 major VOCs: Alpha, Beta, Gamma, and Omicron.[61,78] Similarly, in domestic cats, a consensus mutation at Spike protein, H655Y, has been detected, which is also found in the Gamma and Omicron VOCs.[79] In addition, SARS-CoV-2 transmission among minks is associated with a mutation at Spike Y453F, suggesting adaptation to mink ACE2.[80,81] A very recent study evaluating free-ranging white-tail deer in Ohio, US has demonstrated a shockingly 35.8% SARS-CoV-2 nucleic acid detection rate from nasal swabs between January and March 2021. This study further identified multiple independent human-to-dear transmission events based on the phylogenetic analysis from sequences obtained from human and deer at different locations and timepoints.[82] Surprisingly, certain mutations that are rare in humans (<0.5%–0.05% globally) are seen in deer, including $\Delta141$ to 144 and E484D[82]; this indicates a possibility of deer-to-deer transmission and independent evolution. The significance of animal reservoirs of SARS-CoV-2 remains to be determined but has important implications for our efforts to eradicate the pandemic and prevent the emergence of new variants.

Upper and Lower Respiratory Tract Infection and Replication

SARS-CoV-2 replication follows different virological dynamics in upper and lower respiratory tracts. The biological mechanism behind this finding could be due to different levels of ACE2 and entry factors expression in upper and lower airways. In an early study synthesizing multiple preexisting single-cell RNA sequencing (scRNA-seq) datasets generated from healthy donors, Sungnak and colleagues[83] demonstrated that ACE2 and TMPRSS2 expression levels are higher in cells derived from nasal cavity than lungs and bronchi. This finding is further confirmed by a study using a more sensitive technique, RNA-in situ hybridization, demonstrating that upper airway epithelial cells express higher levels of ACE2 and TMPRSS2 compared with lower respiratory tract.[84] In this study, in vitro cell line models from both upper and lower respiratory tracts, and autopsy results demonstrating patchy segmental/subsegmental viral infection, further suggest that SARS-CoV-2 viral replication starts from the upper respiratory tract followed by aspiration and subsequent lower respiratory tract infection.[84] This theory is further supported by an animal model study in which only intranasal challenge was conducted in rhesus macaque.[85] In this study, an early peak of viral load in the upper respiratory system at days 2 to 6 postinfection was noted, in comparison to peak viral load at day 9 in the lower respiratory tract.[85] In a clinical cohort where the date of infection was known and only mild cases were included, Wölfel and colleagues[86] described that viral level peaked later in sputum sample compared with upper respiratory tract swab; in addition, 2 participants with lower respiratory tract involvement showed prolonged viral persistence in sputum, significant delay in viral level peak in sputum compared with the upper respiratory sample, and more than one viral level peaks in sputum.[86] These findings indicate ongoing replication in the lower respiratory tract that is disconnected from upper airway viral replication.[86] Similarly, in a cohort study of 196 hospitalized participants, the viral level from upper respiratory tract peaked within 7 days after symptom onset, whereas sputum viral level peaked between 7 and 14 days after symptom onset, highlighting the temporal and spatial gradient of SARS-CoV-2 viral spread and replication in different respiratory compartments.[87]

Systemic Dissemination and Disease Severity

Plasma viremia can be detected in several respiratory viral infections including SARS-CoV-1,[88] influenza virus,[89] respiratory syncytial virus,[90] and adenovirus[91] infection and has been associated with more severe disease. In contrast to SARS-CoV-1 infection, where almost 80% of patients have viremia within first 3 days of symptom onset,[88] a lower proportion of patients with COVID-19 have had detectable SARS-CoV-2 RNA in the blood,[92–94] although rates of plasma viremia detection may be affected by disease severity, duration of symptoms, and sensitivity of the tests. The authors' group and other investigators have demonstrated that SARS-CoV-2 viremia (or referenced as RNAemia in other literature) is associated with worse disease outcomes including ARDS and death.[92,94–97] Furthermore, those hospitalized in critical care settings have higher odds of having viremia than in noncritical care settings.[92,95,97,98] Similarly, lower respiratory tract viral loads tend to correlate with disease severity[97,99]; this is in stark contrast with viral levels in the upper respiratory tract, which does not seem to correlate well with severity of symptoms and disease.[97,100–102] As discussed in the previous section, SARS-CoV-2 may have comparable replication levels in upper respiratory tract across different severity spectrum due to expression of high levels of ACE2 and other entry factors, but the determinant of severe disease is mainly due to lower respiratory tract infection and subsequent hematogenous dissemination. This hypothesis is further supported by a proteomic study showing that SARS-CoV-2 viremia is associated with severe disease and death, along with higher levels of lung damage–related proteins, fibrosis markers, and extrapulmonary organ damage markers from gastrointestinal (GI) system, and vasculature- and coagulation-related factors.[92] Several autopsy studies have also demonstrated detection of SARS-CoV-2 RNA in multiple extrapulmonary tissues, including tissues from the GI, cardiovascular, endocrine, lymphatic, urinary, bone marrow, reproductive, and central nervous systems.[35,103,104] This extrapulmonary dissemination theory is further supported by mounting evidence of SARS-CoV-2 replication and virion detection in in vitro organoid models[105] and ultimately clinical samples including GI tract,[106,107] pancreatic islets,[108] placenta,[109] kidney tissue,[110] and endothelium.[111] However, caution is warranted when interpreting some of the transmission electron microscopy (TEM) results, as some subcellular structures can be misconstrued as virions and further clarification methods are warranted.[112,113] In addition to extrapulmonary involvement, several studies have shown that SARS-CoV-2 viremia is further associated with complement system activation and elevated proinflammatory cytokine levels.[92,94,98]

Given that SARS-CoV-2 infection can cause extrapulmonary involvement and dissemination from lungs, an ongoing question is the mechanism by which SARS-CoV-2 disseminates. A few studies have shown that SARS-CoV-2 virions, rather than just RNA fragments, can be detected in the blood vessels and blood. Ackermann and colleagues[111] first reported prominent endothelial injury and inflammation in COVID-19 lung autopsy compared with influenza-infected lung tissue; furthermore, SARS-CoV-2 virions are visible in endothelial cells through TEM. This result suggests that SARS-CoV-2 can infect the endovascular system, leading to systemic dissemination. From plasma samples, Jacobs and colleagues[114] demonstrated that SARS-CoV-2 virions can be detected via TEM and further confirmed by immunostaining. These findings further support the theory that SARS-CoV-2 may first gain entry to the circulatory system from the pulmonary vasculature due to extensive lung damage, followed by infection of endothelial cells, leading to systemic dissemination of virions. However, it remains elusive whether SARS-CoV-2 virions are carried within certain cellular or acellular components in the blood during dissemination (ie, monocytes,[115,116] platelets,[114] and so forth) and how they infect extrapulmonary tissues.

SUMMARY

Understanding the virology behind SARS-CoV-2 infection has provided key insights into our efforts to develop antiviral agents and control the pandemic. However, there remains substantial gaps in our knowledge of SARS-CoV-2 biology and pathogenesis. Studies are needed to further dissect the functions of each nonstructural and accessory proteins and how they contribute to the pathogenesis of SARS-CoV-2. In addition, we need to understand the roles of the multiple mutations in the newly emergent variants (eg, Omicron variant) and how they contribute to increased transmission and immune evasion. There are also increasing questions on the role of systemic viral dissemination in the pathogenesis of severe disease and the detection of viremia as a prognostic marker. Furthermore, we know relatively little about the animal reservoirs of SARS-CoV-2 and their potential to fuel the emergence of new variants. The answers to these questions will be crucial as we devise improved vaccine strategies and antiviral therapies.

CLINICS CARE POINTS

- Immunocompromised patients are at higher risk of developing immune escape mutations and prolonged SARS-CoV-2 infection.
- SARS-CoV-2 has different replication dynamics in the upper and lower respiratory tracts.

- SARS-CoV-2 viremia and dissemination are associated with worse outcomes.

FUNDING SOURCES

Massachusetts Consortium for Pathogen Readiness (to J.Z. Li) and Harvard University Center for AIDS Research (NIAID 5P30AI060354 to J.Z. Li).

DISCLOSURE

J.Z.Li has consulted for Abbvie and Recovery Therapeutics.

REFERENCES

1. Lu R, Zhao X, Li J, et al. Genomic characterisation and epidemiology of 2019 novel coronavirus: implications for virus origins and receptor binding. Lancet 2020;395(10224):565–74.
2. Huang C, Wang Y, Li X, et al. Clinical features of patients infected with 2019 novel coronavirus in Wuhan, China. Lancet 2020;395(10223):497–506.
3. Wiersinga WJ, Rhodes A, Cheng AC, et al. Pathophysiology, transmission, diagnosis, and treatment of coronavirus disease 2019 (COVID-19): a review. JAMA 2020;324(8):782–93.
4. Thompson HA, Mousa A, Dighe A, et al. SARS-CoV-2 setting-specific transmission rates: a systematic review and meta-analysis. Clin Infect Dis 2021;73(3): e754–64.
5. The pandemic's true death toll. 2022. Available at: https://www.economist.com/graphic-detail/coronavirus-excess-deaths-estimates. [Accessed 16 January 2022]. Accessed.
6. Zhou P, Yang XL, Wang XG, et al. A pneumonia outbreak associated with a new coronavirus of probable bat origin. Nature 2020;579(7798):270–3.
7. Lam TT-Y, Jia N, Zhang Y-W, et al. Identifying SARS-CoV-2-related coronaviruses in Malayan pangolins. Nature 2020;583(7815):282–5.
8. Zhou H, Ji J, Chen X, et al. Identification of novel bat coronaviruses sheds light on the evolutionary origins of SARS-CoV-2 and related viruses. Cell 2021; 184(17):4380–91.e14.
9. Delaune D, Hul V, Karlsson EA, et al. A novel SARS-CoV-2 related coronavirus in bats from Cambodia. Nat Commun 2021;12(1):6563.
10. Suryawanshi RK, Koganti R, Agelidis A, et al. Dysregulation of cell signaling by SARS-CoV-2. Trends Microbiol 2021;29(3):224–37.
11. Thoms M, Buschauer R, Ameismeier M, et al. Structural basis for translational shutdown and immune evasion by the Nsp1 protein of SARS-CoV-2. Science 2020;369(6508):1249.
12. Robson F, Khan KS, Le TK, et al. Coronavirus RNA proofreading: molecular basis and therapeutic targeting. Mol Cell 2020;80(6):1136–8.
13. Redondo N, Zaldívar-López S, Garrido JJ, et al. SARS-CoV-2 accessory proteins in viral pathogenesis: knowns and unknowns. Front Immunol 2021;12: 2698.
14. Lei X, Dong X, Ma R, et al. Activation and evasion of type I interferon responses by SARS-CoV-2. Nat Commun 2020;11(1):3810.
15. Xia H, Cao Z, Xie X, et al. Evasion of type I interferon by SARS-CoV-2. Cell Rep 2020;33(1):108234.

16. Zhang Y, Chen Y, Li Y, et al. The ORF8 protein of SARS-CoV-2 mediates immune evasion through down-regulating MHC-I. Proc Natl Acad Sci USA 2021;118(23).
17. Gordon DE, Jang GM, Bouhaddou M, et al. A SARS-CoV-2 protein interaction map reveals targets for drug repurposing. Nature 2020;583(7816):459–68.
18. Hillen HS, Kokic G, Farnung L, et al. Structure of replicating SARS-CoV-2 polymerase. Nature 2020;584(7819):154–6.
19. Beigel JH, Tomashek KM, Dodd LE, et al. Remdesivir for the treatment of Covid-19 - final report. N Engl J Med 2020;383(19):1813–26.
20. Gottlieb RL, Vaca CE, Paredes R, et al. Early remdesivir to prevent progression to severe Covid-19 in outpatients. N Engl J Med 2022;386(4):305–15.
21. Lee J, Worrall LJ, Vuckovic M, et al. Crystallographic structure of wild-type SARS-CoV-2 main protease acyl-enzyme intermediate with physiological C-terminal autoprocessing site. Nat Commun 2020;11(1):5877.
22. Owen Dafydd R, Allerton Charlotte MN, Anderson Annaliesa S, et al. An oral SARS-CoV-2 Mpro inhibitor clinical candidate for the treatment of COVID-19. Science 2021;eabl4784.
23. FDA. Fact sheet for healthcare providers: emergency use authorization for paxlovid. Available at: https://www.fda.gov/media/155050/download. [Accessed 17 January 2021]. Accessed.
24. Peacock TP, Goldhill DH, Zhou J, et al. The furin cleavage site in the SARS-CoV-2 spike protein is required for transmission in ferrets. Nat Microbiol 2021;6(7):899–909.
25. Walls AC, Park Y-J, Tortorici MA, et al. Structure, function, and antigenicity of the SARS-CoV-2 spike glycoprotein. Cell 2020;181(2):281–92.e286.
26. Johnson BA, Xie X, Bailey AL, et al. Loss of furin cleavage site attenuates SARS-CoV-2 pathogenesis. Nature 2021;591(7849):293–9.
27. Shang J, Wan Y, Luo C, et al. Cell entry mechanisms of SARS-CoV-2. Proc Natl Acad Sci 2020;117(21):11727.
28. Weinreich DM, Sivapalasingam S, Norton T, et al. REGN-COV2, a neutralizing antibody cocktail, in outpatients with Covid-19. N Engl J Med 2021;384(3):238–51.
29. Dougan M, Nirula A, Azizad M, et al. Bamlanivimab plus etesevimab in mild or moderate Covid-19. N Engl J Med 2021;385(15):1382–92.
30. Rona G, Zeke A, Miwatani-Minter B, et al. The NSP14/NSP10 RNA repair complex as a Pan-coronavirus therapeutic target. Cell Death Differ 2021;29(2):285–92.
31. Rausch JW, Capoferri AA, Katusiime MG, et al. Low genetic diversity may be an Achilles heel of SARS-CoV-2. Proc Natl Acad Sci 2020;117(40):24614.
32. Lythgoe KA, Hall M, Ferretti L, et al. SARS-CoV-2 within-host diversity and transmission. Science 2021;372(6539):eabg0821.
33. Siqueira JD, Goes LR, Alves BM, et al. SARS-CoV-2 genomic analyses in cancer patients reveal elevated intrahost genetic diversity. Virus Evol 2021;7(1):veab013.
34. Choudhary MC, Crain CR, Qiu X, et al. SARS-CoV-2 sequence characteristics of COVID-19 persistence and reinfection. Clin Infect Dis 2022;74(2):237–45.
35. Choi B, Choudhary MC, Regan J, et al. Persistence and Evolution of SARS-CoV-2 in an Immunocompromised Host. N Engl J Med 2020;383(23):2291–3.
36. Clark SA, Clark LE, Pan J, et al. SARS-CoV-2 evolution in an immunocompromised host reveals shared neutralization escape mechanisms. Cell 2021;184(10):2605–17.e2618.

37. Starr TN, Greaney AJ, Addetia A, et al. Prospective mapping of viral mutations that escape antibodies used to treat COVID-19. Science 2021;371(6531):850–4.
38. Hensley MK, Bain WG, Jacobs J, et al. Intractable COVID-19 and prolonged SARS-CoV-2 replication in a CAR-T-cell therapy recipient: a case study. Clin Infect Dis 2021;73(3):e815–21.
39. Drouin AC, Theberge MW, Liu SY, et al. Successful clearance of 300 day SARS-CoV-2 infection in a subject with B-cell depletion associated prolonged (B-DEAP) COVID by REGEN-COV anti-spike monoclonal antibody cocktail. Viruses 2021;13(7):1202.
40. Gandhi S, Klein J, Robertson A, et al. De novo emergence of a remdesivir resistance mutation during treatment of persistent SARS-CoV-2 infection in an immunocompromised patient: A case report. medRxiv 2021.
41. Korber B, Fischer WM, Gnanakaran S, et al. Tracking changes in SARS-CoV-2 spike: evidence that D614G increases infectivity of the COVID-19 virus. Cell 2020;182(4):812–27.e819.
42. Plante JA, Liu Y, Liu J, et al. Spike mutation D614G alters SARS-CoV-2 fitness. Nature 2021;592(7852):116–21.
43. Gobeil SMC, Janowska K, McDowell S, et al. D614G Mutation Alters SARS-CoV-2 Spike conformation and enhances protease cleavage at the S1/S2 junction. Cell Rep 2021;34(2):108630.
44. Cai Y, Zhang J, Xiao T, et al. Distinct conformational states of SARS-CoV-2 spike protein. Science 2020;369(6511):1586.
45. Li Q, Wu J, Nie J, et al. The impact of mutations in SARS-CoV-2 spike on viral infectivity and antigenicity. Cell 2020;182(5):1284–94.e1289.
46. Elbe S, Buckland-Merrett G. Data, disease and diplomacy: GISAID's innovative contribution to global health. Glob challenges (Hoboken, NJ) 2017;1(1):33–46.
47. GISAID. Available at: https://www.gisaid.org/. Accessed 01/16/2021.
48. Lopez Bernal J, Andrews N, Gower C, et al. Effectiveness of Covid-19 vaccines against the B.1.617.2 (Delta) variant. New Engl J Med 2021;385(7):585–94.
49. Liu Z, VanBlargan LA, Bloyet LM, et al. Identification of SARS-CoV-2 spike mutations that attenuate monoclonal and serum antibody neutralization. Cell Host Microbe 2021;29(3):477–88.e474.
50. Planas D, Veyer D, Baidaliuk A, et al. Reduced sensitivity of SARS-CoV-2 variant Delta to antibody neutralization. Nature 2021;596(7871):276–80.
51. Edara V-V, Pinsky BA, Suthar MS, et al. Infection and vaccine-induced neutralizing-antibody responses to the SARS-CoV-2 B.1.617 variants. New Engl J Med 2021;385(7):664–6.
52. Zhang H, Deng S, Ren L, et al. Profiling CD8+ T Cell Epitopes of COVID-19 convalescents reveals reduced cellular immune responses to SARS-CoV-2 variants. Cell Rep 2021;36(11):109708.
53. Motozono C, Toyoda M, Zahradnik J, et al. SARS-CoV-2 spike L452R variant evades cellular immunity and increases infectivity. Cell Host Microbe 2021;29(7):1124–36.e1111.
54. Zhang J, Xiao T, Cai Y, et al. Membrane fusion and immune evasion by the spike protein of SARS-CoV-2 Delta variant. Science 2021;374(6573):1353–60.
55. Syed Abdullah M, Taha Taha Y, Tabata T, et al. Rapid assessment of SARS-CoV-2 evolved variants using virus-like particles. Science 2021;374(6575):1626–32.
56. Ong SWX, Chiew CJ, Ang LW, et al. Clinical and virological features of SARS-CoV-2 variants of concern: a retrospective cohort study comparing B.1.1.7 (Alpha), B.1.315 (Beta), and B.1.617.2 (Delta). Clin Infect Dis 2021;ciab721.

57. Teyssou E, Delagrèverie H, Visseaux B, et al. The Delta SARS-CoV-2 variant has a higher viral load than the Beta and the historical variants in nasopharyngeal samples from newly diagnosed COVID-19. J Infect 2021;83(4):e1–3.
58. Liu Y, Rocklöv J. The reproductive number of the Delta variant of SARS-CoV-2 is far higher compared to the ancestral SARS-CoV-2 virus. J Travel Med 2021; 28(7):taab124.
59. Brown CM, Vostok J, Johnson H, et al. Outbreak of SARS-CoV-2 Infections, Including COVID-19 vaccine breakthrough infections, associated with large public gatherings - barnstable county, massachusetts, July 2021. MMWR Morb Mortal Wkly Rep 2021;70(31):1059–62.
60. Shamier MC, Tostmann A, Bogers S, et al. Virological characteristics of SARS-CoV-2 vaccine breakthrough infections in health care workers. medRxiv 2021.
61. Nextstrain. Genomic epidemiology of novel coronavirus - Global subsampling. Available at: https://nextstrain.org/ncov/gisaid/global. Accessed 1/6/2022.
62. Cao YR, Wang J, Jian F, et al. Omicron escapes the majority of existing SARS-CoV-2 neutralizing antibodies. Nature 2021.
63. Cathcart AL, Havenar-Daughton C, Lempp FA, et al. The dual function monoclonal antibodies VIR-7831 and VIR-7832 demonstrate potent in vitro and in vivo activity against SARS-CoV-2. bioRxiv 2021.
64. Garcia-Beltran WF, St. Denis KJ, Hoelzemer A, et al. mRNA-based COVID-19 vaccine boosters induce neutralizing immunity against SARS-CoV-2 Omicron variant. Cell 2022;185(3):457–66.e4.
65. Liu L, Iketani S, Guo Y, et al. Striking antibody evasion manifested by the omicron variant of SARS-CoV-2. Nature 2021.
66. Wilhelm A, Widera M, Grikscheit K, et al. Reduced Neutralization of SARS-CoV-2 Omicron Variant by Vaccine Sera and monoclonal antibodies. medRxiv 2021.
67. Dejnirattisai W, Shaw RH, Supasa P, et al. Reduced neutralisation of SARS-CoV-2 omicron B.1.1.529 variant by post-immunisation serum. Lancet 2022; 399(10321):234–6.
68. Nemet I, Kliker L, Lustig Y, et al. Third BNT162b2 vaccination neutralization of SARS-CoV-2 omicron infection. N Engl J Med 2021.
69. Liu J, Chandrashekar A, Sellers D, et al. Vaccines elicit highly cross-reactive cellular immunity to the SARS-CoV-2 omicron variant. medRxiv 2022.
70. Naranbhai V, Nathan A, Kaseke C, et al. T cell reactivity to the SARS-CoV-2 Omicron variant is preserved in most but not all prior infected and vaccinated individuals. medRxiv 2022.
71. Bojkova D, Widera M, Ciesek S, et al. Reduced interferon antagonism but similar drug sensitivity in Omicron variant compared to Delta variant SARS-CoV-2 isolates. bioRxiv 2022.
72. McMahan K, Giffin V, Tostanoski LH, et al. Reduced Pathogenicity of the SARS-CoV-2 Omicron Variant in Hamsters. bioRxiv 2022.
73. Bentley EG, Kirby A, Sharma P, et al. SARS-CoV-2 Omicron-B.1.1.529 Variant leads to less severe disease than Pango B and Delta variants strains in a mouse model of severe COVID-19. bioRxiv 2021.
74. Meng B, Ferreira IATM, Abdullahi A, et al. SARS-CoV-2 Omicron spike mediated immune escape, infectivity and cell-cell fusion. bioRxiv 2021.
75. Maslo C, Friedland R, Toubkin M, et al. Characteristics and Outcomes of Hospitalized Patients in South Africa During the COVID-19 Omicron Wave Compared With Previous Waves. JAMA 2022;327(6):583–4.
76. Conceicao C, Thakur N, Human S, et al. The SARS-CoV-2 Spike protein has a broad tropism for mammalian ACE2 proteins. PLOS Biol 2020;18(12):e3001016.

77. Gu H, Chen Q, Yang G, et al. Adaptation of SARS-CoV-2 in BALB/c mice for testing vaccine efficacy. Science 2020;369(6511):1603–7.
78. Tzou PL, Tao K, Nouhin J, et al. Coronavirus antiviral research database (Cov-RDB): an online database designed to facilitate comparisons between candidate anti-coronavirus compounds. Viruses 2020;12(9):1006.
79. Braun KM, Moreno GK, Halfmann PJ, et al. Transmission of SARS-CoV-2 in domestic cats imposes a narrow bottleneck. PLoS Pathog 2021;17(2):e1009373.
80. Oude Munnink BB, Sikkema RS, Nieuwenhuijse DF, et al. Transmission of SARS-CoV-2 on mink farms between humans and mink and back to humans. Science 2021;371(6525):172.
81. Bayarri-Olmos R, Rosbjerg A, Johnsen LB, et al. The SARS-CoV-2 Y453F mink variant displays a pronounced increase in ACE-2 affinity but does not challenge antibody neutralization. J Biol Chem 2021;296:100536.
82. Hale VL, Dennis PM, McBride DS, et al. SARS-CoV-2 infection in free-ranging white-tailed deer. Nature 2022;602(7897):481–6.
83. Sungnak W, Huang N, Bécavin C, et al. SARS-CoV-2 entry factors are highly expressed in nasal epithelial cells together with innate immune genes. Nat Med 2020;26(5):681–7.
84. Hou YJ, Okuda K, Edwards CE, et al. SARS-CoV-2 reverse genetics reveals a variable infection gradient in the respiratory tract. Cell 2020;182(2):429–46.e414.
85. Zheng H, Li H, Guo L, et al. Virulence and pathogenesis of SARS-CoV-2 infection in rhesus macaques: a nonhuman primate model of COVID-19 progression. PLOS Pathog 2020;16(11):e1008949.
86. Wölfel R, Corman VM, Guggemos W, et al. Virological assessment of hospitalized patients with COVID-2019. Nature 2020;581(7809):465–9.
87. Regan J, Flynn JP, Rosenthal A, et al. Viral load kinetics of SARS-CoV-2 in hospitalized individuals with COVID-19. Open Forum Infect Dis 2021;8(8):ofab153.
88. Grant PR, Garson JA, Tedder RS, et al. Detection of SARS coronavirus in plasma by real-time RT-PCR. N Engl J Med 2003;349(25):2468–9.
89. Choi SM, Xie H, Campbell AP, et al. Influenza viral RNA detection in blood as a marker to predict disease severity in hematopoietic cell transplant recipients. J Infect Dis 2012;206(12):1872–7.
90. Waghmare A, Campbell AP, Xie H, et al. Respiratory syncytial virus lower respiratory disease in hematopoietic cell transplant recipients: viral RNA detection in blood, antiviral treatment, and clinical outcomes. Clin Infect Dis 2013;57(12):1731–41.
91. Taniguchi K, Yoshihara S, Tamaki H, et al. Incidence and treatment strategy for disseminated adenovirus disease after haploidentical stem cell transplantation. Ann Hematol 2012;91(8):1305–12.
92. Li Y, Schneider AM, Mehta A, et al. SARS-CoV-2 viremia is associated with distinct proteomic pathways and predicts COVID-19 outcomes. J Clin Invest 2021;131(13):e148635.
93. Prebensen C, Hre PLM, Jonassen C, et al. SARS-CoV-2 RNA in plasma is associated with ICU admission and mortality in patients hospitalized with COVID-19. Clin Infect Dis 2020;73(3):e799–802.
94. Gutmann C, Takov K, Burnap SA, et al. SARS-CoV-2 RNAemia and proteomic trajectories inform prognostication in COVID-19 patients admitted to intensive care. Nat Commun 2021;12(1):3406.
95. Chen X, Zhao B, Qu Y, et al. Detectable serum severe acute respiratory syndrome Coronavirus 2 viral load (RNAemia) is closely correlated with drastically

elevated interleukin 6 level in critically Ill patients with coronavirus disease 2019. Clin Infect Dis 2020;71(8):1937–42.

96. Eberhardt KA, Meyer-Schwickerath C, Heger E, et al. RNAemia corresponds to disease severity and antibody response in hospitalized COVID-19 patients. Viruses 2020;12(9):1045.

97. Fajnzylber J, Regan J, Coxen K, et al. SARS-CoV-2 viral load is associated with increased disease severity and mortality. Nat Commun 2020;11(1):5493.

98. Bermejo-Martin JF, González-Rivera M, Almansa R, et al. Viral RNA load in plasma is associated with critical illness and a dysregulated host response in COVID-19. Crit Care 2020;24(1):691.

99. Buetti N, Wicky P-H, Le Hingrat Q, et al. SARS-CoV-2 detection in the lower respiratory tract of invasively ventilated ARDS patients. Crit Care 2020;24(1):610.

100. Lee S, Kim T, Lee E, et al. Clinical course and molecular viral shedding among asymptomatic and symptomatic patients with SARS-CoV-2 infection in a community treatment center in the republic of Korea. JAMA Intern Med 2020; 180(11):1447–52.

101. Ra SH, Lim JS, Kim G-u, et al. Upper respiratory viral load in asymptomatic individuals and mildly symptomatic patients with SARS-CoV-2 infection. Thorax 2021;76(1):61.

102. Chew KW, Moser C, Daar ES, et al. Bamlanivimab reduces nasopharyngeal SARS-CoV-2 RNA levels but not symptom duration in non-hospitalized adults with COVID-19. medRxiv 2021.

103. Yao X-H, Luo T, Shi Y, et al. A cohort autopsy study defines COVID-19 systemic pathogenesis. Cell Res 2021;31(8):836–46.

104. Nie X, Qian L, Sun R, et al. Multi-organ proteomic landscape of COVID-19 autopsies. Cell 2021;184(3):775–91.e714.

105. Lamers MM, Beumer J, van der Vaart J, et al. SARS-CoV-2 productively infects human gut enterocytes. Science 2020;369(6499):50–4.

106. Qian Q, Fan L, Liu W, et al. Direct evidence of active SARS-CoV-2 replication in the intestine. Clin Infect Dis 2020.

107. Das Adhikari U, Eng G, Farcasanu M, et al. Fecal SARS-CoV-2 RNA is associated with decreased COVID-19 survival. Clin Infect Dis 2021;ciab623.

108. Steenblock C, Richter S, Berger I, et al. Viral infiltration of pancreatic islets in patients with COVID-19. Nat Commun 2021;12(1):3534.

109. Facchetti F, Bugatti M, Drera E, et al. SARS-CoV2 vertical transmission with adverse effects on the newborn revealed through integrated immunohistochemical, electron microscopy and molecular analyses of Placenta. EBioMedicine 2020;59:102951.

110. Su H, Yang M, Wan C, et al. Renal histopathological analysis of 26 postmortem findings of patients with COVID-19 in China. Kidney Int 2020;98(1):219–27.

111. Ackermann M, Verleden SE, Kuehnel M, et al. Pulmonary vascular endothelialitis, thrombosis, and angiogenesis in Covid-19. N Engl J Med 2020;383(2): 120–8.

112. Akilesh S, Nicosia RF, Alpers CE, et al. Characterizing viral infection by electron microscopy: lessons from the coronavirus disease 2019 pandemic. Am J Pathol 2021;191(2):222–7.

113. Bullock HA, Goldsmith CS, Miller SE. Best practices for correctly identifying coronavirus by transmission electron microscopy. Kidney Int 2021;99(4):824–7.

114. Jacobs JL, Staines B, Bain W, et al., SARS-CoV-2 Viremia is Associated with COVID-19 Severity and Predicts Clinical Outcomes, Clin Infect Dis, 2021; ciab686 [Online ahead of print]

115. Dias SSG, Soares VC, Ferreira AC, et al. Lipid droplets fuel SARS-CoV-2 repli-cation and production of inflammatory mediators. PLoS Pathog 2020;16(12): e1009127.
116. Junqueira C, Crespo Ã, Ranjbar S, et al. SARS-CoV-2 infects blood monocytes to activate NLRP3 and AIM2 inflammasomes, pyroptosis and cytokine release. Res Sq 2021.
117. Baum A, Fulton BO, Wloga E, et al. Antibody cocktail to SARS-CoV-2 spike pro-tein prevents rapid mutational escape seen with individual antibodies. Science 2020;369(6506):1014.
118. McCarthy KR, Rennick LJ, Nambulli S, et al. Recurrent deletions in the SARS-CoV-2 spike glycoprotein drive antibody escape. Science 2021;371(6534): 1139.
119. Pegu A, O'Connell S, Schmidt SD, et al. Durability of mRNA-1273 vaccine-induced antibodies against SARS-CoV-2 variants. Science 2021;373(6561): 1372–7.
120. Krause PR, Fleming TR, Longini IM, et al. SARS-CoV-2 variants and vaccines. New Engl J Med 2021;385(2):179–86.
121. Tada T, Zhou H, Dcosta BM, et al. SARS-CoV-2 lambda variant remains suscep-tible to neutralization by mRNA vaccine-elicited antibodies and convalescent serum. bioRxiv 2021.
122. Uriu K, Kimura I, Shirakawa K, et al. Neutralization of the SARS-CoV-2 Mu Variant by convalescent and vaccine serum. New Engl J Med 2021;385(25):2397–9.
123. Abdel Latif A, Mullen JL, Alkuzweny M, et al. Center for viral systems biology. Lineage Comparison *Outbreakinfo Available at*. https://outbreak.info/. Accessed date 1/12/2022.

SARS-Cov-2 Transmission and Prevention in the Era of the Delta Variant

Eric A. Meyerowitz, MD[a],*, Aaron Richterman, MD, MPH[b]

KEYWORDS

- COVID-19 • SARS-CoV-2 • Delta • Transmission • Vaccination • Aerosol
- Superspreading • Overdispersion

KEY POINTS

- Severe acute respiratory syndrome coronavirus 2 has an intense but discrete infectious period.
- Respiratory transmission is the dominant mode of transmission, with viral particles suspended on fine aerosols emitted from the respiratory tract. Risk for transmission is highest at close distance and in poorly ventilated indoor settings.
- Viral factors are associated with increased transmissibility.
- Transmission dynamics are heterogeneous, with the majority of secondary cases arising from a small minority of index cases and most index cases leading to no secondary transmissions.
- Vaccines dramatically decrease transmission by decreasing the risk of infection among the vaccinated and by decreasing the chance of transmission from vaccinated individuals who become infected.

INTRODUCTION

Understanding the transmission characteristics of severe acute respiratory syndrome coronavirus 2 (SARS-CoV-2) is essential to designing effective mitigation strategies. The virus spreads predominantly through shared air between an index and a secondary case during a relatively brief period of infectiousness.[1] Detailed assessments of transmission have revealed deep flaws in the droplet–aerosol dichotomy that has been emphasized for decades as a model for transmission of respiratory pathogens.[2] Host, viral, and environmental factors all influence risk of transmission of SARS-CoV-2, with marked heterogeneity a key feature of its spread.

In the first year of the pandemic, ancestral SARS-CoV-2 virus that emerged in Wuhan, China (termed Wuhan-Hu-1), was slowly replaced by virus containing the

[a] Montefiore Medical Center, 111 East 210th Street, Bronx, NY 10467, USA; [b] Hospital of the University of Pennsylvania, 3400 Spruce Street, Philadelphia, PA 19104, USA
* Corresponding author.
E-mail address: emeyerowit@montefiore.org

Infect Dis Clin N Am 36 (2022) 267–293
https://doi.org/10.1016/j.idc.2022.01.007
0891-5520/22/© 2022 Elsevier Inc. All rights reserved.
id.theclinics.com

D614G mutation.[3] In experimental models, the D614G-containing virus replicates more efficiently and transmits more rapidly than ancestral virus.[4,5] As D614 G became dominant, experts predicted other variants with a competitive advantage were likely to emerge thereafter.

All RNA viruses accrue mutations, and mutations that confer a fitness advantage are likely to expand at a population level.[6] The base mutation rate for SARS-CoV-2 is 4×10^{-4} nucleotide substitutions per site per year, or approximately 1 to 2 mutations per month based on its large genome size and the presence of a proofreading exoribonuclease that ensures relatively high fidelity transcription.[7,8] Although active viral replication in an immunocompetent human host occurs for a relatively short period, prolonged infection is well-described in some hosts, particularly those with severe B-cell immunodeficiencies.[9–11] In these immunocompromised hosts, mutations may accumulate more rapidly than expected owing to the significantly higher amount of viral replication, and it is thought that this is the context in which more transmissible variants may have emerged.[12]

A variant of concern eventually called alpha was first recognized in the United Kingdom in December of 2020.[13] It was defined by 17 mutations, including 8 in the spike protein, and it rapidly became dominant in the UK and much of the world, with researchers estimating it was 43% to 90% more transmissible than its predecessor virus.[14] A Japanese study found that the secondary attack rate in households was significantly higher for alpha versus prior SARS-CoV-2 lineages (38.7% vs 19.3%; $P<.001$).[15]

The delta variant of concern was first identified in the state of Maharashtra, India, in late 2020 and subsequently spread rapidly around the globe, causing large surges of cases and hospitalizations.[16] It has a higher replication efficiency than alpha in experimental human airway epithelial systems.[17] In India, where alpha and delta first competed, small outbreaks associated with alpha were followed by much larger delta outbreaks in the same regions, and delta was estimated to be 1.3 to 1.7 times more transmissible than alpha.[18] In a matched household cluster study later conducted in the UK, including a total of 2586 delta and 3390 alpha index cases, the adjusted odds ratio of household transmission was 1.70 for delta compared with alpha (95% confidence interval [CI], 1.48–1.95).[19] Delta dominated across the vast majority of the world for the majority of 2021 and has been associated with large outbreaks, even in settings with relatively high vaccine coverage.

In this review, we describe the important factors influencing SARS-CoV-2 transmission, with particular attention to unique features of the delta era. We outline modes of transmission and determinants of infectiousness of SARS-CoV-2. We also review the nature of the heterogeneity that defines the transmission dynamics of this virus. We describe the role of vaccines in preventing transmission both directly, by decreasing cases, and indirectly, by decreasing the likelihood of secondary transmission when a vaccinated individual develops infection. Finally, we review the evidence for other transmission mitigation strategies, including masking, social distancing, rapid case identification and contact tracing, and improved ventilation.

MODES OF TRANSMISSION

The modes of transmission of SARS-CoV-2 have been elucidated through detailed case contact studies in a variety of contexts. Although there was initial concern about the potential role of fomite or indirect transmission, this mechanism of spread is not important for SARS-CoV-2, if it occurs at all.[1] Although SARS-CoV-2 remains viable for hours on contaminated surfaces under ideal experimental conditions, in real-world settings replication-competent virus is only rarely recovered from surfaces and then only at extremely low levels.[20–22] In the few case reports where fomite transmission has been suggested, respiratory transmission cannot be excluded.[1]

Respiratory transmission, with SARS-CoV-2 carried on tiny particles emitted from the respiratory tract of an index case to a contact, is the clear and dominant route of spread.[1] From early in the pandemic, it has been evident that proximity is a key determinant of transmission risk. For instance, a contact tracing study of train passengers in China before universal masking that included 2334 index cases and 72,093 close contacts found that the risk of transmission was directly related to the distance between the seats and the amount of shared time on the train.[23] A detailed contact tracing study of the Diamond Princess cruise ship outbreak found that passengers with SARS-CoV-2 infection were either infected in shared public spaces in close contact or in their cabins when they were lodging with another infected passenger, but did not find evidence of transmissions between rooms.[24] In an outbreak of 14 confirmed and 6 probable cases on a plane in Japan, being seated within 2 rows of the index case was associated with an adjusted odds ratio for infection of 7.47 (95% CI, 2.06–27.2).[25]

Before the COVID-19 pandemic, respiratory transmission of respiratory viruses and bacteria was categorized widely in a dichotomous way, with some pathogens, like tuberculosis, spread on smaller particles called aerosols and others spread on larger particles called droplets.[26–28] Pathogens spread on larger droplets were not thought to reach individuals more than about 6 feet away because they would fall to the ground owing to gravitation effect, whereas smaller aerosols could remain suspended over longer distances and times. Designating a pathogen as droplet or aerosol spread implied the relative importance of different personal protective equipment, with surgical masks thought to suffice in the context of pathogens with droplet transmission (droplet precautions) and respirators needed to prevent aerosol transmission (airborne precautions). Because proximity was so important and surgical masks reasonably effective at preventing spread (particularly in hospital settings), droplet spread within the traditional model was initially presumed to be the most important mechanism of transmission.[29,30] However, it has become clear that the predominant mode of transmission of SARS-CoV-2 (as well as most other respiratory pathogens) is aerosol transmission, with short range aerosols the most important.[31] The risk of aerosol transmission is greatest at short range because the concentration, and therefore infectious dose, is highest there, whereas aerosols are diluted over larger distances.[32] Confusion about this topic has led some experts to call for a change in the terminology used to describe transmission of respiratory pathogens, and for a shift to focusing on inhalation as the major mode of transmission (**Table 1**).[33]

Evidence supporting the importance of aerosol transmission of SARS-CoV-2 includes numerous experimental and clinical studies.[31] For instance, a mathematical model showing the high risk associated with distances of less than 6 feet,[36] a study showing that viral RNA was found in fine aerosols (particles ≤ 5 μm) 85% of the time rather than larger particles,[37] and real-world and experimental animal studies showing transmission is possible through the air at distances far greater than 6 feet.[38–40] In health care settings, there are now many well-documented human-to-human transmissions at distances of more than 6 feet, for instance in shared patient hospital rooms.[41] Longer range transmissions tend to occur in poorly ventilated settings or when the air flow is directed from an index case to secondary cases.[42,43] In a very detailed description of an outbreak at a hospital in Boston, positive pressure in patient rooms relative to a nursing station on the unit was a proposed as a mechanism of spread beyond a patient room.[41] A detailed cluster report with sequencing of virus

Table 1 Traditional versus updated understanding of airborne transmission		
	Traditional: droplet vs aerosol dichotomy	Updated: inhalation
Relative importance of droplets and aerosols	Droplets are thought to be responsible for most transmission of respiratory viruses; aerosols are important for certain pathogens like tuberculosis or measles.[32]	Both droplets and aerosols contribute to transmission, though short range aerosols are the most important vehicle for most respiratory viruses.[33]
Role of proximity	Most aerosol transmissions are thought to happen at longer distances.	Proximity is important for droplets and aerosols, with concentrations decreased by gravity and dilution for droplets and dilution for aerosols.
Role of masking	Surgical masking is sufficient for preventing droplet transmission; respirator/N95 masks are needed to prevent aerosol transmission.[34]	Surgical masks (especially when worn by source) provide some (but not complete) protection against aerosols.[35] There is a theoretic benefit to a respirator/N95, although the incremental benefit has not been clearly demonstrated in clinical trials or real-world studies to date.
Role of ventilation	Not necessary for droplet spread; needed for aerosols or pathogens primarily transmitted via droplets when index cases undergo aerosol generating procedures.	An important tool that can be used to decrease risk of most respiratory pathogens through dilutional mechanism.

genomes at an isolation facility in New Zealand with closed circuit television monitoring found 3 linked secondary cases who were never in the same room an d always more than 2 m away from the index case, with aerosol transmission the only plausible mechanism of spread.[44,45] As discussed elsewhere in this article, despite the overwhelming evidence for the predominance of aerosol transmission, the benefit of higher filtration masks over routine surgical masks in the community and in health care settings has yet to be demonstrated conclusively.

DETERMINANTS OF INFECTIOUSNESS

Host, virologic, and environmental factors all impact infectiousness of SARS-CoV-2. Apart from vaccination, which we discuss elsewhere in this review, the clearest host factor impacting transmission risk is whether the index case eventually develops symptoms. Several studies and systematic reviews have shown that persistently asymptomatic index cases are much less likely to lead to secondary cases compared with symptomatic index cases. For example, a household contact study from the original outbreak in Wuhan that included 27,101 affected households found that asymptomatic index cases were much less likely to transmit, with an adjusted odds ratio of 0.21 (95% CI, 0.14–0.31).[46] A study from Singapore of 628 people with SARS-

CoV-2 infection and 3790 close contacts found the transmission risk was 3.85 times higher for symptomatic versus asymptomatic index cases (95% CI, 2.1–7.2).[47] A systematic review found the secondary attack rate was lower for people with persistently asymptomatic infection (relative risk, 0.35; 95% CI, 0.10–1.27).[48] To date, there are no detailed studies of transmission risk by symptom status of individuals harboring the delta variant.

The respiratory tract viral load in the host at the time of an exposure is also clearly associated with infectiousness, with higher viral loads associated with greater likelihood of transmission.[49] In a pre-delta era cohort study in Spain that included 282 index cases and 753 close contacts, secondary attack rate was directly related to the respiratory tract viral load of the index case at diagnosis.[50] A study of 1058 students with SARS-CoV-2 infection at the University in Colorado, 860 of whom lived in multiple occupancy rooms, found that the average viral load in the 116 index cases who transmitted to a roommate was 6.5 times higher compared with the 414 who did not.[51] In a Danish household contact study that included 66,311 index cases and 213,576 household contacts, the risk of transmission was also directly related to the viral load.[52]

Other host factors that may impact infectiousness include immune status and the age of the index case. Certain immunocompromised hosts may be more likely to transmit, but few studies have quantified this risk. A household contact study of 58 households in the United States found that immunocompromised index cases had a higher risk of transmission; however, just 2 of the 58 index cases were considered immunocompromised.[53] Early in the pandemic, there was some evidence suggesting that young children aged less than 10 years were less susceptible to infection by ancestral SARS-CoV-2.[1,54,55] Whether this decreased susceptibility persists in the era of the delta variant is currently unknown, although it is notable that large numbers of unvaccinated children have developed delta infection in settings where many adults are vaccinated like the United States and United Kingdom.[56,57] A household study of delta transmission in Singapore found that older age was associated with a greater likelihood of transmission, although this finding may relate to contact patterns within households rather than inherent host factors.[58]

Viral factors also impact infectiousness. As described, the in vitro replication rate of delta is higher than that for alpha.[16] The spike protein of delta more efficiently binds to the host cell membrane angiotensin-conerting enzyme 2 protein, which is the key host cell entry receptor.[59] This may correlate with significantly higher in vivo respiratory tract viral loads for delta. In an outbreak of delta in Guangdong province in China, the peak viral load was much higher compared with the ancestral virus with a median peak cycle threshold of 20.6 for delta infections versus 34.0 for a historical cohort ($P<.001$).[60] Although the increased transmissibility and fitness of delta compared with prior variants is not disputed, studies have been mixed about whether the peak viral load is in fact higher for delta.[61–65] Additional mutations outside of the spike region may enhance viral replication in other ways. Researchers showed that mutations in the nucleocapsid protein found in delta and other more transmissible variants enhance messenger RNA (mRNA) delivery and packaging into virions and are associated with a more rapid viral replication.[66]

A number of environmental factors also predict the likelihood of transmission. The most important is ventilation, with outdoor transmission almost never identified.[1,67] Indoor environments were noted to be important very early after the emergence of SARS-CoV-2 based on associations with clusters of transmission in Japan during its first wave.[68] Environmental factors like lower ambient temperatures and higher relative humidity may also be associated with an increased transmission risk.[69] Socioeconomic deprivation has repeatedly been shown to be associated with an increased risk for infection, likely because it is associated with an increased probability of more frequent and higher risk exposures.[70-74]

THE PERIOD OF INFECTIOUSNESS AND SERIAL INTERVAL

A person with SARS-COV-2 infection has a discrete period of infectiousness that has been well-defined for immunocompetent hosts. After an individual is exposed, there is an incubation period, defined as the time from exposure to symptom onset. Two key early papers examining the early cases in Wuhan, China, in the pre-delta era estimated the incubation period as 5.2 days (95% CI, 4.1–7.0) with 97.5% developing symptoms by 12.5 days (when reviewing the first 425 known cases)[75] and 5.1 days (95% CI, 4.5–5.8 days), with 97.5% developing symptoms by 11.5 days after exposure (for 181 cases with a known exposure and symptom onset) (**Fig. 1**).[76] The incubation period for delta seems to be significantly shorter than for prior SARS-CoV-2 viruses (**Table 2**).[60] An analysis of 68 infections from 24 clusters from a contained delta outbreak in Guangdong, China, found the mean incubation period was 4.4 days (95% CI, 3.9–5.0).[77] The incubation period for SARS-CoV-2, including the delta variant, is significantly longer and more variable than the incubation period for influenza. In 1 example, the incubation period for pandemic H1N1 influenza A virus in 2009 was approximately 2 days, with a standard deviation of approximately 2 days.[78]

Because 20% to 30% of people never develop symptoms, the latent period, which is the period from exposure to first detectable polymerase chain reaction (PCR), is also useful for understanding the transmission risk.[48,79] Among 101 confirmed delta cases from the Guangdong outbreak, the mean latent period was 4.0 days (95% CI, 3.5–4.4), with 95% of cases having detectable viral RNA by 8.2 days (95% CI, 7.1–9.3).[80] This interval is shorter than the mean latent period estimated in the pre-delta period, which was 5.5 days (95% CI, 5.1–5.9), with 95% of cases having detectable viral RNA by 10.6 days (95% CI, 9.6–11.6).[79]

These viral characteristics lead to the observed serial interval, or the time between symptom onset in a primary and secondary case. A meta-analysis in the pre-delta era estimated the serial interval as 5.4 days (95% CI, 5.19–5.61).[81] Some studies have

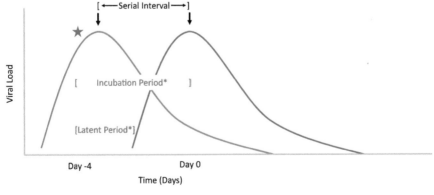

Fig. 1. Virologic characteristics of a transmission.

Table 2
Incubation period, latent period, and serial interval for Wuhan-Hu-1 and the delta variant

	Prior SARS-CoV-2 Viruses	Delta
Mean incubation period	5.2 d (95% CI, 4.1–7.0)[75]	4.4 d (95% CI, 3.9–5.0)[77]
Mean latent period	5.5 d (95% CI, 5.1–5.9)[79]	4.0 d (95% CI, 3.5–4.4)[80]
Serial interval	5.4 d (95% CI, 5.2–5.6)[81]	Not yet well defined

observed a shorter serial interval for delta compared with earlier variants,[77,80,82] although others have not.[83] The long and variable incubation period and significant proportion of presymptomatic transmission make it difficult to estimate a mean serial interval for recently emerged variants, because it takes data from numerous well-defined transmission pairs to generate a reliable estimate. The degree to which a possible shorter serial interval contributes to the more rapid spread of delta, which is also more transmissible than prior SARS-CoV-2 viruses (discussed in the section on Transmissibility and heterogeneity), is not known at this time.

For those who develop symptoms, the infectious period begins before symptom onset, with presymptomatic transmission a major driver of the COVID-19 pandemic (see **Fig. 1**). A detailed study of 25,381 people with SARS-CoV-2 infection in Germany from February 2020 through March 2021 found that, among those who develop symptoms, the respiratory tract viral load peaked 1 to 3 days before symptom onset with higher viral loads among sicker patients.[64] Detailed viral load data from an analysis of the delta outbreak in Guangdong suggest that viral loads peak around the time of symptom onset[60] and researchers estimated that 73.9% of transmissions may have occurred before symptom onset in the index case.[80]

Although individuals may remain PCR positive for weeks after infection, late transmissions occur very rarely, if at all. An early rigorous contact tracing study from Taiwan in the pre-delta era that included nearly 3000 close contacts of 100 cases found no linked cases from exposures occurring after an index case had symptoms for 6 days.[84] The National Basketball Association had a closed environment for their 2020 season, with systematic and frequent testing, allowing for detailed descriptions of transmission in this setting that included nearly 4000 individuals.[85] Their policies allowed individuals with infection to discontinue isolation at 10 days after symptom onset or first positive PCR test. They found no secondary infections after that time, despite 36 individuals remaining persistently PCR positive on nasopharyngeal testing.

The period of infectiousness is related to SARS-CoV-2 viral load dynamics, which are quite different than those of other severe coronavirus infections like SARS-CoV-1 and MERS-CoV. As noted elsewhere in this article, index case viral load is a key determinant of transmission risk.[49,50] For SARS-CoV-2, transmissions occur starting 1 to 2 days before symptom onset as the viral load increases and peaks around or just after symptoms onset, before decreasing thereafter.[9] The viral load, therefore, peaks well before most people with severe cases of SARS-CoV-2 are hospitalized and explains why more SARS-CoV-2 aerosols are found in homes of index cases than critical care wards for affected patients.[86] In contrast, in both SARS-CoV-1 and MERS-CoV, the respiratory tract viral load peaks after inevitable symptom onset (neither are known to have asymptomatic cases), peaking around day 10 for SARS-CoV-1 and days 7 to 10 for MERS-CoV.[9] The transmission risk is greater later in infection, after symptom onset for SARS-CoV-1 and MERS-CoV, making transmission mitigation of those infections easier than for SARS-CoV-2.

TRANSMISSIBILITY AND HETEROGENEITY

The basic reproductive number (R_0) of an infectious disease is a measure of its transmissibility. The R_0 is defined as the mean number of secondary infections resulting from an infected person in a susceptible population. The R_0 is influenced by the rate of contacts within a given population, the probability of transmission during a given contact, and the duration of infectiousness. Infectious diseases with an R_0 of greater than 1 can result in epidemics depending in part on the degree of population immunity. Estimates of the R_0 are, thus, useful for a general understanding of the epidemic threat of a given pathogen, but vary significantly by setting and the methodology used for estimation.[87] For SARS-CoV-2, approximations of the R_0 have increased as the dominant virus has evolved from the ancestral strain ($R_0 \approx 3$) to the alpha variant ($R_0 \approx 4.5$) to the delta variant ($R_0 \approx 8$) (**Table 3**).[88–90]

Because the R_0 is an average, it does not describe individual variation in transmission. This individual variation, or heterogeneity, can be an important feature of some infectious diseases, with implications for epidemic control. Heterogeneity is typically described using the dispersion parameter of a negative binomial distribution, or k.[100] When the k is very small, transmission displays overdispersion, meaning that a relatively high proportion of secondary infections result from a relatively low proportion of index cases. Highly overdispersed pathogens are characterized by superspreading events—discrete transmission events with unusually large numbers of secondary cases. Investigations early during the pandemic using a variety of methodologies documented high degrees of overdispersion with SARS-CoV-2 transmission, with 10% to 20% of index cases leading to approximately 80% of secondary infections,[101–104] and numerous examples of superspreading events (**Fig. 2**).[105–110] Despite the delta variant's increased overall transmissibility, manifested by an increased R_0, there is early evidence that transmission continues to display a similar degree of heterogeneity.[82,111] Superspreading events continue to be identified in the delta era, including in highly vaccinated populations.[112] Although superspreading occurs for other highly transmissible respiratory pathogens like influenza and the measles, it is generally thought to be less important as compared with SARS-CoV-2, with higher dispersion parameters for these other pathogens (**Table 4**).[113] Note that increased overdispersion for measles has been reported in the postvaccination era, likely owing to heterogeneity of susceptibility.[114,115]

Many factors can contribute to the likelihood of a superspreading event, including those related to the virus (eg, timing relative to peak viral load), host (eg, presence

Table 3
Basic reproductive number (R_0) for various pathogens

Pathogen	Approximate Basic R_0
MERS-CoV[91,92]	0.7–1.3
Ebola[93,94]	1.6–2.0
Pandemic influenza 2009[95]	1.8
Pandemic influenza 1918[96]	2.0
SARS-CoV-1[97]	2.2–3.6
Original SARS-CoV-2[88]	3.0
SARS-CoV-2 alpha variant[89]	4.5
SARS-CoV-2 delta variant[89,90]	8.0
Measles[98,99]	10.0–18.0

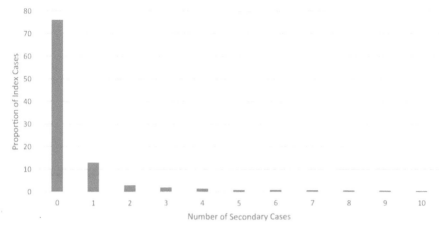

Fig. 2. Example of proportion of secondary cases from SARS-CoV-2 index cases.

of symptoms), environment (eg, ventilation, proximity), and behavior (eg, singing, masking).[117] Transmission heterogeneity is also heavily driven by the concentration of exposure risk factors within specific networks, including among frontline and low-wage workers, and in congregate settings such as nursing homes, prisons, and homeless shelters.[118] The heterogeneity of transmission clusters can be visualized when transmission chains are depicted pictorially (**Fig. 3**).

Although superspreading events are rare, they make an outsized contribution to epidemic growth. As a result, public health interventions that reduce superspreading events (so-called cutting the tail interventions) can meaningfully decrease transmission, with modeling suggesting that elimination of transmission events with greater than 10 secondary infections could result in a reduction in the R_0 of ancestral virus from 3.00 to 1.09.[119]

TRANSMISSION PREVENTION WITH VACCINATION

Prevention of SARS-CoV-2 through vaccination can be achieved through direct protection (prevention of infection or disease among vaccinated individuals) and indirect protection (prevention of infection among all community members through decreases in transmission). In the early months after vaccination and before the delta era, randomized controlled trials and large-scale observational studies demonstrated high degrees of direct protection from vaccines using a variety of platforms, particularly against symptomatic and severe disease.[120,121] Similarly, infection-acquired immunity showed substantial protection against reinfection of at least 80%.[122]

Table 4
Estimated dispersion parameter (k) for selected highly transmissible respiratory pathogens

Respiratory pathogen	Dispersion
SARS-CoV-2 (Wuhan-Hu-1 strain)	0.1 (95% CI 0.05–0.2)[102]
Measles (prevaccination era)	0.83 (95% CI 0.70–0.94)[114]
Measles (postvaccination era)	0.40 (95% CI 0.19–1.99)[115]
Pandemic influenza H1N1 (1918)	0.94 (95% CI 0.59–1.72)[116]

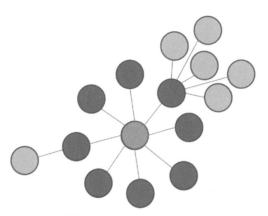

Fig. 3. Chains and clustering of SARS-CoV-2 transmission.

Indirect protection can be generated through 2 distinct mechanisms. First, vaccines may decrease the overall risk of infection by protecting against both symptomatic and asymptomatic infections—put simply, if a person never becomes infected, they cannot transmit the virus to another person. Second, a vaccine may decrease the transmission potential of a vaccinated person who does become infected, leading to a lower secondary attack rate compared with unvaccinated people with infection. During the early months of the vaccine roll out, before the global dominance of delta, the sum of the evidence from well-designed studies using a variety of methodologies suggested a large decrease in transmission through both of these mechanisms.[49] Although the exact amount of the decrease varied by vaccine and transmission context, the overall protection against infection was at least 50%, and the decrease in transmission potential among the vaccinated relative to the unvaccinated was also 50% or greater, equivalent to an approximate transmission reduction of at least 75%.[49] In the delta era, however, we must consider 2 additional factors that may influence the effects of vaccines on transmission—that is, the impact of the delta variant itself and changes in immunity over time since vaccination.

Delta's Impact on Vaccine Protection against Transmission

When compared with alpha, direct protection by the vaccines against symptomatic delta infections seems to be modestly decreased—by about 10% to 20%—with no change in the relative protection against severe outcomes.[123,124] An increased risk of symptomatic reinfection also seems to be greater with delta compared with alpha, with surveillance data from the United Kingdom showing an adjusted odds ratio of 1.46 (95% CI, 1.03–2.05) for symptomatic reinfection for delta compared with alpha.[125] Importantly, even though the relative protection by vaccines against illness and severe disease is largely preserved when compared with pre-delta viruses, the increased overall transmissibility seen with delta results in a substantially increased absolute risk of these outcomes among vaccinated people.

Understanding how vaccine effectiveness against all infections changes in the context of delta is critical to informing expectations about the vaccines' continued indirect protection. To reliably estimate this change, observational studies must use systematic or regular testing regardless of symptom status. To date, the most rigorous study to use this approach was a population representative survey of randomly selected households in the United Kingdom that included 384,543 individuals, conducted scheduled PCR testing of participants, and adjusted for a number of important potential confounding variables.[126] After 2 doses of the ChAdOx1 vaccine, they found a lower vaccine effectiveness against infection of 67% (95% CI, 62%–71%) during a period dominated by delta, relative to 79% (95% CI, 56%–90%) during a period dominated by alpha. For the mRNA-1273 vaccine, they found no difference in protection against infection by delta compared with alpha, with an 82% vaccine effectiveness (95% CI, 75%–87%) during the delta period and 77% vaccine effectiveness (95% CI, 66%–84%) during the alpha period. One other study of 4217 frontline workers in the United States similarly used regular testing and control of confounders, finding a combined vaccine effectiveness against overall infection for mRNA-1273, BNT162b2, and (to a much lesser extent) Ad26.COV2.S, against overall infection of 91% (95% CI, 81%–96%) before delta dominance and 66% (95% CI, 26%–84%) during a period of delta dominance.[127] The limited reliable data to date thus suggest substantial preservation in relative vaccine effectiveness against all infections by delta, with a decrease of 0% to 25% compared with pre-delta viruses. As before, this metric needs to be distinguished from the absolute risk of delta infection for vaccinated people, which is considerably increased because of delta's increased overall transmissibility relative to earlier variants.

The impact of delta's emergence on the second component of indirect protection—the decrease in transmission potential among vaccinated people who become infected—has been scrutinized intensely ever since it was shown that the amount of SARS-CoV-2 viral RNA present at diagnosis (as measured semiquantitatively by the cycle threshold of PCR assays) did not differ by vaccination status for people with delta infection.[128] For pre-delta viruses, the cycle threshold value at diagnosis had been consistently found to be higher (meaning lower viral levels) for vaccinated people,[49] so this finding suggested that the transmission potential had possibly become more similar between vaccinated and unvaccinated people in the context of delta. However, a subsequent study in Singapore used longitudinal sampling to show that, although cycle threshold values at diagnosis were similar between vaccinated and unvaccinated people, there was a much more rapid decay in the cycle threshold value among those who had been vaccinated,[129] a finding that has since been replicated.[63] They also found that vaccinated people with delta infection had far fewer symptoms relative to unvaccinated people, which has also been associated with reduced transmission potential.[47,130] Several studies have attempted to examine whether the relationship between cycle threshold values and presence of replication-competent virus differs by vaccination status, with mixed findings.[131,132] One study of 24,706 health care workers found that infectious virus was present in 69% of 162 infections after vaccination (91% of which were delta), relative to 85% of infections among the unvaccinated.[132] There was a significantly lower probability of culture positivity with vaccination after adjusting for the cycle threshold value. Another study found infectious virus in 37 of 39 vaccinated people (95%) infected with delta, relative to 15 of 17 specimens (88%) from unvaccinated people, with both groups having similar cycle threshold values at diagnosis.[131]

Regardless of these virologic findings, rigorously designed contact tracing studies provide the most direct evidence about the transmission potential of people with delta infection after vaccination. The largest such study used contact tracing data from England and included 108,498 index cases with 146,243 contacts.[133] After adjusting for potential confounders, investigators found that 2 BNT162b2 doses (adjusted risk ratio, 0.;, 95% CI, 0.39–0.65) and 2 ChAdOx1 doses (adjusted risk ratio, 0.76; 95% CI, 0.70–0.83) reduced delta transmission, but that this was less than for alpha transmission (BNT162b2 adjusted risk ratio, 0.32; 95% CI, 0.21–0.48; ChAdOx1 adjusted risk ratio,

0.48; 95% CI, 0.30–0.78). Of note, these estimated decreases were early after vaccination and transmission reduction attenuated over time, as we discuss elsewhere in this review. Another household contact tracing study of 4921 index cases and 7771 contacts in the Netherlands found a decrease in the transmission potential for delta after full vaccination of the index case of 63% (95% CI, 46%–75%).[124] A much smaller contact tracing study of a delta outbreak in China similarly found a decrease in transmission after 2 doses of an inactivated SARS-CoV-2 vaccine (65% decrease; 95% CI, 16%–88%).[80] In contrast, a contact tracing study of 1024 household contacts linked to 301 index cases in Singapore did not find a significant difference in the transmission risk based on index case vaccination status (adjusted odds ratio, 0.73; 95% CI, 0.38–1.40), although the confidence interval was relatively wide.[58] Finally, a contact tracing study of 471 delta index cases and 602 contacts in the United Kingdom that collected daily upper respiratory tract samples for up to 20 days found similar secondary attack rates in contacts of vaccinated (25%; 95% CI, 15%–35%) and unvaccinated (23%; 95% CI, 15%–31%) index cases.[63] The discrepant findings between this study and the larger contact tracing studies may relate to its smaller sample size, intensive sampling strategy, and/or greater time since vaccination among the index cases.

Importantly, these contact tracing studies are likely to underestimate the reduction in transmission potential resulting from vaccination for people infected with delta for 2 reasons. First, index cases with a greater number and severity of symptoms are more likely to be identified and included in these studies. Because vaccines decrease the severity of symptoms, and more severe symptoms are associated with an increased risk of transmission, there is likely to be selection bias present. Second, some contacts may have been infected outside the household, potentially even during the same exposure as the index case.[134]

Transmission Risk in the Context of Waning Immunity

Although the majority of observational analyses assessing changes in vaccine protection over time since vaccination are highly vulnerable to biases inherent to their study design,[135] there are several reliable lines of evidence showing modest decreases in protection against symptomatic and overall infection over time, as well as an attenuation over time in the reduction in transmission potential after vaccination. The strongest evidence comes from the randomized controlled trials of mRNA-1273 and BNT162b2, which continued to follow participants after the placebo group crossed over to receive the vaccine about 5 to 6 months after the trials began, resulting in early and late vaccinated groups. Symptomatic infection rates were modestly higher in the early vaccine group for both vaccines nearly 1 year after initial vaccination, when the delta variant was dominant in the United States. Vaccine efficacy against symptomatic infection at close to 1 year after vaccination can be approximated after considering the change in protection caused by delta for the more recently vaccinated group (**Table 5**).

Further evidence for waning protection against infection regardless of symptom status comes from the previously described community-based study in the United Kingdom, which used representative population sampling and systematic testing.[126] These investigators found a modest decrease in vaccine effectiveness against infection (as above, the critical outcome for transmission prevention) from 14 to 90 days after the second dose for BNT162b2 (85% at 14 days [95% CI, 79%–90%]; 75% at 90 days [95% CI, 70%–80%]) and ChAdOx1 (68% at 14 days [95% CI, 61%–73%]; 61% at 90 days [95% CI, 53%–68%]). The previously described study of 4217 frontline workers in the United States who underwent regular testing found a vaccine effectiveness after full vaccination of 85% (95% CI, 68%–93%) at 14 to 119 days, 81% (95%

Table 5

Vaccine efficacy against symptomatic delta

Assumed baseline vaccine efficacy vs symptomatic delta[124]	Vaccine efficacy vs symptomatic delta, 10–12 mo after vaccination, BNT162b2[136]	Vaccine efficacy vs symptomatic delta, 10–12 mo after vaccination, mRNA-1273[137]
0.9	0.87	0.84
0.85	0.8	0.76
0.8	0.73	0.69
0.75	0.66	0.61
0.7	0.6	0.53
0.65	0.53	0.45

CI, 34%–95%) at 120 to 149 days, and 73% (95% CI, 49%–86%) at 150 days or more.[127]

The decrease in the transmission potential resulting from vaccination among people who become infected also seems to attenuate over time, as shown by the detailed contact tracing study of 108,498 index cases and 146,243 contacts in England.[133] This analysis found no transmission decrease at 12 weeks after vaccination for index cases vaccinated with ChAdOx1 (2%, 95% CI, –2% to 6%) and a significantly attenuated decrease for those vaccinated with BNT162b2 (24%, 95% CI, 20%–28%). This finding is further supported by virologic data from Israel, where viral loads at diagnosis were found to be lower among vaccinated individuals with delta infection within 2 months of vaccination relative to unvaccinated people, but that this difference disappeared by 6 months after vaccination.[138]

In summary, the considerable indirect protection seen during the early months of the vaccine roll out, although still substantial in the delta era, has likely been diminished to some extent because of a modest decrease in the relative protection against infection and increased transmission potential of vaccinated individuals who become infected. The durable impact of booster doses on transmission remains to be seen, though they have shown early promise in short-term follow-up.[138–141]

TRANSMISSION PREVENTION

Extensive accumulated evidence supports multiple additional strategies for effective transmission prevention. Of note, most of the evidence supporting these strategies comes from the pre-delta era. Besides vaccination, the other major tools to prevent transmission of SARS-CoV-2 include ventilation, physical distancing, rapid case contact tracing and isolating, and effective personal protective equipment.

The role of improved ventilation in preventing transmission of SARS-CoV-2 has been shown in a variety of ways. In a crossover study looking at the effect of portal air/UV filtration devices in hospital wards with patients with COVID-19, SARS-CoV-2 was detected in aerosols when the filters were not in use, but not when the devices were turned on.[142] In a study of household transmission in China, opening a window to allow for better ventilation was associated with a decreased infection risk.[143] In a study that included 169 primary schools in the state of Georgia, schools that had improved ventilation had a lower incidence of SARS-CoV-2 cases, with an adjusted relative risk of 0.61 (95% CI, 0.43–0.87).[144] Dilution methods alone, including opening doors and windows, or combining dilution with filtration (with installation of HEPA air filters) were protective against incident SARS-CoV-2 infections. The importance of ventilation in decreasing transmission of respiratory pathogens was widely recognized even before the COVID-19 pandemic; for example, opening windows in hospitals and homes was found to provide excellent ventilation and decrease tuberculosis transmission risk.[145,146]

The protective role of masking has been shown in multiple settings. In community settings, a large, prospective, cluster randomized controlled trial including nearly 350,000 people from 600 villages in Bangladesh from November 2020 through April 2021 found 11.2% lower cases (estimated via history of symptoms with a positive serology) in villages randomized to surgical masks.[147] In the trial, people living in towns in the intervention arms were given free masks and information about the importance of masking, and observed masking was 13.3% in control villages and 42.3% in treatment villages, with a regression adjusted increase of 28.8% increase in masking associated with the intervention (95% CI, 27%–31%). The investigators found no statistically significant benefit for their primary outcome in villages randomized to cloth masking. The only other randomized control trial of community masking individually randomized 4862 Danish participants to recommendations to wear surgical masks outside the home or not and found that 1.8% of the mask group and 2.1% of the control group developed infection in the following month, a difference that was not statistically significant.[148] The broader importance of this study is limited by individual randomization (because of the hypothesized importance of masks for source control) and the low prevalence of infection. A systematic review of 6 studies evaluating the impact of face masking found that wearing a mask was associated with a significantly decreased risk of SARS-CoV-2 infection with an adjusted odds ratio of 0.19 (95% CI, 0.11–0.33).[149] Another systematic review that assessed the effect of masking on severe coronavirus infections from SARS-CoV-2, SARS-CoV-1, or MERS-CoV found that face masks were associated with a reduced risk of infection (adjusted odds ratio, 0.15; 95% CI, 0.07–0.34).[150] Observational studies of mask mandate policies have also suggested a benefit to community masking.[151] A study comparing 15 counties in Kansas with a mask mandate with 68 counties without mask mandates found a mean 60% decrease in cases and hospitalizations and a 65% decrease in deaths in counties with mask mandates.[152] These observational studies must be interpreted with caution because of secular trends and other policies that were implemented concurrently.

Universal masking in health care settings has also played an important role in decreasing transmission in health care settings, which have the potential to be important sites of SARS-CoV-2 transmission.[30] A systematic review found masking in health care settings may have decreased the infection risk by 70% (unadjusted odds ratio, 0.29; 95% CI, 0.18–0.44).[149] Universal masking policies were also associated with fewer health care worker infections at large hospital systems.[153–155] An outbreak at a Veterans Affairs hospital ended after the implementation of universal masking.[156]

Despite the clear dominance of aerosol transmission for SARS-CoV-2 and other respiratory viruses, the benefit of N95 masks over surgical masks has not been shown conclusively for preventing transmission. In the pre–COVID-19 era, a cluster randomized trial of nearly 3000 health care workers did not find a benefit for the prevention of influenza A infections for those who used N95 versus surgical masks.[157] A meta-analysis examining masking for SARS-CoV-2 and other viral infections found greater benefits with N95 versus surgical masks, though the interaction was not significant ($P = .09$).[150] In an unadjusted analysis of transmissions at a large hospital system in Michigan between April and May 2020, those wearing an N95 at time of exposure to a patient with COVID-19 were significantly less likely to be seropositive (10.2%) compared with those wearing surgical or cloth masks (13.1%) or no mask (17.5%).[158]

Observational studies in health care settings have suggested that eye protection may incrementally increase protection for health care workers. A systematic review of 13 studies from SARS-CoV-1, MERS-CoV, and SARS-CoV-2 found that eye protection was associated with a lower risk of infection (unadjusted relative risk, 0.34; 95% CI, 0.22–0.52).[150] Numerous case and cluster reports have also suggested a potential role for eye protection, including in a detailed outbreak investigation at a hospital in Boston where staff members who developed infection were less likely to have worn eye protection during encounters with index cases, although the difference was not statistically significant (30% vs 67%; prevalence ratio, 0.44; 95% CI, 0.18–1.08).[159]

Although universal masking policies seem to be effective at substantially reducing the risk of transmission in health care settings, it does not bring the risk to zero. Most residual cases occur in settings where masking is impractical or not possible, like break rooms, shared work rooms, or shared patient rooms or open wards.[30,41,160] However, a few cases of well-documented transmission between a masked source patient and masked health care worker wearing eye protection have been described.[161] These cases seem to occur with prolonged exposure at close proximity with source patients with very high respiratory tract viral loads at the time of contact.

Rapid case identification and contact tracing with testing and isolation has been used to help control the COVID-19 pandemic. During the initial outbreak in South Korea, the roll out of rapid contact tracing with testing before symptom onset brought the effective R_0 from 1.3 to 0.6 compared with the preceding period, when testing was symptom driven.[162] In another pre-delta study, the launch of an immediate trace and test program on the Isle of Wight in the UK was associated with a decrease in the R_0 from 1.3 to 0.5.[163] In contrast a retrospective study in Portugal that compared 98 cases identified through contact tracing with 453 found through routine testing did not find a difference in the secondary attack rate (13.3% vs 17.2%; $P = .406$).[164] A mathematical model suggests that although contact tracing can be helpful early in an outbreak, the benefit is lost once cases outnumber contact tracing capacity by more than 10 to 1.[165]

Given the efficiency with which SARS-CoV-2 can be transmitted, multiple mitigation strategies are typically used at times of outbreaks, including improving ventilation and encouraging physical distancing and indoor universal masking, as well as additional layers of protection for people in certain high-risk environments like health care settings.

PRELIMINARY UNDERSTANDING OF TRANSMISSION DYNAMICS OF THE OMICRON VARIANT

In November 2021 the omicron variant, with more than 50 total mutations including 15 in the spike protein's receptor binding domain, was identified in South Africa.[166] It rapidly spread throughout South Africa and the globe, leading to massive surges in infections. Evidence of the characteristic features of omicron transmission are rapidly emerging but remain highly preliminary as of this writing.

Initial estimates suggested a 5.4-fold (95% CI, 3.1- to 10.0-fold) weekly growth advantage for omicron over delta.[166] Although omicron's R_0 is estimated to be 3.19 (95% CI, 2.82–3.61) times greater than delta, much of the transmission advantage seems to be driven by an increased risk of infection among people with existing immunity.[167] This finding is supported by a large Danish household transmission study, which found similar attack rates among unvaccinated people living in households with an omicron or delta index case, but much higher risk of infection for fully vaccinated and boosted household members for omicron compared with delta (adjusted odds ratio, 2.61 [95% CI, 2.34–2.90] and 3.66 [95% CI, 2.65–5.05], respectively).[168] This finding corroborates in vitro data showing a substantially attenuated neutralization of omicron with sera from vaccinated or convalesced individuals.[169,170] Whether omicron has intrinsically increased transmissibility over prior variants is unknown at this time.

Another characteristic feature of early omicron outbreak reports is a shorter incubation period of about 3 days, with very high rates of symptoms among vaccinated people.[171,172] Viral load increases, peaks, and decreased over a period of about 10 days, similar to findings from prior variants, with somewhat lower peak viral loads compared with delta.[173,174] Preliminary evidence from Japan suggests that the peak viral load may occur 3 to 6 days after symptom onset, which may be later than was seen with prior variants.[175] Occasional long-range transmission continues to be documented along with superspreading events, although additional data are needed.[168,171,176]

These preliminary reports suggest that omicron is more rapidly transmitted than delta with a shorter incubation period and marked immune evasion that greatly increases risk of infection among vaccinated and recovered individuals. Very preliminary reports suggest that the viral load may peak later for omicron infections compared with those from prior variants. More data are needed to confirm these findings and to determine whether there are changes in the infectious period of each case and the exact degree of overdispersion characterizing transmission of omicron.

SUMMARY

The SARS-CoV-2 delta variant transmits more rapidly and efficiently than prior SARS-CoV-2 viruses. The predominant mode of transmission of SARS-CoV-2 is via short-range aerosols. Vaccines prevent transmission both by blocking cases and by decreasing the risk of secondary cases from a vaccinated index case. However, the effect of vaccination on transmission reduction has been attenuated owing to the significantly increased transmissibility of the delta variant and waning protection for individuals remotely vaccinated. Besides vaccination, ventilation, masking, eye protection, and rapid case identification with contact tracing and isolation have all been shown to decrease transmission.

DISCLOSURE

The authors have no relevant financial or commercial disclosures. There were no funding sources for this article.

REFERENCES

1. Meyerowitz EA, Richterman A, Gandhi RT, et al. Transmission of SARS-CoV-2: a review of viral host, and environmental factors. Ann Intern Med 2021;174:69–79.
2. Fang FC, Benson CA, Del Rio C, et al. COVID-19-lessons learned and questions remaining. Clin Infect 2021;72:2225–40.
3. Plante JA, Liu Y, Liu J, et al. Spike mutation D614G alters SARS-CoV-2 fitness. Nature 2021;592:116–21.
4. Zhou B, Thao TTN, Hoffmann D, et al. SARS-CoV-2 spike D614G change enhances replication and transmission. Nature 2021;592:122–7.
5. Hou YJ, Chiba S, Halfmann P, et al. SARS-CoV-2 D614G variant exhibits efficient replication ex vivo and transmission in vivo. Science 2020;370:1464–8.

6. Kepler L, Hamins-Puertolas M, Rasmussen DA. Decomposing the sources of SARS-CoV-2 fitness variation in the United States. Virus Evol 2021;7. https://doi.org/10.1093/ve/veab073.

7. Majumdar P, Niyogi S. SARS-CoV-2 mutations: the biological trackway towards viral fitness. Epidemiol Infect 2021;149. https://doi.org/10.1017/s0950268 821001060.

8. Liu C, Shi W, Becker ST, et al. Structural basis of mismatch recognition by a SARS-CoV-2 proofreading enzyme. Science 2021;373:1142–6.

9. Cevik M, Tate M, Lloyd O, et al. SARS-CoV-2, SARS-CoV, and MERS-CoV viral load dynamics, duration of viral shedding, and infectiousness: a systematic review and meta-analysis. Lancet Microbe 2021;2:e13–22.

10. Choi B, Choudhary MC, Regan J, et al. Persistence and Evolution of SARS-CoV-2 in an Immunocompromised Host. N Engl J Med 2020;383:2291–3.

11. D'Abramo A, Vita S, Maffongelli G, et al. Prolonged and severe SARS-CoV-2 infection in patients under B-cell-depleting drug successfully treated: a tailored approach. Int J Infect Dis 2021;107:247–50.

12. Corey L, Beyrer C, Cohen MS, et al. SARS-CoV-2 Variants in Patients with Immunosuppression. N Engl J Med 2021;385:562–6.

13. Galloway SE, Paul P, MacCannell DR, et al. Emergence of SARS-CoV-2 B.1.1.7 Lineage - United States, December 29, 2020-January 12, 2021. MMWR Morb Mortal Wkly Rep 2021;70:95–9.

14. Davies NG, Abbott S, Barnard RC, et al. Estimated transmissibility and impact of SARS-CoV-2 lineage B.1.1.7 in England. Science 2021;372. https://doi.org/10.1126/science.abg3055.

15. Tanaka H, Hirayama A, Nagai H, et al. Increased Transmissibility of the SARS-CoV-2 Alpha Variant in a Japanese Population. Int J Environ Res Public Health 2021;18. https://doi.org/10.3390/ijerph18157752.

16. Mlcochova P, Kemp SA, Dhar MS, et al. SARS-CoV-2 B.1.617.2 Delta variant replication and immune evasion. Nature 2021;599:114–9. https://doi.org/10.1038/s41586-021-03944-y.

17. Li H, Liu T, Wang L, et al. SARS-CoV-2 Delta variant infects ACE2(low) primary human bronchial epithelial cells more efficiently than other variants. J Med Virol 2021. https://doi.org/10.1002/jmv.27372.

18. Dhar MS, Marwal R, Vs R, et al. Genomic characterization and epidemiology of an emerging SARS-CoV-2 variant in Delhi, India. Science 2021. https://doi.org/10.1126/science.abj9932.

19. Allen H, Vusirikala A, Flannagan J, et al. Household transmission of COVID-19 cases associated with SARS-CoV-2 delta variant (B.1.617.2): national case-control study. Lancet Reg Health Eur 2021. https://doi.org/10.1016/j.lanepe.2021.100252.

20. van Doremalen N, Bushmaker T, Morris DH, et al. Aerosol and Surface Stability of SARS-CoV-2 as Compared with SARS-CoV-1. N Engl J Med 2020;382:1564–7.

21. Rocha ALS, Pinheiro JR, Nakamura TC, et al. Fomites and the environment did not have an important role in COVID-19 transmission in a Brazilian mid-sized city. Sci Rep 2021;11:15960.

22. Harvey AP, Fuhrmeister ER, Cantrell ME, et al. Longitudinal Monitoring of SARS-CoV-2 RNA on High-Touch Surfaces in a Community Setting. Environ Sci Technol Lett 2021;8:168–75.

23. Hu M, Lin H, Wang J, et al. Risk of coronavirus disease 2019 transmission in train passengers: an epidemiological and modeling study. Clin Infect Dis 2021;72:604–10.

24. Xu P, Jia W, Qian H, et al. Lack of cross-transmission of SARS-CoV-2 between passenger's cabins on the Diamond Princess cruise ship. Build Environ 2021; 198:107839.

25. Toyokawa T, Shimada T, Hayamizu T, et al. Transmission of SARS-CoV-2 during a 2-h domestic flight to Okinawa, Japan, March 2020. Influenza Other Respir Viruses 2021. https://doi.org/10.1111/irv.12913.

26. Xie X, Li Y, Chwang AT, et al. How far droplets can move in indoor environments–revisiting the Wells evaporation-falling curve. Indoor Air 2007;17:211–25. https://doi.org/10.1111/j.1600-0668.2007.00469.x.

27. Riley RL. What nobody needs to know about airborne infection. Am J Respir Crit Care Med 2001;163:7–8. https://doi.org/10.1164/ajrccm.163.1.hh11-00.

28. Riley RL, Mills CC, O'Grady F, et al. Infectiousness of air from a tuberculosis ward. Ultraviolet irradiation of infected air: comparative infectiousness of different patients. Am Rev Respir Dis 1962;85:511–25. https://doi.org/10.1164/arrd.1962.85.4.511.

29. Klompas M, Baker MA, Rhee C. Airborne transmission of SARS-CoV-2: theoretical considerations and available evidence. JAMA 2020;324:441–2. https://doi.org/10.1001/jama.2020.12458.

30. Richterman A, Meyerowitz EA, Cevik M. Hospital-acquired SARS-CoV-2 infection: lessons for public health. JAMA 2020;324:2155–6. https://doi.org/10.1001/jama.2020.21399.

31. Wang CC, Prather KA, Sznitman J, et al. Airborne transmission of respiratory viruses. Science 2021;373 2021–08/28. https://doi.org/10.1126/science.abd9149.

32. Klompas M, Milton DK, Rhee C, et al. Current insights into respiratory virus transmission and potential implications for infection control programs: a narrative review. Ann Intern Med 2021. https://doi.org/10.7326/m21-2780.

33. Marr LC, Tang JW. A paradigm shift to align transmission routes with mechanisms. Clin Infect Dis 2021. https://doi.org/10.1093/cid/ciab722.

34. Meyerowitz EA, Richterman A. A defense of the classical model of transmission of respiratory pathogens. Clin Infect Dis 2021;73:1318. https://doi.org/10.1093/cid/ciab016.

35. Dharmadhikari AS, Mphahlele M, Stoltz A, et al. Surgical face masks worn by patients with multidrug-resistant tuberculosis: impact on infectivity of air on a hospital ward. Am J Respir Crit Care Med 2012;185:1104–9. https://doi.org/10.1164/rccm.201107-1190OC.

36. Li Y, Cheng P, Jia W. Poor ventilation worsens short-range airborne transmission of respiratory infection. Indoor Air 2021. https://doi.org/10.1111/ina.12946.

37. Coleman KK, Tay DJW, Sen Tan K, et al. Viral load of SARS-CoV-2 in respiratory aerosols emitted by COVID-19 patients while breathing, talking, and singing. Clin Infect Dis 2021. https://doi.org/10.1093/cid/ciab691.

38. Kutter JS, de Meulder D, Bestebroer TM, et al. SARS-CoV and SARS-CoV-2 are transmitted through the air between ferrets over more than one meter distance. Nat Commun 2021;12:1653.

39. Chaintoutis SC, Thomou Z, Mouchtaropoulou E, et al. Outbreaks of SARS-CoV-2 in naturally infected mink farms: impact, transmission dynamics, genetic patterns, and environmental contamination. Plos Pathog 2021;17:e1009883.

40. Port JR, Yinda CK, Avanzato VA, et al. Increased aerosol transmission for B.1.1.7 (alpha variant) over lineage A variant of SARS-CoV-2. bioRxiv 2021. https://doi.org/10.1101/2021.07.26.453518.

41. Karan A, Klompas M, Tucker R, et al. The risk of SARS-CoV-2 transmission from patients with undiagnosed Covid-19 to roommates in a large academic medical center. Clin Infect Dis 2021. https://doi.org/10.1093/cid/ciab564.

42. Kwon K-S, Park J-I, Park YJ, et al. Evidence of long-distance droplet transmission of SARS-CoV-2 by direct air flow in a restaurant in Korea. J Korean Med Sci 2020;35.

43. Lu J, Gu J, Li K, et al. COVID-19 outbreak associated with air conditioning in restaurant, Guangzhou, China, 2020. Emerg Infect Dis 2020;26:1628–31.

44. Fox-Lewis A, Williamson F, Harrower J, et al. Airborne transmission of SARS-CoV-2 delta variant within tightly monitored isolation facility, New Zealand (Aotearoa). Emerg Infect Dis 2021;28:2021.

45. Wong SC, Au AK, Chen H, et al. Transmission of omicron (B.1.1.529) - SARS-CoV-2 variant of concern in a designated quarantine hotel for travelers: a challenge of elimination strategy of COVID-19. Lancet Reg Health West Pac 2021. https://doi.org/10.1016/j.lanwpc.2021.100360.

46. Li F, Li YY, Liu MJ, et al. Household transmission of SARS-CoV-2 and risk factors for susceptibility and infectivity in Wuhan: a retrospective observational study. Lancet Infect Dis 2021;21:617–28.

47. Sayampanathan AA, Heng CS, Pin PH, et al. Infectivity of asymptomatic versus symptomatic COVID-19. Lancet 2021;397:93–4.

48. Buitrago-Garcia D, Egli-Gany D, Counotte MJ, et al. Occurrence and transmission potential of asymptomatic and presymptomatic SARS-CoV-2 infections: a living systematic review and meta-analysis. Plos Med 2020;17:e1003346.

49. Richterman A, Meyerowitz EA, Cevik M. Indirect protection by reducing transmission: ending the pandemic with SARS-CoV-2 vaccination. Open Forum Infect Dis 2021. https://doi.org/10.1093/ofid/ofab259.

50. Marks M, Millat-Martinez P, Ouchi D, et al. Transmission of COVID-19 in 282 clusters in Catalonia, Spain: a cohort study. Lancet Infect Dis 2021;21:629–36.

51. Bjorkman KK, Saldi TK, Lasda E, et al. Higher viral load drives infrequent severe acute respiratory syndrome coronavirus 2 transmission between asymptomatic residence hall roommates. J Infect Dis 2021;224:1316–24.

52. Lyngse FP, Mølbak K, Træholt Frank K, et al. Association between SARS-CoV-2 transmission risk, viral load, and age: a nationwide study in Danish households. medRxiv 2021;2028. https://doi.org/10.1101/2021.02.28.21252608.

53. Lewis NM, Chu VT, Ye D, et al. Household transmission of severe acute respiratory syndrome coronavirus-2 in the United States. Clin Infect Dis 2021;73: 1805–13.

54. Goldstein E, Lipsitch M, Cevik M. On the effect of age on the transmission of SARS-CoV-2 in households, schools, and the community. J Infect Dis 2021; 223:362–9. https://doi.org/10.1093/infdis/jiaa691.

55. Davies NG, Klepac P, Liu Y, et al. Age-dependent effects in the transmission and control of COVID-19 epidemics. Nat Med 2020;26:1205–11.

56. Tonzel JL, Sokol T. COVID-19 outbreaks at youth summer camps - Louisiana, June-July 2021. MMWR Morb Mortal Wkly Rep 2021;70:1425–6.

57. Lam-Hine T, McCurdy SA, Santora L, et al. Outbreak associated with SARS-CoV-2 B.1.617.2 (Delta) variant in an elementary school - Marin County, California, May-June 2021. MMWR Morb Mortal Wkly Rep 2021;70:1214–9.

58. Ng OT, Koh V, Chiew CJ, et al. Impact of delta variant and vaccination on SARS-CoV-2 secondary attack rate among household close contacts. Lancet Reg Health West Pac 2021;17. https://doi.org/10.1016/j.lanwpc.2021.100299.

59. Zhang J, Xiao T, Cai Y, et al. Membrane fusion and immune evasion by the spike protein of SARS-CoV-2 delta variant. Science 2021. https://doi.org/10.1126/science.abl9463.

60. Wang Y, Chen R, Hu F, et al. Transmission, viral kinetics and clinical characteristics of the emergent SARS-CoV-2 Delta VOC in Guangzhou, China. EClinicalMedicine 2021;40. https://doi.org/10.1016/j.eclinm.2021.101129.

61. Luo CH, Morris CP, Sachithanandham J, et al. Infection with the SARS-CoV-2 delta variant is associated with higher infectious virus loads compared to the alpha variant in both unvaccinated and vaccinated individuals. medRxiv 2021. https://doi.org/10.1101/2021.08.15.21262077.

62. Teyssou E, Delagrèverie H, Visseaux B, et al. The delta SARS-CoV-2 variant has a higher viral load than the beta and the historical variants in nasopharyngeal samples from newly diagnosed COVID-19 patients. J Infect 2021;83:e1–3.

63. Singanayagam A, Hakki S, Dunning J, et al. Community transmission and viral load kinetics of the SARS-CoV-2 delta (B.1.617.2) variant in vaccinated and unvaccinated individuals in the UK: a prospective, longitudinal, cohort study. Lancet Infect Dis 2021. https://doi.org/10.1016/S1473-3099(21)00648-4.

64. Jones TC, Biele G, Mühlemann B, et al. Estimating infectiousness throughout SARS-CoV-2 infection course. Science 2021;373 2021–05/27.

65. Li B, Deng A, Li K, et al. Viral infection and transmission in a large, well-traced outbreak caused by the SARS-CoV-2 Delta variant. medRxiv 2021;21260122. https://doi.org/10.1101/2021.07.07.21260122.

66. Syed AM, Taha TY, Tabata T, et al. Rapid assessment of SARS-CoV-2 evolved variants using virus-like particles. Science 2021. https://doi.org/10.1126/science.abl6184.

67. Dixon BC, Fischer RSB, Zhao H, et al. Contact and SARS-CoV-2 infections among college football athletes in the southeastern conference during the COVID-19 pandemic. JAMA Netw Open 2021;4:e2135566. https://doi.org/10.1001/jamanetworkopen.2021.35566.

68. Furuse Y, Sando E, Tsuchiya N, et al. Clusters of coronavirus disease in communities, Japan, January-April 2020. Emerg Infect Dis 2020;26:2176–9.

69. Raines KS, Doniach S, Bhanot G. The transmission of SARS-CoV-2 is likely co-modulated by temperature and by relative humidity. PLoS One 2021;16:e0255212. https://doi.org/10.1371/journal.pone.0255212.

70. Cevik M, Marcus JL, Buckee C, et al. Severe acute respiratory syndrome coronavirus 2 (SARS-CoV-2) transmission dynamics should inform policy. Clin Infect Dis 2021;73:S170–6. https://doi.org/10.1093/cid/ciaa1442.

71. Esaryk EE, Wesson P, Fields J, et al. Variation in SARS-CoV-2 infection risk and socioeconomic disadvantage among a Mayan-Latinx population in Oakland, California. JAMA Netw Open 2021;4:e2110789. https://doi.org/10.1001/jamanetworkopen.2021.10789.

72. Mazzilli S, Chieti A, Casigliani V, et al. Risk of SARS-CoV-2 infection and disease severity in people at socioeconomic disadvantage in Italy. Eur J Public Health 2021;31. https://doi.org/10.1093/eurpub/ckab164.552.

73. Allan-Blitz LT, Goldbeck C, Hertlein F, et al. Association of lower socioeconomic status and SARS-CoV-2 positivity in Los Angeles, California. J Prev Med Public Health 2021;54:161–5.

74. Rodriguez-Diaz CE, Guilamo-Ramos V, Mena L, et al. Risk for COVID-19 infection and death among Latinos in the United States: examining heterogeneity in transmission dynamics. Ann Epidemiol 2020;52:46–53.

75. Li Q, Guan X, Wu P, et al. Early Transmission Dynamics in Wuhan, China, of Novel Coronavirus-Infected Pneumonia. N Engl J Med 2020;382:1199–207.

76. Lauer SA, Grantz KH, Bi Q, et al. The Incubation Period of Coronavirus Disease 2019 (COVID-19) From Publicly Reported Confirmed Cases: Estimation and Application. Ann Intern Med 2020;172:577–82. https://doi.org/10.7326/m20-0504.

77. Meng Z, Jianpeng X, Aiping D, et al. Notes from the Field: Transmission Dynamics of an Outbreak of the COVID-19 Delta Variant B.1.617.2 — Guangdong Province, China, May–June 2021. China CDC Weekly 2021;3:584–6.

78. Tom BD, Van Hoek AJ, Pebody R, et al. Estimating time to onset of swine influenza symptoms after initial novel A(H1N1v) viral infection. Epidemiol Infect 2011;139:1418–24.

79. Xin H, Li Y, Wu P, et al. Estimating the latent period of coronavirus disease 2019 (COVID-19). Clin Infect Dis 2021. https://doi.org/10.1093/cid/ciab746.

80. Kang M, Xin H, Yuan J, et al. Transmission dynamics and epidemiological characteristics of Delta variant infections in China. medRxiv 2021;2021:21261991. https://doi.org/10.1101/2021.08.12.21261991.

81. Rai B, Shukla A, Dwivedi LK. Estimates of serial interval for COVID-19: A systematic review and meta-analysis. Clin Epidemiol Glob Health 2021;9:157–61. https://doi.org/10.1016/j.cegh.2020.08.007.

82. Hari H, Jun-Sik L, Sun-Ah S, et al. Transmission dynamics of the delta variant of SARS-CoV-2 infections in Daejeon, South Korea. Res Square 2021. https://doi.org/10.21203/rs.3.rs-934350/v1.

83. Pung R, Mak TM, Kucharski AJ, et al. Serial intervals in SARS-CoV-2 B.1.617.2 variant cases. Lancet 2021;398:837–8.

84. Cheng HY, Jian SW, Liu DP, et al. Contact Tracing Assessment of COVID-19 Transmission Dynamics in Taiwan and Risk at Different Exposure Periods Before and After Symptom Onset. JAMA Intern Med 2020;180:1156–63.

85. Mack CD, DiFiori J, Tai CG, et al. SARS-CoV-2 Transmission Risk Among National Basketball Association Players, Staff, and Vendors Exposed to Individuals With Positive Test Results After COVID-19 Recovery During the 2020 Regular and Postseason. JAMA Intern Med 2021;181:960–6.

86. de Man P, Ortiz M, Bluyssen PM, et al. Airborne SARS-CoV-2 in home- and hospital environment investigated with a high-powered air sampler. J Hosp Infect 2021. https://doi.org/10.1016/j.jhin.2021.10.018.

87. Delamater PL, Street EJ, Leslie TF, et al. Complexity of the Basic Reproduction Number (R(0)). Emerg Infect Dis 2019;25:1–4.

88. Billah MA, Miah MM, Khan MN. Reproductive number of coronavirus: A systematic review and meta-analysis based on global level evidence. PLoS One 2020; 15:e0242128.

89. Xia F, Yang X, Cheke RA, et al. Quantifying competitive advantages of mutant strains in a population involving importation and mass vaccination rollout. Infect Dis Model 2021;6:988–96. https://doi.org/10.1016/j.idm.2021.08.001.

90. Dagpunar J. Interim estimates of increased transmissibility, growth rate, and reproduction number of the Covid-19 B.1.617.2 variant of concern in the United Kingdom. medRxiv 2021;21258293. https://doi.org/10.1101/2021.06.03.21258293.

91. Breban R, Riou J, Fontanet A. Interhuman transmissibility of Middle East respiratory syndrome coronavirus: estimation of pandemic risk. Lancet 2013;382: 694–9.

92. Cauchemez S, Fraser C, Van Kerkhove MD, et al. Middle East respiratory syndrome coronavirus: quantification of the extent of the epidemic, surveillance biases, and transmissibility. Lancet Infect Dis 2014;14:50–6.

93. Fisman D, Khoo E, Tuite A. Early epidemic dynamics of the West African 2014 Ebola outbreak: estimates derived with a simple two-parameter model. Plos Curr 2014;6. https://doi.org/10.1371/currents.outbreaks.89c0d3783f36958d96 ebbae97348d571.

94. Khan A, Naveed M, Dur EAM, et al. Estimating the basic reproductive ratio for the Ebola outbreak in Liberia and Sierra Leone. Infect Dis Poverty 2015;4. https://doi.org/10.1186/s40249-015-0043-3.

95. Balcan D, Hu H, Goncalves B, et al. Seasonal transmission potential and activity peaks of the new influenza A(H1N1): a Monte Carlo likelihood analysis based on human mobility. BMC Med 2009;7. https://doi.org/10.1186/1741-7015-7-45.

96. Andreasen V, Viboud C, Simonsen L. Epidemiologic characterization of the 1918 influenza pandemic summer wave in Copenhagen: implications for pandemic control strategies. J Infect Dis 2008;197:270–8.

97. Lipsitch M, Cohen T, Cooper B, et al. Transmission dynamics and control of severe acute respiratory syndrome. Science 2003;300:1966–70. https://doi.org/10.1126/science.1086616.

98. Guerra FM, Bolotin S, Lim G, et al. The basic reproduction number (R(0)) of measles: a systematic review. Lancet Infect Dis 2017;17:e420–8. https://doi.org/10.1016/s1473-3099(17)30307-9.

99. Anderson RM, May RM. Directly transmitted infections diseases: control by vaccination. Science 1982;215:1053–60.

100. Lloyd-Smith JO, Schreiber SJ, Kopp PE, et al. Superspreading and the effect of individual variation on disease emergence. Nature 2005;438:355–9.

101. Miller D, Martin MA, Harel N, et al. Full genome viral sequences inform patterns of SARS-CoV-2 spread into and within Israel. Nat Commun 2020;11:5518. https://doi.org/10.1038/s41467-020-19248-0.

102. Endo A, Abbott S, Kucharski AJ, et al. Estimating the overdispersion in COVID-19 transmission using outbreak sizes outside China. Wellcome Open Res 2020; 5:67. https://doi.org/10.12688/wellcomeopenres.15842.3.

103. Adam DC, Wu P, Wong JY, et al. Clustering and superspreading potential of SARS-CoV-2 infections in Hong Kong. Nat Med 2020;26:1714–9.

104. Bi Q, Wu Y, Mei S, et al. Epidemiology and transmission of COVID-19 in 391 cases and 1286 of their close contacts in Shenzhen, China: a retrospective cohort study. Lancet Infect Dis 2020;20:911–9.

105. Lemieux JE, Siddle KJ, Shaw BM, et al. Phylogenetic analysis of SARS-CoV-2 in Boston highlights the impact of superspreading events. Science 2021;371. https://doi.org/10.1126/science.abe3261.

106. Park SY, Kim YM, Yi S, et al. Coronavirus Disease Outbreak in Call Center, South Korea. Emerg Infect Dis 2020;26:1666–70.

107. Yusef D, Hayajneh W, Awad S, et al. Large Outbreak of Coronavirus Disease among Wedding Attendees, Jordan. Emerg Infect Dis 2020;26:2165–7.

108. Hamner L, Dubbel P, Capron I, et al. High SARS-CoV-2 Attack Rate Following Exposure at a Choir Practice - Skagit County, Washington, March 2020. MMWR Morb Mortal Wkly Rep 2020;69:606–10.

109. Szablewski CM, Chang KT, Brown MM, et al. SARS-CoV-2 Transmission and Infection Among Attendees of an Overnight Camp - Georgia, June 2020. MMWR Morb Mortal Wkly Rep 2020;69:1023–5.
110. Payne DC, Smith-Jeffcoat SE, Nowak G, et al. SARS-CoV-2 Infections and Serologic Responses from a Sample of U.S. Navy Service Members - USS Theodore Roosevelt, April 2020. MMWR Morb Mortal Wkly Rep 2020;69:714–21.
111. Ryu S, Kim D, Lim J-S, et al. Serial interval and transmission dynamics during the SARS-CoV-2 Delta variant predominance in South Korea. medRxiv 2021;21262166. https://doi.org/10.1101/2021.08.18.21262166.
112. Siddle KJ, Krasilnikova LA, Moreno GK, et al. Evidence of transmission from fully vaccinated individuals in a large outbreak of the SARS-CoV-2 Delta variant in Provincetown, Massachusetts. medRxiv 2021. https://doi.org/10.1101/2021.10.20.21265137.
113. Chen PZ, Koopmans M, Fisman DN, et al. Understanding why superspreading drives the COVID-19 pandemic but not the H1N1 pandemic. Lancet Infect Dis 2021;21:1203–4.
114. Becker AD, Birger RB, Teillant A, et al. Estimating enhanced prevaccination measles transmission hotspots in the context of cross-scale dynamics. Proc Natl Acad Sci U S A 2016;113:14595–600.
115. Ackley SF, Hacker JK, Enanoria WTA, et al. Genotype-Specific Measles Transmissibility: A Branching Process Analysis. Clin Infect Dis 2018;66:1270–5. https://doi.org/10.1093/cid/cix974.
116. Fraser C, Cummings DA, Klinkenberg D, et al. Influenza transmission in households during the 1918 pandemic. Am J Epidemiol 2011;174:505–14.
117. Frieden TR, Lee CT. Identifying and Interrupting Superspreading Events-Implications for Control of Severe Acute Respiratory Syndrome Coronavirus 2. Emerg Infect Dis 2020;26:1059–66.
118. Cevik M, Baral SD. Networks of SARS-CoV-2 transmission. Science 2021;373:162–3.
119. Althouse BM, Wenger EA, Miller JC, et al. Superspreading events in the transmission dynamics of SARS-CoV-2: Opportunities for interventions and control. Plos Biol 2020;18:e3000897.
120. Dagan N, Barda N, Kepten E, et al. BNT162b2 mRNA Covid-19 Vaccine in a Nationwide Mass Vaccination Setting. N Engl J Med 2021;384:1412–23.
121. McDonald I, Murray SM, Reynolds CJ, et al. Comparative systematic review and meta-analysis of reactogenicity, immunogenicity and efficacy of vaccines against SARS-CoV-2. NPJ Vaccin 2021;6. https://doi.org/10.1038/s41541-021-00336-1.
122. Kojima N, Shrestha N, Klausner J. A Systematic Review of the Protective Effect of Prior SARS-CoV-2 Infection on Repeat Infection. medRxiv 2021;21262741. https://doi.org/10.1101/2021.08.27.21262741.
123. Cevik M, Grubaugh ND, Iwasaki A, et al. COVID-19 vaccines: Keeping pace with SARS-CoV-2 variants. Cell 2021;184:5077–81.
124. de Gier B, Andeweg S, Joosten R, et al. Vaccine effectiveness against SARS-CoV-2 transmission and infections among household and other close contacts of confirmed cases, the Netherlands. Euro Surveill 2021;26. https://doi.org/10.2807/1560-7917.Es.2021.26.31.2100640.
125. England PH. SARS-CoV-2 variants of concern and variants under investigation in England: Technical briefing 19. Available at: https://assets.publishing.service.gov.uk/government/uploads/system/uploads/attachment_data/file/1005517/Technical_Briefing_19.pdf. Accessed October 1, 2021.

126. Pouwels KB, Pritchard E, Matthews PC, et al. Effect of Delta variant on viral burden and vaccine effectiveness against new SARS-CoV-2 infections in the UK. Nat Med 2021. https://doi.org/10.1038/s41591-021-01548-7.

127. Fowlkes A, Gaglani M, Groover K, et al. Effectiveness of COVID-19 Vaccines in Preventing SARS-CoV-2 Infection Among Frontline Workers Before and During B.1.617.2 (Delta) Variant Predominance - Eight U.S. Locations, December. MMWR Morb Mortal Wkly Rep 2021;70:1167–9.

128. Brown CM, Vostok J, Johnson H, et al. Outbreak of SARS-CoV-2 Infections, Including COVID-19 Vaccine Breakthrough Infections, Associated with Large Public Gatherings - Barnstable County, Massachusetts. MMWR Morb Mortal Wkly Rep 2021;70:1059–62.

129. Chia PY, Xiang Ong SW, Chiew CJ, et al. Virological and serological kinetics of SARS-CoV-2 Delta variant vaccine-breakthrough infections: a multi-center cohort study. medRxiv 2021;21261295. https://doi.org/10.1101/2021.07.28. 21261295.

130. Qiu X, Nergiz AI, Maraolo AE, et al. The role of asymptomatic and pre-symptomatic infection in SARS-CoV-2 transmission-a living systematic review. Clin Microbiol Infect 2021;27:511–9.

131. Riemersma KK, Grogan BE, Kita-Yarbro A, et al. Shedding of Infectious SARS-CoV-2 Despite Vaccination. medRxiv 2021;21261387. https://doi.org/10.1101/ 2021.07.31.21261387.

132. Shamier MC, Tostmann A, Bogers S, et al. Virological characteristics of SARS-CoV-2 vaccine breakthrough infections in health care workers. medRxiv 2021;21262158. https://doi.org/10.1101/2021.08.20.21262158.

133. Eyre DW, Taylor D, Purver M, et al. Effect of Covid-19 Vaccination on Transmission of Alpha and Delta Variants. N Engl J Med 2022. https://doi.org/10.1056/ NEJMoa2116597.

134. Accorsi EK, Qiu X, Rumpler E, et al. How to detect and reduce potential sources of biases in studies of SARS-CoV-2 and COVID-19. Eur J Epidemiol 2021;36: 179–96.

135. Scott J, Richterman A, Cevik M. Covid-19 vaccination: evidence of waning immunity is overstated. Bmj 2021;374:n2320. https://doi.org/10.1136/bmj.n2320.

136. U.S. Food & Drug Administration (2021) Vaccines and Related Biological Products Advisory Committee Meeting September 17, 2021: Application for licensure of a booster dose for COMIRNATY (COVID-19 Vaccine, mRNA). FDA Briefing Document.

137. Baden LR, El Sahly HM, Essink B, et al. Phase 3 Trial of mRNA-1273 during the Delta-Variant Surge. N Engl J Med 2021. https://doi.org/10.1056/ NEJMc2115597.

138. Levine-Tiefenbrun M, Yelin I, Alapi H, et al. Viral loads of Delta-variant SARS-CoV-2 breakthrough infections after vaccination and booster with BNT162b2. Nat Med 2021. https://doi.org/10.1038/s41591-021-01575-4.

139. Bar-On YM, Goldberg Y, Mandel M, et al. Protection of BNT162b2 Vaccine Booster against Covid-19 in Israel. N Engl J Med 2021;385:1393–400.

140. Barda N, Dagan N, Cohen C, et al. Effectiveness of a third dose of the BNT162b2 mRNA COVID-19 vaccine for preventing severe outcomes in Israel: an observational study. Lancet 2021. https://doi.org/10.1016/s0140-6736(21) 02249-2.

141. Pfizer. Pfizer and BioNTech announce phase 3 trial data showing high efficacy of a booster dose of their covid-19 vaccine. Available at: *https://wwwpfizercom/*

news/press-release/press-release-detail/pfizer-and-biontech-announce-phase-3-trial-data-showing 2021.

142. Conway Morris A, Sharrocks K, Bousfield R, et al. The removal of airborne SARS-CoV-2 and other microbial bioaerosols by air filtration on COVID-19 surge units. Clin Infect Dis 2021. https://doi.org/10.1093/cid/ciab933.

143. Wang Y, Tian H, Zhang L, et al. Reduction of secondary transmission of SARS-CoV-2 in households by face mask use, disinfection and social distancing: a cohort study in Beijing, China. BMJ Glob Health 2020;5. https://doi.org/10.1136/bmjgh-2020-002794.

144. Gettings J, Czarnik M, Morris E, et al. Mask Use and Ventilation Improvements to Reduce COVID-19 Incidence in Elementary Schools - Georgia, November 16-December 11, 2020. MMWR Morb Mortal Wkly Rep 2021;70:779–84.

145. Escombe AR, Oeser CC, Gilman RH, et al. Natural ventilation for the prevention of airborne contagion. Plos Med 2007;4. https://doi.org/10.1371/journal.pmed.0040068.

146. Lygizos M, Shenoi SV, Brooks RP, et al. Natural ventilation reduces high TB transmission risk in traditional homes in rural KwaZulu-Natal, South Africa. BMC Infect Dis 2013;13. https://doi.org/10.1186/1471-2334-13-300.

147. Abaluck J, Kwong LH, Styczynski A, et al. The Impact of Community Masking on COVID-19. A Cluster Randomized Trial in Bangladesh 2021;31:2021. https://doi.org/10.3386/w28734.

148. Bundgaard H, Bundgaard JS, Raaschou-Pedersen DET, et al. Effectiveness of Adding a Mask Recommendation to Other Public Health Measures to Prevent SARS-CoV-2 Infection in Danish Mask Wearers : A Randomized Controlled Trial. Ann Intern Med 2021;174:335–43.

149. Li Y, Liang M, Gao L, et al. Face masks to prevent transmission of COVID-19: A systematic review and meta-analysis. Am J Infect Control 2021;49:900–6.

150. Chu DK, Akl EA, Duda S, et al. Physical distancing, face masks, and eye protection to prevent person-to-person transmission of SARS-CoV-2 and COVID-19: a systematic review and meta-analysis. Lancet 2020;395:1973–87.

151. Lyu W, Wehby GL. Community Use Of Face Masks And COVID-19: Evidence From A Natural Experiment Of State Mandates In The US. Health Aff (Millwood) 2020;39:1419–25.

152. Ginther DK, Zambrana C. Association of Mask Mandates and COVID-19 Case Rates, Hospitalizations, and Deaths in Kansas. JAMA Netw Open 2021;4:e2114514. https://doi.org/10.1001/jamanetworkopen.2021.14514.

153. Baker MA, Fiumara K, Rhee C, et al. Low Risk of Coronavirus Disease 2019 (COVID-19) Among Patients Exposed to Infected Healthcare Workers. Clin Infect Dis 2021;73:e1878–80.

154. Rhee C, Baker M, Vaidya V, et al. Incidence of Nosocomial COVID-19 in Patients Hospitalized at a Large US Academic Medical Center. JAMA Netw Open 2020;3:e2020498. https://doi.org/10.1001/jamanetworkopen.2020.20498.

155. Kociolek LK, Patel AB, Hultquist JF, et al. Viral whole-genome sequencing to assess impact of universal masking on SARS-CoV-2 transmission among pediatric healthcare workers. Infect Control Hosp Epidemiol 2021;1–5. https://doi.org/10.1017/ice.2021.415.

156. Thompson ER, Williams FS, Giacin PA, et al. Universal masking to control healthcare-associated transmission of severe acute respiratory coronavirus virus 2 (SARS-CoV-2). Infect Control Hosp Epidemiol 2021;1–7. https://doi.org/10.1017/ice.2021.127.

157. Radonovich LJ Jr, Simberkoff MS, Bessesen MT, et al. N95 Respirators vs Medical Masks for Preventing Influenza Among Health Care Personnel: A Randomized Clinical Trial. Jama 2019;322:824–33.

158. Sims MD, Maine GN, Childers KL, et al. Coronavirus Disease 2019 (COVID-19) Seropositivity and Asymptomatic Rates in Healthcare Workers Are Associated with Job Function and Masking. Clin Infect Dis 2021;73:S154–62.

159. Klompas M, Baker MA, Rhee C, et al. A SARS-CoV-2 Cluster in an Acute Care Hospital. Ann Intern Med 2021;174:794–802.

160. Lindsey BB, Villabona-Arenas CJ, Campbell F, et al. Characterising within-hospital SARS-CoV-2 transmission events: a retrospective analysis integrating epidemiological and viral genomic data from a UK tertiary care setting across two pandemic waves. medRxiv 2021;2021:21260537. https://doi.org/10.1101/2021.07.15.21260537.

161. Klompas M, Baker MA, Griesbach D, et al. Transmission of Severe Acute Respiratory Syndrome Coronavirus 2 (SARS-CoV-2) From Asymptomatic and Presymptomatic Individuals in Healthcare Settings Despite Medical Masks and Eye Protection. Clin Infect Dis 2021;73:1693–5.

162. Park Y, Huh IS, Lee J, et al. Application of Testing-Tracing-Treatment Strategy in Response to the COVID-19 Outbreak in Seoul, Korea. J Korean Med Sci 2020;35:e396. https://doi.org/10.3346/jkms.2020.35.e396.

163. Kendall M, Milsom L, Abeler-Dörner L, et al. Epidemiological changes on the Isle of Wight after the launch of the NHS Test and Trace programme: a preliminary analysis. Lancet Digit Health 2020;2:e658–66. https://doi.org/10.1016/s2589-7500(20)30241-7.

164. Malheiro R, Figueiredo AL, Magalhães JP, et al. Effectiveness of contact tracing and quarantine on reducing COVID-19 transmission: a retrospective cohort study. Public Health 2020;189:54–9. https://doi.org/10.1016/j.puhe.2020.09.012.

165. Gardner BJ, Kilpatrick AM. Contact tracing efficiency, transmission heterogeneity, and accelerating COVID-19 epidemics. Plos Comput Biol 2021;17:e1009122. https://doi.org/10.1371/journal.pcbi.1009122.

166. Viana R, Moyo S, Amoako DG, et al. Rapid epidemic expansion of the SARS-CoV-2 Omicron variant in southern Africa. medRxiv 2021;21268028. https://doi.org/10.1101/2021.12.19.21268028.

167. Ito K, Piantham C, Nishiura H. Relative Instantaneous Reproduction Number of Omicron SARS-CoV-2 variant with respect to the Delta variant in Denmark. J Med Virol 2021. https://doi.org/10.1002/jmv.27560.

168. Lyngse FP, Mortensen LH, Denwood MJ, et al. SARS-CoV-2 Omicron VOC Transmission in Danish Households. medRxiv 2021;2021:21268278. https://doi.org/10.1101/2021.12.27.21268278.

169. Carreño JM, Alshammary H, Tcheou J, et al. Activity of convalescent and vaccine serum against SARS-CoV-2 Omicron. Nature 2021. https://doi.org/10.1038/s41586-022-04399-5.

170. Schmidt F, Muecksch F, Weisblum Y, et al. Plasma Neutralization of the SARS-CoV-2 Omicron Variant. New Engl J Med 2021. https://doi.org/10.1056/NEJMc2119641.

171. Brandal LT, MacDonald E, Veneti L, et al. Outbreak caused by the SARS-CoV-2 Omicron variant in Norway, November to December 2021. Euro Surveill 2021. https://doi.org/10.2807/1560-7917.Es.2021.26.50.2101147.

172. Helmsdal G, Hansen OK, Møller LF, et al. Omicron outbreak at a private gathering in the Faroe Islands, infecting 21 of 33 triple-vaccinated healthcare workers. medRxiv 2021;21268021. https://doi.org/10.1101/2021.12.22.21268021.
173. Hay JA, Kissler SM, Fauver JR, et al. Viral dynamics and duration of PCR positivity of the SARS-CoV-2 Omicron variant. medRxiv 2022;22269257. https://doi.org/10.1101/2022.01.13.22269257.
174. Puhach O, Adea K, Hulo N, et al. Infectious viral load in unvaccinated and vaccinated patients infected with SARS-CoV-2 WT, Delta and Omicron. medRxiv 2022. https://doi.org/10.1101/2022.01.10.22269010.
175. Torjesen I. Covid-19: Peak of viral shedding is later with omicron variant, Japanese data suggest. Bmj 2022;376. https://doi.org/10.1136/bmj.o89.
176. Gu H, Krishnan P, Ng DYM, et al. Probable Transmission of SARS-CoV-2 Omicron Variant in Quarantine Hotel, Hong Kong, China, November 2021. Emerg Infect Dis 2021;28. https://doi.org/10.3201/eid2802.212422.

Awakening

The Unveiling of Historically Unaddressed Social Inequities During the COVID-19 Pandemic in the United States

Michele P. Andrasik, PhD, EdM[a,*], Alika K. Maunakea, PhD[b],
Linda Oseso, MPH[a], Carlos E. Rodriguez-Diaz, PhD, MPH[c],
Stephaun Wallace, PhD[a], Karina Walters, PhD[d],
Michi Yukawa, MD, MPH[e,f]

KEYWORDS

- Race • Ethnicity • LGBTQ • Inequities • COVID-19 • Disparities

KEY POINTS

- Violence and victimization brought by colonization and slavery and justified for over a century by race-based science have resulted in enduring inequities for Black, Indigenous and People of Color (BIPOC) across the United States.
- The seeds planted from the rhetoric and policies of colonization and race-based science have strong and enduring roots ensuring that biases persist across societal domains.
- These biases have resulted in ongoing and pervasive discriminatory economic, social, and structural practices placing BIPOC individuals, families and communities at increased risk for violence, victimization, mass incarceration, trauma, and negative health outcomes.
- Intersecting marginalized identities weave together systems of discrimination or social disadvantages and amplify the impact of negative health outcomes, poverty, trauma, and other social ills.
- What is critical are the actions taken by organizations and institutions to reconcile and repair the harm that has been perpetrated for more than a century.

[a] Vaccine and Infectious Disease Division, Fred Hutchinson, 1100 Eastlake Avenue, E3-300, Seattle, WA 98109, USA; [b] Department of Anatomy, Biochemistry, and Physiology, John A. Burns School of Medicine, University of Hawaii, 651 Ilalo Street, BSB-222K, Honolulu, HI 96813, USA; [c] Department of Prevention and Community Health, Milken Institute School of Public Health, The George Washington University, 950 New Hampshire Avenue NW, Suite 300, Washington, DC 20052, USA; [d] Indigenous Wellness Research Institute, University of Washington, 4101 15th Avenue NE Box 354900, Seattle, WA 98105, USA; [e] Division of Geriatrics, University of California San Francisco, San Francisco, CA 94121, USA; [f] Geriatric Palliative and Extended Care, San Francisco VA Medical Center, 490 Illinois Street, Floor 8, UCSF BOX 1265, San Francisco, CA 94143, USA
* Corresponding author.
E-mail address: mandrasik@fredhutch.org

Infect Dis Clin N Am 36 (2022) 295–308
https://doi.org/10.1016/j.idc.2022.01.009
0891-5520/22/© 2022 Elsevier Inc. All rights reserved.

id.theclinics.com

INTRODUCTION

Racial and ethnic biases have resulted in ongoing and pervasive discriminatory economic, social, and structural practices placing Black, Indigenous and People of Color (BIPOC) (people of color includes Asian Americans, Native Hawaiians [NH], and Pacific Islanders [PI]), their families, and communities at increased risk for violence, victimization, mass incarceration, trauma, and negative health outcomes. The violence and victimization brought by colonization and slavery, and justified for over a century by race-based science,[1,2] have resulted in enduring inequities for BIPOC across the United States; this is particularly true if BIPOC individuals have other intersecting devalued identities. Herein, we highlight how such longstanding inequities paved the way for the disproportionate burdens of coronavirus disease 2019 (COVID-19) among BIPOC across the United States and other countries that share a colonial legacy. We also provide recommendations on how to improve COVID-19 mitigation strategies with the goal of eliminating disparities.

US settler colonialism and[3,4] the "discovery" of the "new world" sought to erase Indigenous people from the land through massacres, enslavement, and forced relocations so that the land could be reconfigured as settler property and settler "origin" stories could be inserted to uphold settler rationalizations for ongoing colonial violence in the service of colonial progress. US settler colonialism also included the theft and enslavement of African peoples from their "homelands to become the property of settlers to labor on stolen land[5]" as well as the creation of racialized migrant "others" imported to serve as a source of easily accessible, manipulatable, and expendable labor.[6,7]

US settler colonialism is a structure that resulted in the death of more than 100 million native and Indigenous peoples as far back as 1607 (ie, the first colony founded at Jamestown, Virginia) with transgenerational adverse impacts persisting to the present day.[8] Native peoples were subject to community massacres, enslavement, pandemics from the introduction of new disease, and genocidal policies such as the "Kill the Indian, Save the man" policy (1879 to ~1935) resulting in the forced removal of children from their homes into boarding schools where they were subjected to rampant sexual and physical abuse. First Indigenous peoples and then African slaves were made inhuman or "othered" to obtain their labor and land. Creating structures of racial subordination through erasing and "racing" "others" and hiding behind narratives of progress and Western superiority to gain access to land and exploitable labor were critical to consolidating the settler state, augmenting settler wealth and power, obscuring the conditions of its own production and reproduction, and freeing future generations from accountability.[5,7,9,10]

In the 1820s race-based science was introduced by US southern physicians seeking to legitimize slavery[1,2]; it purported an inherent inferiority based on race and soon became the prominent scientific paradigm in the country and throughout Europe. At its foundation was a nondata- and pseudoscience-driven justification of a system of inhumane forced labor, first, for enslaved Africans, later for Chinese, Japanese, Mexican, and Central American immigrant laborers, and continuously among residents of US unincorporated territories. Job scarcity during the Great Depression led to the "discovery" that white individuals did not differ from their BIPOC counterparts in their heat adaptability or pain tolerance.[11] The seeds planted from the rhetoric and policies of colonization and race-based science have strong and enduring roots ensuring that biases persist across societal domains. The implementation of public health initiatives in the United States is a product of this history and has been fundamentally exclusionary and racist.[12–14]

Intersectionality

Intersectionality can be defined as the interconnected nature of social categories like class, gender, and race. These interconnected identities weave together systems of discrimination or social disadvantages to amplify the impact of negative health outcomes, poverty, trauma, and other social ills.[15] The social and structural devaluation of gender, sex, sexuality, and racial minority groups is anchored in societal and political attitudes and beliefs that have been nourished over settler colonial policies over generations. This coupled with contemporary and historical experiences of discrimination and bias results in a constant assault on the health, lives, and personhood of marginalized communities. For most infectious diseases, including COVID-19, the most extreme burden of disease is experienced by society's most vulnerable, most often, people who experience multiple forms of social disadvantage.

Lesbian, Gay, Transgender, and Queer Populations

It is well established that people who identify as lesbian, gay, bisexual, transgender, or queer (LGBTQ) experience elevated levels of discrimination and bias, social disadvantages, and physical and mental health disparities. These disparities are exacerbated by the social isolation and trauma from the COVID-19 pandemic.[16–18] When these disparities are overlain with racism, LGBTQ communities of color carry a greater burden of vulnerability due to these same systems of oppression.

During the COVID-19 pandemic, LGBTQ communities have been disadvantaged by longstanding and new challenges associated with employment and financial stability, negative experiences with health care, limited or no health insurance, and effects of physical distancing and social isolation on mental health.[19] LGBTQ youth experience greater proportions of homelessness, violence, and suicide compared with their cisgender and heterosexual counterparts, increasing their vulnerability to a range of negative health and psychological threats.[20] Older LGBTQ adults face unique challenges because they experience high rates of systemic discrimination in housing and health care that increases risk for poverty. Transgender older adults experience higher rates of sexual assault, violence, family rejection, and social isolation than any other group within the LGBTQ community.[21] In addition, for some older adult LGBTQ people, the COVID-19 pandemic is reminiscent of the earlier days of the human immunodeficiency virus (HIV) epidemic when death and despair were pervasive, and the initial HIV response ignored the nuanced impact it had on communities with intersectional identities.[22] The elevated health threats to LGBTQ persons, including youth and adults, coupled with the COVID-19 pandemic result in alarming increases in vulnerabilities. Although these examples of susceptibility are not unique to LGBTQ communities, the intersection of invisibility,[23] homophobia, transphobia, racism, sexism, and other forms of discrimination ensures that LGBTQ populations, particularly those who are also BIPOC, are disproportionately impacted by COVID-19. The disparities LGBTQ communities face, illuminated by the COVID-19 pandemic, represent a failure to address these same determinants of health that impact HIV burden in these communities.[24]

American Indian/Alaska Native

American Indian and Alaska Native (AIAN) populations number 9.7 million people representing 2.9% of the US population.[25] There are 574 federally recognized AIAN nations and villages as well as more than 63 state-recognized tribes representing linguistically and culturally diverse Indigenous populations across the United States. AIANs are dying of COVID-19 at higher rates and at younger ages than other populations.[26,27] As of February 10, 2021, AIANs have the highest age-adjusted COVID-19 mortality rate of any other population (265 of 100,000 vs 108–249 of 100,00 across Asian, white, black, and Hispanic/Latino populations respectively).[28] As of November 22, 2021, risk for COVID-19 death remained highest among AIAN populations (ratios of age-adjusted rates: 2.2× vs 0.9–2.1×).[29] Moreover, although COVID-19 mortality rates increase with age across all populations, AIANs aged 20 to 29 years, 30 to 39 years, and 40 to 49 years are 10.5 times, 11.6 times, and 8.2 times more likely to die than white persons in the same age groups, respectively.[27] Findings from the Native American COVID-19 Alliance national needs assessment study (March, 2021; N = 8549) found that the crude estimate of COVID-19 AIAN deaths of 765 of 100,000 was three times that of current estimates.[30] Finally, as of February 17, 2022, AIAN populations continue to have the highest rates of age-adjusted, laboratory confirmed COVID-19 hospitalizations (1943.6 of 100,000) than any other population (496.9-1538.1 of 100,000).[31]

Raising the visibility of Native experiences is critical during the COVID-19 pandemic, because AIAN communities have been hit hard and yet remain largely invisible, under-counted, or misclassified in COVID-19 public health surveillance data.[30,32] Deficient and inaccurate systems of reporting, data collection methods, and data analytical ap-proaches have led to invisibility and erasure of AIAN health needs as well as significant gaps in understanding the lived experiences and impact of COVID-19 on AIAN popu-lations, communities, and families.[30] As noted earlier, erasure is a hallmark of US settler colonialism, and the chronic and pervasive invisibility in systems of data report-ing do not simply reflect shoddy systems, but rather, reflect colonial structures' inten-tion or complacency in upholding data colonialism. Coupled with ongoing structural data inequities that place AIANs at risk for not adequately receiving economic and structural health supports are the chronic socioeconomic-environmental structural in-equities that have been a harbinger of poor health and health inequities in Indian country.

The convergence of socioeconomic and environmental inequities combined with "pre-existing chronic disease conditions create a potentially perilous interacting syn-ergistic epidemic –known as a syndemic– accelerating the hazardous impact of COVID-19"[7,30] on AIAN populations. The multiple, interacting network of health, so-cial, and structural conditions works synergistically to accelerate poor AIAN popula-tion health, particularly during pandemics and environmental disasters.[30]

AIAN communities know all too well that COVID-19 is exacerbating existing health inequities across the country; however, the high rate of vaccine uptake in many tribal communities, despite justifiable mistrust of medical and vaccine systems, reveals a story of hope and motivation to persevere despite pandemic outbreaks, discrimina-tion, and persistent inequities, and is a testament to the strength of AIAN commitment to the health and well-being of the present and future generations[30]; this is because the COVID-19 vaccines are not just about personal safety, but about protecting family, community, and elders, and ultimately protecting culture, ceremonies, language, and lifeways, for the present and future generations.[30]

Asian/Asian Americans

First-generation immigrant Asian and Asian Americans are a diverse nonmonolithic group, and yet the "Asian" category is only 1 of 5 race/ethnicity data collected by fed-eral agencies.[33] The 6 major subgroups (in the United States) are Chinese, Indian, Fili-pino, Vietnamese, Korean, and Japanese, but there is more ethnic diversity. For example, South Asian Americans include Afghani, Bangladeshi, Indian, Nepalese, Pakistani, and Sri Lankan ethnicities.[33] The Centers of Disease Control and Prevention and Kaiser Family Foundation COVID-19 vaccination data do not disaggregate Asian

Americans.[34,35] Lack of specific race determination among Asian Americans has led to inequitable resource allocation.[36] Case in point, South Philadelphia's Southeast Asian community did not have adequate supply of vaccine, and vaccination sites were not located within walking distance for older Southeast Asian adults.[36] Owing to language barriers, these older adults could not take public transportation to vaccination sites outside of South Philadelphia[36]; this is reflected in Kaiser Family Foundation COVID-19 vaccination data, which showed that only 33% of Asian Americans were vaccinated in Pennsylvania, and in South Dakota, only 10% of Asian Americans had been vaccinated by November 2021.[35] Diverse languages within Asian American populations may have hindered dissemination of information about vaccine safety and efficacy. Vietnamese Americans have the lowest rate of English proficiency, followed by Filipino and Korean Americans.[33] Information about COVID-19 vaccines needs to be translated into multiple languages beyond the 6 major subgroups identified as the dominant groups.

Perception that Asian Americans are compliant and would accept COVID-19 vaccination has not been entirely true. Survey studies found that Asian Americans had concerns about side effects, safety, and effectiveness of the COVID-19 vaccine, similar to African Americans and Hispanic/Latinos/as/x.[37,38] In Los Angeles's Chinatown, community health workers and community leaders diligently urged people to be vaccinated, especially the older adults.[4] Their effort was hindered as Asian Americans were targeted and assaulted, bearing the blame that COVID-19 infection originated from China.[33] Older Chinese Americans were beaten and harassed, whereas younger Asian Americans were denied services at stores or shunned at school or at work.[33,36] A disproportionate number of Asian American businesses closed during the early COVID pandemic, leading to food insecurity and difficulties accessing health care.[33] This racial discrimination is reminiscent of Japanese American internment camps during World War II, when Japanese Americans were suddenly treated as enemies and as a national security threat.[39] Throughout American history, Asian Americans have been treated as foreigners and outsiders, whereas European immigrants were generally more accepted in the American culture. The Chinese Exclusion Act of 1882 prohibited immigration of Chinese into the United States, and the National Origins Act of 1924 prevented Japanese immigration.[39] Despite racial violence, Asian American community leaders and neighborhood health center workers continue to reach out to their community and campaign for COVID-19 vaccinations. Owing to their efforts, Asian Americans in most states reached 50% to 80% fully vaccination rates by the beginning of November 2021.[35]

Black/African Americans

The current racial disparities[40] in infant and maternal mortality, pain management, poor patient provider relations, and many other examples, including COVID-19, trace back to race-based pseudoscience.[41] Throughout US history the relationship between medical science and the black body has often been precarious at best and horrifying at worst. Black people can easily point to the long history of experimentation on black bodies, the US Public Health Service Syphilis study at Tuskegee,[42] Henrietta Lacks,[43] and the list goes on. At the same time, it is effortless to identify invalidating, demeaning, and egregious behaviors experienced in medical encounters in the not-so-distant past and ongoing at present. These experiences have cemented the view of medical providers and the larger medical and research enterprise as being untrustworthy. The dominant discourse is that black people have mistrust and are vaccine hesitant, ignoring the more difficult discussions focused on institutional and individual provider efforts—or lack thereof—to build reputations of trustworthiness among black people and the larger black community.[44]

Decades of housing and economic discrimination (black codes, apprenticeship laws, antienticement measures, Jim Crow laws, sundown towns, restrictive covenants, redlining, government "projects," creation of "ghettos," gentrification, and so forth) have created precarious situations for many black communities. Black people are more likely to live in areas with high housing density, pollution, and food insecurity[45,46]; they are also more likely to be in employment circumstances that do not allow for work from home, and do not offer insurance, unpaid sick leave, or childcare.[47–49] For foreign-born black people in the United States, anti-immigrant sentiment and language access challenges are additional critical factors impacting disparities. Black people generally experience higher levels of police violence and criminalization.[50] Across the United States, these factors have resulted in increased risk of exposure to SARS-CoV-2. It is these unaddressed social and structural factors that have consistently placed black Americans at increased risk for infectious diseases and chronic disease. COVID-19 is the most recent in this long list of disease outcomes that disproportionately impact black people. As with other disease outcomes, black Americans are overrepresented in COVID-19 cases, hospitalizations, and deaths, experiencing the highest COVID death rate[51] of any racial group in the country.

Black Americans have also faced many challenges in their efforts to engage in preventative care, and these challenges contribute to the lagging rates of vaccination among black people. When testing and vaccines are available at large venues with increased police presence, this may increase discomfort and create barriers to access. Employment circumstances may prohibit taking time off without losing pay during vaccination timeframes. Access to technology may impair the ability to schedule appointments, and vaccination locations may require transportation and time, which may not be available. These factors and others contribute to the fact that African Americans and black people have low rates of COVID-19 vaccine uptake.[34]

Hispanic/Latino/a/x

Hispanic/Latino/a/x populations have historically experienced displacement, exploitation, discrimination, racism, and stigma. Furthermore, they have been used to test medical interventions without consent, affecting the health and quality of life of multiple generations across the United States and its territories.[52–54] As of 2020, Hispanic/Latino/a/x populations represented 18.7% of the US total population and account for more than half (51.1%) of the country's population growth.[55] Hispanic/Latinos/as/x are not a monolithic group. When described as an "ethnic group" in federally managed data, Hispanic/Latinos/as/x include any person of Cuban, Mexican, Puerto Rican, South or Central American, or other Spanish culture origin, regardless of race. Hispanic/Latino groups have transnational experiences that intersect with their lived experiences in the United States and their countries of origin.[56] The largest Hispanic/Latino/a/x group in the United States is Mexicans (61.4%), followed by Puerto Ricans (9.6%), and Central Americans (9.8%). Most Hispanic/Latinos/as/x (71.7%) speak a language other than English at home and have lower educational attainment and median household income when compared with non-Hispanic whites. Among all racial and ethnic groups within the United States, Hispanic/Latinos/as/x have the highest health uninsured rates. Furthermore, they are overrepresented within service occupations[57].

Since early in the COVID-19 pandemic, it was documented that Hispanic/Latino/a/x populations were overrepresented in the US morbidity and motality rates. With data from the first 3 months of the COVID-19 pandemic, it was already established that SARS-CoV-2 infections among Hispanic/Latinos/as/x were associated with being monolingual Spanish speakers, being employed, less social distancing, and preexisting chronic diseases. Similarly, COVID-19 deaths among Hispanic/Latinos/as/x were associated with household occupancy density, air pollution, and being employed.[58] Over the course of the pandemic, we have had ample evidence of these factors affecting multiple Hispanic/Latino/a/x groups with intersectional experiences.[16,59,60] Many have advocated to improve the systemic ability to capture specific data that could help point to root causes of these disparities and therefore improve COVID-19 prevention, testing, and care. For Hispanic/Latinos/as/x, the negative outcomes being experienced during the COVID-19 pandemic reflect historic experiences of living in places with high levels of pollution, working in high-risk occupations, experiencing housing instability, and interacting with a health care system and providers who are not culturally appropriate or accessible. As these structural issues have not been systematically addressed, the vaccine acceptability and completion rates reflect these challenges for these populations.[61,62] Being Hispanic/Latino/a/x, or of any other racial or ethnic group, is not an intrinsic risk factor for negative health outcomes. The cause of these inequities is the living conditions and general health inequities faced by these populations.

Native Hawaiian/Pacific Islanders

Native Hawaiians and other Pacific Islanders (NHOPI) comprise 0.2% of the US population and have been disproportionately impacted by COVID-19,[63] yet understanding disparities in incidence, mortality, and COVID-19 vaccination coverage within this group has been hindered by inadequacies in data reporting and disaggregation.[64] Identifying vulnerable populations by geography, ethnicity, age, and socioeconomic group is a requisite to deploying community-contextualized, culturally-specific COVID-19 mitigation strategies, which thus far remain insufficient. Although NH comprise approximately 60% of the NHOPI category (under the 20 US Code § 7517, the term "Native Hawaiian" means any individual who is a citizen of the United States and a descendant of the aboriginal people who, before 1778, occupied and exercised sovereignty in the area that now comprises the State of Hawaii. In 1997, the US Office of Management and Budget reclassified Native Hawaiians under the category of "Native Hawaiian or Other Pacific Islander." Although this recategorization resolved issues with data bias in their former category, Native Hawaiians remain aggregated along with Guamanians, Samoans, Carolinian, Fijian, Kosraean, Melanesian, Micronesian, Northern Mariana Islander, Palauan, Papua New Guinean, Ponapean [Pohnpelan], Polynesian, Solomon Islander, Tahitian, Tarawa Islander, Tokelauan, Tongan, Trukese [Chuukese], and Yapese),[65] Indigenous Pacific peoples are distinct, each with their own linguistic, cultural, and sociodemographic backgrounds; migration histories; and genetic origins.[66] Such heterogeneity may confound interpretation of aggregated NHOPI data and thereby hinder appropriate responses to address COVID-19-related health disparities.

NHOPIs have a history of encountering, and overcoming, infectious diseases introduced by foreign contact that have decimated these populations in their ancestral islands. The population of Native citizens of the Kingdom of Hawaii was decimated by imported infectious diseases before the US-aided overthrow of the Kingdom in 1893.[67] Immigrant laborers were then brought in to augment the depleted workforce, causing drastic socioeconomic changes, and relegating NH to a minority population within their own, previously sovereign nation.[68] The longstanding social inequities and health disparities currently faced by NHOPIs render these populations particularly vulnerable to increased rates of SARS-CoV-2 infection and severe COVID-19 disease.[69-71] In Hawaii, NHOPIs comprise 25% of the population, yet currently account for 38% of all COVID-19 cases,[72] demonstrating an intensification of prepandemic health disparities.[73,74]

Glaring gaps in vaccine coverage, historically derived sentiments of distrust in government, and the emergence of more infectious SARS-CoV-2 variants altogether fuel widening disparities even within the NHOPI population. Early into the pandemic (March to December 2020), NH and PIs accounted for 19% and 25% of all COVID-19 cases despite comprising 21% and 4% of Hawaii's population, respectively.[75] Yet with the emergence of the Delta and Omicron variants, NHs and PIs accounted for 29% and 8% of COVID-19 cases, respectively, over June to November 2021.[75] Despite widespread access to vaccines, recent vaccination data from the state indicate that whereas PIs are fairly represented at 4.5%, the vaccination rate among NHs remains underrepresented at 13.5%,[75] indicating vaccine hesitancy as a major contributor to the disproportionately higher rates of COVID-19 among NHs in Hawaii. A recent finding of a dual and opposing role of trust as a mediator of vaccine hesitancy[76] among NHOPIs offers insight into addressing this disparity.

Box 1
Recommendations for working with black, Indigenous and people of color communities to increase the uptake and acceptability of preventive interventions (eg, vaccines)

1. Interventions that foster trust

2. Interventions that increase health literacy

3. Equitable partnerships with communities

4. Appropriate data reporting and disaggregation by geography, ethnicity, sexual orientation, gender identity, age, and socioeconomic status

5. Improve data collection to adequately differentiate specific communities within Asian American and Hispanic/Latino/a/x populations to improve understanding of the impact and identify methods to equitably allocate resources

6. Address language barriers to disseminate information and provide services equally and enable ease in accessing public resources

7. Prevent racial violence

8. Develop and support structural changes such as policies and guidelines to address the social and structural determinants of health inequities

9. Interventions to address homophobia, transphobia, xenophobia, sexism, and anti-black racism at all levels in our societies

10. Restructure our civil systems to ensure we are fervently pursuing equity in all aspects of our societies

11. Improving safety nets for people living in poverty to reduce additional burdens (eg, missing workdays to complete paperwork, inability to subsist on single employment, affordable housing)

12. Provide comprehensive training to medical, nursing, health services, and public health students about bias, historic oppression, and trauma

13. Develop culturally appropriate tools and interventions to improve health care encounters

14. Provide resources to communities and populations to sustain effective grassroot interventions

15. Support community-based research that fosters collaborations between scientists and communities with common experience of vulnerability and marginalization.

DISCUSSION

Health is recognized as a human right, but not everyone enjoys the right to health equally. The COVID-19 pandemic has brought to the surface some of the many root causes of health inequities in the United States and globally. Public health is intrinsically political,[77] and although the historical inequities causing health disparities among racial and ethnic groups are evident, very few systemic actions are being taken toward an antiracist and anticolonial approach to health. Recently, the American Psychological Association acknowledged its failure and accepted responsibility for its role and the role of the discipline of psychology in contributing to systemic racism.[78] Acknowledgment, recognition, and apology are the first critical steps in addressing the inequities underlying health disparities. Actions taken by organizations and institutions to reconcile and repair the harm that has been perpetrated for more than a century are critical; this will require diversifying the health care workforce, addressing social determinants of health such as housing and employment, and efforts to actively reduce stigma, bias, and discrimination. There is much to be done.

In the absence of a proper political response to address the structural inequities experienced by marginalized populations during the COVID-19 pandemic, it is important to support grassroot initiatives and communities that are demonstrating effective responses to their population's needs. Experienced persons identifying with these priority populations should lead the services needed for these communities. Furthermore, there is a need to support BIPOC people conducting research and providing information to their communities. As racial equity is not the problem of only one group, collaboration and partnership should lead the next efforts to improve the health and livelihoods of all BIPOC and other minoritized populations.[79,80] We end this discussion with a table putting forth specific recommendations for working with BIPOC communities to increase the uptake and acceptability of interventions related to COVID-19 health promotion (**Box 1**).

CLINICS CARE POINTS

- Appropriate data reporting and disaggregation by geography, ethnicity, sexual orientation, gender identity, age, and socioeconomic status

- Develop and support structural changes such as policies and guidelines to address the social and structural determinants of health inequities

- Provide comprehensive training to medical, nursing, health services, and public health students about bias, historic oppression, and trauma

- Develop culturally appropriate tools and interventions to improve health care encounters

- Support community-based research that fosters collaborations between scientist and communities with common experience of vulnerability and marginalization.

DISCLOSURE

The authors have nothing to disclose.

REFERENCES

1. Tidyman P. A Sketch of the Most Remarkable Diseases of the Negroes of the Southern States, With an Account of the Method of Treating Them, Accompanied by Physiological Observations. Philadelphia J Med Phys Sci 1826;12(2):306–13.

2. Kendi IX. Stamped from the beginning: the Definitive history of racist Ideas in America. New York, NY: Nation Books; 2016.

3. Jaimes MA, Hu-DeHart E, Wunder D. The state of native America: genocide, colonization, and Resistance (race and Resistance). Boston, Massachusetts: South End Press; 1999.

4. Cavanagh EV L. The Routledge Handbook of the history of settler colonialism. London; New York: Routledge Handbooks; 2017.

5. Rowe AC, Tuck E. Settler Colonialism and Cultural Studies: Ongoing Settlement, Cultural Production, and Resistance. Cult Stud ↔ Crit Methodologies 2017; 17(1):3–13.

6. Saito NT. Settler colonialism, race, and the law: Why Strcutural racism Presists. New York: NYU Press; 2020.

7. Grills C, et al. ApplyingCulturalist Methodologies to Discern COVID-19's Impact on Communities of Color. J Community Psychol 10.1002/jcop.22802

8. The native population of the Americas in 1492. The University of Wisconsin Press; 1992.

9. Veracini L. Settler colonialism: a Theoretical Overview. New York: Palgrave Macmillan; 2010.

10. Glenn EN. Settler Colonialism as Structure: A Framework for Comparative Studies of U.S. Race and Gender Formation. Sociol Race Ethn 2015;1(1):52–72.

11. Talbott JH, Edwards HT, Dill DB, et al. Physiological Responses to High Environmental Temperature. The Am J Trop Med 1933;s1-13(4):381–97.

12. Mendez DD, Scott J, Adodoadji L, et al. Racism as Public Health Crisis: Assessment and Review of Municipal Declarations and Resolutions Across the United States. Front Public Health 2021;9:1142.

13. CDC. Racism and Health. Secondary Racism and Health. 2021. Available at: https://www.cdc.gov/healthequity/racism-disparities/index.html.

14. Came H, Griffith D. Tackling racism as a "wicked" public health problem: Enabling allies in anti-racism praxis. Soc Sci Med 2018;199:181–8.

15. Collins PH, Bilge S. *Intersectionality* Cambridge, UK. Medford, MA, USA.: Polity Press; 2020.

16. Harkness A, Weinstein ER, Atuluru P, et al. Let's Hook Up When the Pandemic is Over:" Latinx Sexual Minority Men's Sexual Behavior During COVID-19. J Sex Res 2021;58(8):951–7.

17. Harkness A, Weinstein ER, Atuluru P, et al. Latinx Sexual Minority Men's Access to HIV and Behavioral Health Services in South Florida During COVID-19: A Qualitative Study of Barriers, Facilitators, and Innovations. J Assoc Nurses AIDS Care 2021;33(1):9–21.

18. Salerno JP, Williams ND, Gattamorta KA. LGBTQ populations: Psychologically vulnerable communities in the COVID-19 pandemic. Psychol Trauma Theor Res Pract Policy 2020;12(S1):S239–42.

19. Campaign HR. The lives and livelihoods of many in the LGBTQ community are at risk amidst COVID-19 crisis, 2020.

20. Mitchell KJ, Ybarra ML, Banyard V, et al. Impact of the COVID-19 Pandemic on Perceptions of Health and Well-Being Among Sexual and Gender Minority Adolescents and Emerging Adults. LGBT Health 2021;9(1):34–42.

21. Wallach S, Garner A, Howell S, et al. Address Exacerbated Health Disparities and Risks to LGBTQ+ Individuals during COVID-19. Health Hum Rights 2020;22(2): 313–6.

22. Quinn KG, Walsh JL, John SA, et al. I Feel Almost as Though I've Lived This Before": Insights from Sexual and Gender Minority Men on Coping with COVID-19. AIDS Behav 2021;25(1):1–8.
23. Cahill S, Grasso C, Keuroghlian A, et al. Sexual and Gender Minority Health in the COVID-19 Pandemic: Why Data Collection and Combatting Discrimination Matter Now More Than Ever. Am J Public Health 2020;110(9):1360–1.
24. Millett GA. New pathogen, same disparities: why COVID-19 and HIV remain prevalent in U.S. communities of colour and implications for ending the HIV epidemic. J Int AIDS Soc 2020;22(11):e25639.
25. American Indians and Alaska Natives - By the Numbers - Fact Sheet In: HHS, ed.: U.S. Department of Health and Human Services | Administrationn for Children & Families, 2021. Available at: https://www.acf.hhs.gov/ana/fact-sheet/american-indians-and-alaska-natives-numbers.
26. Arrazola J, Masiello M, Joshi S, et al. COVID-19 Mortality Among American Indian and Alaska Native Persons — 14 States, January–June 2020. MMWR Morb Mortal Wkly Rep 2020;66(49):1853–6.
27. Williamson LL, Harwell TS, Koch TM, Anderson SL, et al. COVID-19 Incidence and Mortality Among American Indian/Alaska Native and White Persons — Montana, March 13–November 30, 2020. MMWR Morb Mortal Wkly Rep 2021;70(14).
28. CDC. COVID-19 Weekly Cases and Deaths per 100,000 Population by Age, Race/Ethnicity, and Sex. Secondary COVID-19 Weekly Cases and Deaths per 100,000 Population by Age, Race/Ethnicity, and Sex. 2022. Available at: https://covid.cdc.gov/covid-data-tracker/#demographicsovertime.
29. CDC. Risk for COVID-19 Infection, Hospitalization, and Death By Race/Ethnicity. Secondary Risk for COVID-19 Infection, Hospitalization, and Death By Race/Ethnicity 2021. Available at: https://www.cdc.gov/coronavirus/2019-ncov/covid-data/investigations-discovery/hospitalization-death-by-race-ethnicity.html.
30. Walters KL, Fryberg S, Eason AE, et al. National native American COVID-19 Alliance needs assessment Survey: Congressional Report.: the indigenous Wellness research Institute (IWRI) in partnership with the research for indigenous social action and equity center. RISE) report; 2021.
31. CDC. Disparities in COVID-19-Associated Hospitalizations | Racial and Ethnic Health Disparities. Secondary Disparities in COVID-19-Associated Hospitalizations | Racial and Ethnic Health Disparities 2021. Available at: https://www.cdc.gov/coronavirus/2019-ncov/community/health-equity/racial-ethnic-disparities/disparities-hospitalization.html.
32. UIHI. Data genocide of American Indians and Alaska Natives in COVID-19 data. Seattle, WA: Urban Indian Health Institute; 2021.
33. Chin MK, Đoàn LN, Chong SK, et al. Asian American subgroups and the COVID-19 experience: what We know and Still Don't know. Health Affairs Blog; 2021.
34. Demographic CDC. Characteristics of People Receiving COVID-19 Vaccinations in the United States. Secondary Demographic Characteristics of People Receiving COVID-19 Vaccinations in the United States November 14, 2021 2021. Available at: https://covid.cdc.gov/covid-data-tracker/#vaccination-demographic.
35. Ndugga NH, Latoya, Artiga Samantha, et al. Latest Data on COVID-19 Vaccinations by Race/Ethnicity. Secondary Latest Data on COVID-19 Vaccinations by Race/Ethnicity November, 03, 2021 2021. Available at: https://www.kff.org/coronavirus-covid-19/issue-brief/latest-data-on-covid-19-vaccinations-by-race-ethnicity/.

36. Wang C. Asian Americans have high vaccine rates, but it hasn't come easy, nonprofit groups say. NBC News 2021;2021.
37. Ta Park V, Dougan M, Meyer O, et al. Differences in COVID-19 Vaccine Concerns Among Asian Americans and Pacific Islanders: The COMPASS Survey. J Racial Ethn Health Disparities 2021;1–13.
38. Momplaisir FM, Kuter BJ, Ghadimi F, et al. Racial/Ethnic Differences in COVID-19 Vaccine Hesitancy Among Health Care Workers in 2 Large Academic Hospitals. JAMA Netw Open 2021;2574–3805 (Electronic)).
39. Takaki R. *Strangers from A different Shore* Boston. Toronto: London Littel Brown & Co; 1989.
40. 2021, National Healthcare Quality and Disparities Report. Secondary 2021 National Healthcare Quality and Disparities Report 2022. https://www.ahrq.gov/research/findings/nhqrdr/nhqdr21/index.html.
41. Horsman R. Race and Manifest Destiny: the origins of American racial Anglo-Saxonism. Cambridge, MA: Harvard University Press; 1981.
42. Vonderlehr RA, Clark T, Wenger OC, et al. Untreated Syphilis in the Male Negro, Journal of Venereal Disease Information. J Venereal Dis Inf 1936;(17):260–5.
43. Skloot R. The Immortal life of Henrietta lacks. New York, NY: Crown Publishing Group; 2010.
44. Warren RC, Forrow L, Hodge DA, et al. Trustworthiness before Trust — Covid-19 Vaccine Trials and the Black Community. N Engl J Med 2020;383(22):e121.
45. Odoms-Young A. Examining the Impact of Structural Racism on Food Insecurity: Implications for Addressing Racial/Ethnic Disparities. Fam Community Health 2018;41 S3–S6.
46. Bower KM, Thorpe RJ Jr, Rohde C, et al. The Intersection of Neighborhood Racial Segregation, Poverty, and Urbanicity and its Impact on Food Store Availability in the United States. Prev Med 2014;58:33–9.
47. Do DP, Frank R. Unequal burdens: assessing the determinants of elevated COVID-19 case and death rates in New York City's racial/ethnic minority neighbourhoods. J Epidemiol Community Health 2021;75(4):321.
48. Millett GA, Jones AT, Benkeser D, et al. Assessing differential impacts of COVID-19 on black communities. Ann Epidemiol 2020;47:37–44.
49. Poteat T, Millett GA, Nelson LE, et al. Understanding COVID-19 risks and vulnerabilities among black communities in America: the lethal force of syndemics. Ann Epidemiol 2020;47:1–3.
50. Alexander M. The New Jim Crow: mass incarceration in the age of color blindness. New York: United States The New Press; 2010.
51. CDC. Data Tracker Home. Secondary Data Tracker Home 2021. Available at: https://covid.cdc.gov/covid-data-tracker/?CDC_AA_refVal=https%3A%2F%2Fwww.cdc.gov%2Fcoronavirus%2F2019-ncov%2Fcases-updat.
52. Muñoz-Laboy M, Guidry JA, Kreisberg A. Internalised stigma as durable social determinant of HIV care for transnational patients of Puerto Rican ancestry. Glob Public Health 2021;1–20.
53. Cacari-Stone L, Avila M. Rethinking Research Ethics for Latinos: The Policy Paradox of Health Reform and the Role of Social Justice. Ethics Behav 2012; 22(6):445–60.
54. Uperesa FA, Garriga Lopez AM. Contested sovereignties: Puerto Rico and American Samoa. . Sovereign Acts: Contesting colonialism across indigenous nations and Latinx America. Tuscon, AZ, USA: University of Arizona Press; 2017.
55. Jones NM, Rachel S, Ramirez Roberto, et al. Improved Race and Ethnicity Measures Reveal U.S. Population Is Much More Multiracial. Secondary Improved

Race and Ethnicity Measures Reveal U.S. Population Is Much More Multiracial 2021. Available at: https://www.census.gov/library/stories/2021/08/improved-race-ethnicity-measures-reveal-united-states-population-much-more-multiracial.html.

56. Sauceda JA, Brooks RA, Xavier J, et al. From Theory to Application: A Description of Transnationalism in Culturally-Appropriate HIV Interventions of Outreach, Access, and Retention Among Latino/a Populations. J Immigr Minor Health 2019; 21(2):332–45.

57. HHS. Profile: Hispanic/Latino Americans. Secondary Profile: Hispanic/Latino Americans. 2021. https://minorityhealth.hhs.gov/omh/browse.aspx?lvl=3&lvlid=64.

58. Rodriguez-Diaz CE, Guilamo-Ramos V, Mena L, et al. Risk for COVID-19 infection and death among Latinos in the United States: examining heterogeneity in transmission dynamics. Ann Epidemiol 2020;52:46–53.e2.

59. Vilar-Compte M, Gaitán-Rossi P, Félix-Beltrán L, et al. Pre-COVID-19 Social Determinants of Health Among Mexican Migrants in Los Angeles and New York City and Their Increased Vulnerability to Unfavorable Health Outcomes During the COVID-19 Pandemic. J Immigr Minor Health 2021;1–13.

60. Melgoza E, Beltrán-Sánchez H, Bustamante AV. Emergency Medical Service Use Among Latinos Aged 50 and Older in California Counties, Except Los Angeles, During the Early COVID-19 Pandemic Period. Front Public Health 2021;9:660289.

61. Melin K, Zhang C, Zapata JP, et al. Factors Associated with Intention to Receive Vaccination against COVID-19 in Puerto Rico: An Online Survey of Adults. Int J Environ Res Public Health 2021;18(15).

62. Siegel M, Critchfield-Jain I, Boykin M, et al. Racial/Ethnic Disparities in State-Level COVID-19 Vaccination Rates and Their Association with Structural Racism. J Racial Ethn Health Disparities 2021;1–14.

63. Raine S, Liu A, Mintz J, et al. Racial and Ethnic Disparities in COVID-19 Outcomes: Social Determination of Health. Int J Environ Res Public Health 2020; 17(21):8115.

64. Wang D, Gee GC, Bahiru E, et al. Asian-Americans and Pacific Islanders in COVID-19: Emerging Disparities Amid Discrimination. J Gen Intern Med 2020; 35(12):3685–8. https://doi.org/10.1007/s11606-020-06264-5 [published Online First: Epub Date]].

65. Congress US. 20 U.S. Code § 7517 - Definitions, 2015. Available at: https://www.law.cornell.edu/uscode/text/20/7517.

66. Sun H, Lin M, Russell EM, et al. The impact of global and local Polynesian genetic ancestry on complex traits in Native Hawaiians. Plos Genet 2021;17(2):e1009273. https://doi.org/10.1371/journal.pgen.1009273 [published Online First: Epub Date]].

67. 107 STAT. 1510. Public Law 103-150. 103d Congress. Joint Resolution. Secondary 107 STAT. 1510. Public Law 103-150. 103d Congress. Joint Resolution 1993. Available at: https://www.govinfo.gov/content/pkg/STATUTE-107/pdf/STATUTE-107-Pg1510.pdf#page=1.

68. La Croix S. Hawai'i: Eight Hundred Years of political and economic change. University of Chicago Press; 2019.

69. Kaholokula JK, Samoa RA, Miyamoto RES, et al. COVID-19 Special Column: COVID-19 Hits Native Hawaiian and Pacific Islander Communities the Hardest. Hawaii J Health Soc Welf 2020;79(5):144–6.

70. Palafox NA, Best BR, Hixon A, et al. Viewpoint: Pacific Voyages - Ships - Pacific Communities: A Framework for COVID-19 Prevention and Control. Hawaii J Health Soc Welf 2020;79(6 Suppl 2):120–3.

71. Penaia CS, Morey BN, Thomas KB, et al. Disparities in Native Hawaiian and Pacific Islander COVID-19 Mortality: A Community-Driven Data Response. Am J Public Health 2021;111:S49–52.

72. Kaiser Family Foundation. Secondary Kaiser Family Foundation. Available at: https://www.kff.org/coronavirus-covid-19/issue-brief/latest-data-on-covid-19-vaccinations-by-race-ethnicity/.

73. Mau MK, Sinclair K, Saito EP, et al. Cardiometabolic health disparities in native Hawaiians and other Pacific Islanders. Epidemiol Rev 2009;31:113–29.

74. Mokuau N, DeLeon PH, Kaholokula JKA, et al. Challenges and promise of health equity for Native Hawaiians. NAM Perspectives; 2016.

75. Hawaii State Department of Health. Secondary Hawaii State Department of Health. https://health.hawaii.gov/coronavirusdisease2019/current-situation-in-hawaii.

76. COVID-19 PAA. About Pacific Alliance Against COVID-19 | A Community-Driven Approach to Mitigate COVID-19 Disparities in Hawaii's Vulnerable Populations. Secondary About Pacific Alliance Against COVID-19 | A Community-Driven Approach to Mitigate COVID-19 Disparities in Hawaii's Vulnerable Populations 2021. https://www.paac.info/about.

77. Rodríguez-Díaz CE. Health is political: Advocacy and Mobilization for Latinx health. New and emerging issues in Latinx health. Springer International Publishing; 2019. p. 349–61.

78. APA. Apology to People of Color for APA's Role in Promoting Perpetuating, and Failing to Challenge Racism, Racial Discrimination, and Human Hierarchy in U.S. Secondary Apology to People of Color for APA's Role in Promoting Perpetuating, and Failing to Challenge Racism, Racial Discrimination, and Human Hierarchy in U.S. 2021. Available at: https://www.apa.org/about/policy/racism-apology.

79. Andrasik MP, Broder GB, Wallace SE, et al. Increasing Black, Indigenous and People of Color participation in clinical trials through community engagement and recruitment goal establishment. PloS one 2021;16(10):e0258858.

80. Quinn SC, Andrasik MP. Addressing Vaccine Hesitancy in BIPOC Communities — Toward Trustworthiness, Partnership, and Reciprocity. N Engl J Med 2021; 385(2):97–100.

Infection Prevention and Control of Severe Acute Respiratory Syndrome Coronavirus 2 in Health Care Settings

Marisa L. Winkler, MD, PhD[a,b,c,]*, David C. Hooper, MD[a,b,c],
Erica S. Shenoy, MD, PhD[a,b,c]

KEYWORDS

- SARS-CoV-2 • COVID-19 • Infection prevention and control • Hierarchy of controls
- Standard precautions • Transmission-based precautions

KEY POINTS

- Adherence to the Hierarchy of Controls can mitigate the risk of transmission of infectious diseases.
- Nosocomial COVID-19 transmission events often involve multiple lapses in implementation of infection prevention and control.
- Implementation of the Hierarchy of Controls is likely to evolve over the course of the pandemic.

BACKGROUND

Coronaviruses have been known to infect both humans and animals, and most identified human coronaviruses cause mild seasonal respiratory tract infections.[1] Before the current COVID-19 pandemic caused by the severe acute respiratory syndrome coronavirus 2 (SARS-CoV-2), the outbreaks of severe acute respiratory syndrome coronavirus in 2003 to 2004 and of middle east respiratory syndrome coronavirus in 2012 raised concerns regarding the public health implications of coronaviruses emerging from animals to infect humans.[2,3]

[a] Infection Control Unit, Massachusetts General Hospital, 55 Fruit Street, Bulfinch 334, Boston, MA 02114, USA; [b] Division of Infectious Diseases, Massachusetts General Hospital, 55 Fruit Street, Boston, MA, 02114, USA; [c] Harvard Medical School, 25 Shattuck Street, Boston, MA, 02115, USA
* Corresponding author. Massachusetts General Hospital, 55 Fruit Street, Bulfinch 334, Boston, MA, 02114
E-mail address: mlwinkler@partners.org

Infect Dis Clin N Am 36 (2022) 309–326
https://doi.org/10.1016/j.idc.2022.01.001   id.theclinics.com
0891-5520/22/© 2022 Elsevier Inc. All rights reserved.

This article reviews the chain of transmission of infectious agents, including SARS-CoV-2, recommended infection prevention and control (IPC) practices to mitigate the risk of transmission of SARS-CoV-2 in health care settings, including implementation of the Hierarchy of Controls and evaluation and management of potential nosocomial transmission events, and summarizes lessons learned from transmission events in health care settings.

TRANSMISSION OF INFECTIOUS AGENTS

The chain of transmission of an infectious agent is a cycle comprising multiple parts (**Fig. 1**), and including 3 main requirements: a reservoir of infectious agent, a mode of transmission, and a susceptible host.[4] Reservoirs include humans, animals, and inanimate objects. The infectious agent exits the reservoir and is transmitted by direct or indirect contact (ie, fomite), droplet, or airborne transmission, or a combination of modes. A susceptible host with a portal of entry through which the infectious agent can enter at an inoculum sufficient to result in infection is required to complete the chain of transmission. This involves a complicated interplay of host factors, including vaccination status and response to vaccination for vaccine-preventable diseases,

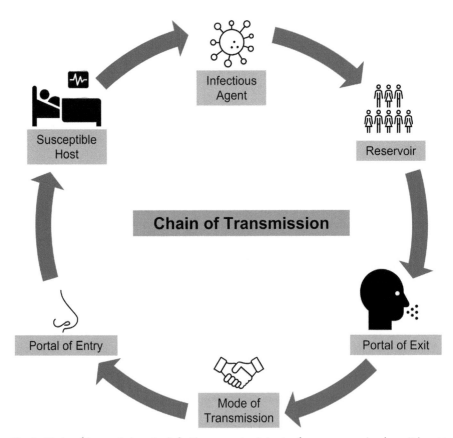

Fig. 1. Chain of transmission: An infectious agent originates from a reservoir where it leaves by a portal of exit, then through a mode of transmission uses a portal of entry in a susceptible host to start a new cycle of infection.

history of prior infection, genetic makeup, and predisposing or immunocompromising conditions.[5,6] One important concept of the chain of transmission is that if any single link in the chain is broken, transmission can be prevented. Interventions within IPC are aimed at multiple links in the chain, providing redundancy, which increases the likelihood of interrupting transmission.

Individuals infected with SARS-CoV-2 can transmit infection while asymptomatic, presymptomatic, and symptomatic. The highest risk of transmission occurs early in infection, before symptom development and within the first 5 days of symptoms, when viral load is highest.[7] Most of the transmission is thought to occur through either deposition of droplet particles on mucous membrane surfaces or inhalation of particles, both in close proximity to the source. Fomite transmission is possible, although not thought to represent a major transmission risk.[8] Despite the ability to culture SARS-CoV-2 from surfaces, the viral particles are easily inactivated by heat or various disinfectants.[9] Proximity of both space and time is a key factor in transmission risk.[9,10] This risk has been demonstrated in studies assessing secondary attack rates, with households reported to have the highest risk, ranging from 17% to 53%.[11–13]

PREVENTION OF TRANSMISSION IN HEALTH CARE SETTINGS: IMPLEMENTATION OF THE HIERARCHY OF CONTROLS

Prevention of transmission in health care settings is focused on breaking links in the chain of transmission, using a layered mitigation approach, often described as the Hierarchy of Controls. This framework was developed by the National Institute of Occupational Safety and Health (NIOSH) to describe interventions to improve workplace safety by reducing workplace hazard risk.[14,15] This framework has been applied to a variety of workplace settings, including health care, during the pandemic to prevent risk of exposure to SARS-CoV-2 (ie, the "hazard"), to health care providers (HCP), patients, and visitors. The framework includes elimination, substitution, engineering controls, administrative controls, and use of personal protective equipment (PPE), in descending order (**Fig. 2**).[14] Generally, interventions at the top of the pyramid are thought to be most effective, and implementation of each level of the pyramid leads to progressively safer environments.

ELIMINATION

During the COVID-19 pandemic, several elimination strategies have been implemented to reduce risk of transmission, including visitor restrictions and use of telemedicine and telework.[16,17] At peak periods of the pandemic, nonessential and elective procedures were canceled, and routine visits were postponed, reducing density in the workplace and clinical areas and also helping manage the volume of patients related to the surge of COVID-related illness. With the first Emergency Use Authorization of COVID-19 vaccines in December 2020, vaccination was added as an elimination strategy. Many employers, including health care facilities, have made employee vaccination for COVID-19 a condition of employment, an approach that has been supported by multiple professional societies and organizations.[18–20] As variants of SARS-CoV-2 evolve, the need for booster vaccinations is likely to be reevaluated, and the definition of full vaccination may change.

Some elimination strategies, notably visitor restrictions, have been associated with negative impacts on patient, HCP, and family well-being in terms of social isolation, reduced quality of life, emotional distress, and difficulty with end-of-life care and have been reconsidered since the initial phase of the pandemic.[21,22] Before the COVID-19 pandemic, studies showed that allowance of visitors did not increase risk

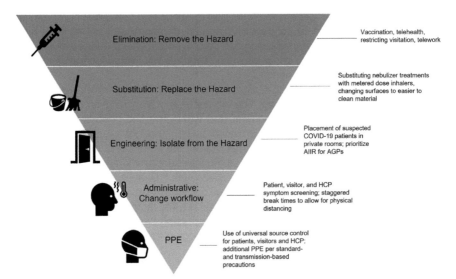

Fig. 2. Following this Hierarchy of Controls normally leads to the implementation of inherently safer systems, where the risk of illness or injury has been substantially reduced. (*Adapted from* Centers for Disease Control and National Institute for Occupational Safety, The National Institute for Occupational Safety and Health (NIOSH): Hierarchy of Controls. Accessed 9/8/2021, https://www.cdc.gov/niosh/topics/hierarchy/default.html)

of infection but did reduce frequency of delirium and anxiety-related symptoms in patients and family satisfaction.[23] The postponement of routine or emergency medical care has led to delayed diagnoses of malignancies and avoidable and ongoing excess morbidity and mortality.[24–26] Although telemedicine can improve access to medical services, it has been found to be less accessible to patients with certain social determinant factors, such as lower income, lower education level, and public insurance.[27,28]

SUBSTITUTION

An example of substitution or replacement of a hazard was a change of nebulizers to metered inhalers, which do not aerosolize secretions and therefore reduce the risk of SARS-CoV-2 transmission.[29,30] Replacing work surfaces with materials that are easier to clean and disinfect is also performed.[31]

ENGINEERING CONTROLS

A variety of engineering controls have been recommended to decrease the risk of SARS-CoV-2 transmission in health care settings. Placement of patients with suspected or confirmed COVID-19, or confirmed exposure during the quarantine period, should be in a standard patient room with the door closed; this room should have a private bathroom.[32] Airborne infection isolation rooms ("negative pressure") are reserved for patients in whom aerosol-generating procedures (AGPs) are anticipated or planned.[32] Patients with confirmed COVID-19 can be grouped together. Appropriate ventilation, filtration, and pressurization of patient care spaces as required by the Facilities Guidelines Institute and public health authorities are essential to prevent infection, reduce contamination, and decrease the number of infectious particles through a combination of air exchanges, occupancy, and cycling time between patient use.[33,34] Eating spaces that allow increased distance between persons were also designed to decrease transmission between employees in the setting of face mask removal.[35]

Administrative Controls

Administrative controls that require changes in workflows constitute a major component of the Hierarchy of Controls. These controls can be some of the most challenging to implement because of their impact on health care operations. Symptom and exposure screening of all HCP, patients, and visitors is recommended. In one study, a sensitivity of 83% was found if at least 2 symptoms of fever, cough, anosmia, dyspnea, oxygen saturation less than 93%, or headache were reported among patients presenting to the emergency department between April and July of 2020.[36] Temperature checks are not a reliable screening tool, as only 19.4% of patients with active COVID-19 infection by polymerase chain reaction (PCR)-based testing platform had a fever $\geq 38°C$.[36,37] Other workflow modifications include bundling of clinical tasks to reduce room entry and exit in caring for patients exposed to or with suspected or confirmed COVID-19, enhanced training for clinicians in correct donning and doffing of PPE, and supporting physical distancing when source control (ie, face masks) are removed during break and mealtimes by scheduling staff in a staggered fashion.[35,38,39] An observational study found that restructuring computer workstations, workrooms, break rooms, use of clear cognitive aids, adjusting shift times, and using virtual conferencing are successful in encouraging physical distancing in health care facilities.[35]

Symptom and exposure screening will fail to identify all infected patients, and thus in addition to testing of all symptomatic and exposed patients for COVID-19, asymptomatic testing has been used in specific situations to further reduce the risk of transmission in health care facilities from an occultly infected patient. For patients admitted to facilities or undergoing AGPs, preadmission and preprocedural testing to identify asymptomatic infected individuals has been implemented.[40] Some institutions have instituted surveillance testing at intervals to identify individuals who test negative at admission but may be in the incubation period.[40] In health care facilities with congregate living arrangements as well as behavioral health treatment facilities where physical distancing and compliance with source control may be suboptimal, more frequent asymptomatic screening may be used particularly in the setting of high community prevalence.[40] The conversion rate from negative to positive with serial testing of inpatients was 1% to 1.9% in 2 studies.[41,42] Specific screening strategies are expected to change over time, based on a combination of factors, including community prevalence and vaccination within the specific community and patient population.

High rates of presenteeism (HCP working while sick) have been documented with symptom monitoring and remains a challenge.[43] Early reports during the COVID-19 pandemic found that 64.6% of infected HCP came to work after developing symptoms.[44] Use of a passive symptom screening tool found that 82% of those who screened positive had not been planning to stay home from work.[43]

HCP should similarly be evaluated if they develop symptoms consistent with COVID-19 or have a confirmed exposure. The role of routine testing of asymptomatic HCP has not been demonstrated to be necessary to support IPC when strategies are in place to limit risk of transmission. Several studies have demonstrated the prevalence of asymptomatic infection in HCP to be less than 1% in 2020.[45] Mass testing of asymptomatic HCP in 1 facility found 15 asymptomatic HCP who tested positive out of 13,703 total tests, with a much lower prevalence of positive results compared with the community.[46] Current Centers for Disease Control and Prevention (CDC) guidance states that testing with either a PCR- or antigen-based test should be performed in the setting of symptoms and can be considered in asymptomatic HCP if community risk and transmission levels are high.[40] As with testing strategies for patients, strategies applied to HCP are expected to change over time, based on the same factors of community prevalence and vaccination among HCP and the community.

PERSONAL PROTECTIVE EQUIPMENT

The final component of the Hierarchy of Controls is the use of PPE. Although correct and consistent use of PPE is a cornerstone of HCP and patient safety, it appears at the bottom of the pyramid, as it is susceptible to human error and requires compliance.[15] In the setting of the COVID-19 pandemic, universal source control (ie, use of a face mask for HCP, patients, and visitors) has been implemented and associated with reduced risk of transmission.[47–51] In addition, use of eye protection (ie, face shields or goggles) is recommended for use by HCP in all clinical encounters during periods of substantial to high community transmission as a barrier to prevent direct mucous membrane inoculation and contamination of the eyes by hands.[52] Patients with suspected or confirmed COVID-19, or confirmed exposures to COVID-19 in the quarantine period, are managed in health care settings using Standard and Transmission-based precautions.[32,53] For these patients, the recommended PPE by the CDC includes an NIOSH-approved fit-tested N95 filtering facepiece respirator or higher, eye protection (face shield or goggles), gown, and gloves. Personal glasses are not considered to be sufficient protective eyewear.[54] Both the CDC and World Health Organization (WHO) state that in the setting of N95 respirator shortages, face masks can be used for patient care outside of AGPs.[55]

The CDC definition of AGP includes suctioning of airways, sputum induction, cardiopulmonary resuscitation, endotracheal intubation and extubation, noninvasive ventilation, bronchoscopy, manual ventilation, nebulizer administration, high-flow oxygen delivery, or procedures involving areas of higher viral load, such as nose and throat, oropharynx, or respiratory tract.[32,56] WHO definition of AGP includes tracheal intubation, noninvasive ventilation, tracheostomy, cardiopulmonary resuscitation, manual ventilation, bronchoscopy, sputum induction using nebulized hypertonic saline, dentistry, and autopsy procedures.[57,58] The definition of an AGP has evolved during the pandemic, and analysis has found that the patient characteristics, such as severe illness with high viral load and significant symptoms, sustained exposure by HCP to the patient, and procedures with close proximity to the respiratory tract are more significant factors leading to transmission events.[59]

Practice in use of face masks or N95 respirators for care of patients with suspected or confirmed COVID-19 or confirmed exposures outside of AGPs has varied; in 1 survey of Veterans Administration facilities, 63% used N95 respirators in all patients with suspected or confirmed COVID-19.[60] A meta-analysis of randomized trials did not find a statistical difference in the risk of acquiring a respiratory infection when wearing a surgical mask or an N95 respirator.[61]

Early in the COVID-19 pandemic, owing to disruption in the supply chain of PPE, crisis and contingency standards of care were implemented under guidance from public health authorities.[62,63] Reuse of PPE, defined as donning for a patient contact then doffing and storing for use with another patient, and extended use, defined as wearing PPE for a prolonged period, including multiple patient contacts before removing and discarding, were used for items that under conventional standards are single use.[62] The implementation of extended use and reuse raises challenges related to the potential for cross- and self-contamination as well as concerns for decrements in filtration efficiency and fit over multiple uses of N95 respirators.[64,65] Supplies have improved over the course of the pandemic, and many health care settings have returned to conventional standards in the use of PPE.[66] The impact of extended use and reuse on effectiveness of PPE has been assessed without failure over up to 12 reuses,[67] but concerns have been raised regarding failure with higher numbers of reuse.[67–69] There is also concern regarding contamination of PPE over multiple uses even in the setting of proper handling technique.[65] Simulation training to increase the understanding of infection control practices in the setting of donning or doffing PPE, resuscitation, airway management, and transportation was performed in some hospitals.[70–72] Some facilities have provided just-in-time education with observed donning and doffing to improve HCP practice.[70]

EVALUATION AND MANAGEMENT OF HEALTH CARE PROVIDER INFECTIONS AND EXPOSURES

Infections in HCP risk spread to other HCP, patients, and visitors. Contact tracing of HCP with infections is important to determine, when possible, the likely source of infection, if breaches in correct practices may have contributed, and to identify potentially exposed HCP, patients, and others. Studies have shown that most HCP infections are attributable to community exposures and not related to occupational exposure, particularly in the setting of appropriate IPC procedures.[73]

Duration of isolation for infected HCP and duration of quarantine for exposed HCP continue to evolve. HCP who are moderately to severely immunocompromised or with severe illness may require either longer duration of isolation when infected or a test-based approach to clearance with consultation with both local infectious disease and occupational health experts.

Exposure definitions in health care differ in important ways with respect to mitigating risk of exposure through use of PPE. In health care settings, exposures that qualify based on duration (cumulative 15 minutes of direct contact) and proximity (within 6 feet) can be mitigated by use of PPE.[74] In the setting of an AGP, if proper PPE is not worn, then an exposure is considered to have occurred regardless of the duration of interaction. The CDC framework for managing HCP exposures is detailed, including vaccination status, postexposure testing, level of staffing, and restrictions from work. Lack of eye protection has been associated with COVID-19 infection following occupational exposure.[52,75,76] Despite implementation of multiple infection prevention interventions, transmission in health care settings has been observed, although it is low in the setting of adherence to IPC methods.[77]

HCP are expected to report community exposures to their occupational health departments to determine the testing protocol and work restriction, and frequently household exposures are managed in a similar manner as high-risk occupational exposures.[74]

TRANSMISSION IN HEALTH CARE SETTINGS AND LESSONS LEARNED

The potential routes of transmission in health care settings include patient-to-HCP, patient-to-patient, HCP-to-HCP, HCP-to-patient, visitor-to-patient, and visitor-to-HCP. Examples of each are discussed later and described in **Table 1**. For the most part, the published exposure and transmission events described occurred before widespread vaccination of HCP and the general public. Transmission has, however, been noted in health care settings in the postvaccination period. Common themes

Table 1
Documented health care facility severe acute respiratory syndrome coronavirus 2 outbreaks, actions attributed to the spread of infection, and facility response to contain infections

Outbreak Setting	Number of Infected People	Attributable Actions	Response to Infection	Citation
Long-term care facilities, skilled nursing facilities, or nursing homes				
Skilled nursing facility	16 HCP, 5 residents	Presenteeism	Closure to new admissions, limited ancillary services, contact tracing, symptom screening, serial respiratory surveys, whole genome sequencing to characterize spread, isolate staff with close contact with confirmed cases, restrict movement between units, uniform masking, use of recommended PPE (isolation gown, N95 respirator, gloves, and eye protection with face shield or reusable goggles) for interactions in units with cases, training for donning and doffing, hand hygiene, and cleaning	93
Ambulatory (including emergency department)				
Emergency department	2 clusters, one with 3 HCP, one with 2 HCP	Close interactions among coworkers without source control	Reinforced uniform masking, increased space between computer workstations, encouraged social distancing and avoiding shared meals	88
Inpatient				
Inpatient stroke ward	14 HCP and 10 patients	Patients moving through ward unmasked, close contact	Increased PPE, quarantined exposed patients, decreased	94

Setting	HCP involved	Contributing factors	Interventions	
Academic cancer center	3 clusters, first with 8 HCP, second with 4 HCP, third with 2 HCP	Presenteeism required between patients and staff, decreased compliance with hand hygiene	Reinforcement of symptom reporting, enhanced cleaning, reinforcement and monitoring of masking, break room closed and gathering prohibited, isolation of all positive HCP, testing of all asymptomatic employees in same area; break room capacity, increased random PPE and cleaning assessments, HCP offered testing	89
Inpatient medical ward	3 HCP	Undiagnosed patient receiving AGPs without appropriate precautions	Early testing and isolation of patients with possible COVID-19, use of eye protection, gowns, N95 respirators, or powered air-purifying respirators in the setting of AGPs	79
Inpatient psychiatry unit	5 HCP and 5 patients	Community-exposed patient with minimal symptoms admitted to double room, slow uptake of PPE by staff, patient behaviors limited appropriate PPE use, physical distancing difficult given need for group sessions and meals, limited testing capacity early in pandemic	Closed to new admissions, universal PPE, observed hand hygiene before meals and group therapy, restricted visitors, staff and patient symptom screening, limited number of patients in shared spaces by staggered group mealtimes, increased cleaning frequency	80
OR staff	24 HCP	Presenteeism, using communal spaces, including break rooms, without appropriate IC practices, other nonoccupational high-risk exposure	Increased cleaning, rapid screening of asymptomatic HCP, reeducation regarding masking, limiting capacity in communal areas, quarantine if symptomatic	95

(continued on next page)

Table 1
(continued)

Outbreak Setting	Number of Infected People	Attributable Actions	Response to Infection	Citation
Integrated health care system	14 (not separated between HCP and patients)	Presenteeism, transport of infectious patients between facilities, no universal masking or use of PPE, no available in-house testing, patients not under isolation while testing pending, shared rooms, variable symptom screening	Implemented universal source control, symptom screening at facility entrance, empiric precautions until test results if patients screen positive for symptoms, restricted visitors, altered testing algorithm, testing all new admissions	81
Acute care hospital	38 HCP, 14 patients	Symptomatic patient with false-negative serial testing receiving AGPs, shared rooms, infectious patients moved several times, positive pressure in index patient room, lack of eye protection among staff, interaction among unmasked staff in nonclinical areas	Mobilized incident command for cluster response, increased testing capacity, serial testing of all patients and exposed staff, preemptive enhanced respiratory isolation for all patients on involved units, positive patients moved to dedicated unit, enhanced cleaning of affected units, occupational health interviews of all positive staff, air changes and airflow patterns assessed	75

Abbreviations: ERI, enhanced respiratory isolation; HCP, healthcare provider; PPE, personal protective equipment; AGP, aerosol-generating procedure, OR, operating room; IC, infection control.

from nosocomial transmission events include HCP presenteeism, lack of compliance with IPC measures including appropriate use of PPE, and unrecognized asymptomatic, presymptomatic, or symptomatic infection in patients who subsequently undergo high-risk activities, such as AGPs.

Despite symptom screening of patients and the use of testing to identify asymptomatic infection, patients who are incubating infection on admission and are missed by such strategies, or patients who acquire infection from another source (roommate, HCP, visitor) during the course of an admission while not isolated, can result in exposures to HCP and other patients.[75,78–81] In one outbreak in an acute care hospital, tracing by epidemiology and genomic sequencing found late-onset infection following admission of the index patient who spread COVID-19 to both other patients and HCP.[75] The initial exposure event was attributed to a symptomatic patient who tested negative for SARS-CoV-2 on 2 serial nasopharyngeal swabs upon admission with subsequent AGPs performed. At the time of the cluster, universal source control with face masks was in place for all HCP and eye protection for all interactions with patients. In response to this cluster, implementation of serial admission screening as well as repeat screening before AGPs was implemented. Studies show an attack rate of 0% to 4.7% for hospital exposures versus 15.2% for community exposures, supporting the efficacy of layered infection control approaches to reduce risk of transmission, including universal source control.[82–84]

Patient-to-patient transmission in the setting of roommates in semiprivate accommodations in health care facilities has been directly studied.[85,86] In one report over 7 months at an acute care hospital, there were 31 exposed patient roommates, 39% of whom ultimately tested positive for SARS-CoV-2.[85] The beds were 5 feet apart side by side and 7 feet apart mid-pillow to mid-pillow with a closed curtain between them. Exposed patients who subsequently became infected were more likely to have roommates with cycle thresholds ≤ 21 by PCR-based testing. A separate study found a secondary attack rate for hospitalized roommates of 18.9% overall and 35.7% in the setting of AGPs.[86] The attack rate in these scenarios mirrors that observed in household settings.[11–13,87] Infections among patients have also been observed in inpatient psychiatric units where it is difficult to promote mask wearing, distancing, and hand hygiene, and group activities are instrumental to treatment.[80] Strategies to reduce the risk of patient-to-patient transmission include serial testing at regular intervals during hospitalization and rapid isolation with positive testing or development of symptoms.

Multiple descriptions of transmission events between HCP resulting in clusters of infections have been reported in the literature. Often the initial source is attributed to community acquisition with subsequent occupational spread in break rooms or other settings where masks are removed and where distance is not maintained. Presenteeism has been featured in several published accounts.[43,44,88,89] Since the widespread adoption of vaccination against SARS-CoV-2, in areas with minimal community transmission, current CDC guidance permits fully vaccinated HCP to be nonmasked and nondistanced for dining or socializing in areas restricted from patient access.[32] However, as evidence of postvaccination infection increases, guidelines regarding this are also evolving.[90,91]

Exposures from infected HCP to patients resulting in transmission appear to be uncommon, especially in the era of universal masking in health care facilities. A study evaluating transmission from infected HCP to patients found 2 transmission events, one where neither the HCP nor patient was wearing a mask and one where the patient was not wearing a mask but also had a household exposure.[92]

Visitors to health care facilities are screened for symptoms and exposure and are required to wear face masks. Transmission from infected visitors is not thought to be common, although can occur, usually in the setting of lack of masking between visitors and the patients they are visiting. One transmission event from a presymptomatic infected spouse visiting daily to a patient infected on hospital day 15 was reported.[42]

In most nosocomial clusters, there may be multiple events arising from a single index source, before recognition of the transmission events and implementation of additional control measures as appropriate.

SUMMARY

IPC approaches to prevention of SARS-CoV-2 transmission in health care settings are grounded in understanding the chain of transmission and implementation of the Hierarchy of Controls. As community prevalence of SARS-CoV-2 waxes and wanes, duration and protection from vaccines continue to be assessed, and effective and accessible therapies and prophylaxis options emerge, the relative importance of various components of mitigation strategies will change. This will mean that public health recommendations and health care facilities strategies will continue to evolve.

CLINICS CARE POINTS

- Transmission of infectious agents in health care settings can be interrupted through application of the Hierarchy of Controls.

- The Hierarchy of Controls involves elimination, substitution, engineering controls, administrative controls, and use of personal protective equipment; implementation of multiple strategies reduces the risk of transmission.

- Observed transmission events in health care settings often involve multiple lapses in control measures, including health care personnel presenteeism, lack of compliance with infection prevention and control measures, and unrecognized infections in patients.

ACKNOWLEDGMENTS

The authors thank Noah Feder for assistance with figure preparation. We would also like to thank Massachusetts General Hospital for support of the Infection Prevention, Healthcare Epidemiology, and Antimicrobial Stewardship training track.

DISCLOSURE

None.

REFERENCES

1. V'Kovski P, Kratzel A, Steiner S, et al. Coronavirus biology and replication: implications for SARS-CoV-2. Nat Rev Microbiol 2021;19(3):155–70.
2. Cui J, Li F, Shi ZL. Origin and evolution of pathogenic coronaviruses. Nat Rev Microbiol 2019;17(3):181–92.
3. Hu B, Guo H, Zhou P, et al. Characteristics of SARS-CoV-2 and COVID-19. Nat Rev Microbiol 2021;19(3):141–54.
4. Dicker RC, Coronado F, Koo D, et al. Principles of epidemiology in public health practice, 3rd edition. An introduction to applied epidemiology and biostatistics, lesson 1: introduction to epidemiology. Section 10: CHAIN OF INfection. Available

at: https://www.cdc.gov/csels/dsepd/ss1978/lesson1/section10.html. Accessed October 25, 2021.

5. Fricke-Galindo I, Falfan-Valencia R. Genetics Insight for COVID-19 susceptibility and severity: a review. Front Immunol 2021;12:622176.

6. Liu X, Zhou H, Zhou Y, et al. Risk factors associated with disease severity and length of hospital stay in COVID-19 patients. J Infect 2020;81(1):e95–7.

7. Delta variant: what we know about the science. Available at: https://www.cdc.gov/coronavirus/2019-ncov/variants/delta-variant.html. Accessed September 6, 2021.

8. Science brief: SARS-CoV-2 and surface (fomite) transmission for indoor community environments. Available at: https://www.cdc.gov/coronavirus/2019-ncov/more/science-and-research/surface-transmission.html. Accessed October 18, 2021.

9. Meyerowitz EA, Richterman A, Gandhi RT, et al. Transmission of SARS-CoV-2: a review of viral, host, and environmental factors. Ann Intern Med 2021;174(1): 69–79.

10. Transmission of SARS-CoV-2: implications for infection prevention precautions. Available at: https://www.who.int/news-room/commentaries/detail/transmission-of-sars-cov-2-implications-for-infection-prevention-precautions. Accessed September 6, 2021.

11. Martinez DA, Klein EY, Parent C, et al. Latino household transmission of SARS-CoV-2. Clin Infect Dis 2021. https://doi.org/10.1093/cid/ciab753.

12. Musa S, Kissling E, Valenciano M, et al. Household transmission of SARS-CoV-2: a prospective observational study in Bosnia and Herzegovina, August - December 2020. Int J Infect Dis 2021. https://doi.org/10.1016/j.ijid.2021.09.063.

13. Grijalva CG, Rolfes MA, Zhu Y, et al. Transmission of SARS-COV-2 Infections in Households - Tennessee and Wisconsin, April-September 2020. MMWR Morb Mortal Wkly Rep 2020;69(44):1631–4.

14. The National Institute for Occupational Safety and Health (NIOSH): hierarchy of controls. Available at: https://www.cdc.gov/niosh/topics/hierarchy/default.html. Accessed September 8, 2021.

15. Kraus A, Awoniyi O, AlMalki Y, et al. Practical solutions for healthcare worker protection during the COVID-19 pandemic response in the ambulatory, emergency, and inpatient settings. J Occup Environ Med 2020;62(11):e616–24.

16. Using telehealth to expand access to essential health services during the COVID-19 pandemic. Available at: https://www.cdc.gov/coronavirus/2019-ncov/hcp/telehealth.html. Accessed September 17, 2021.

17. Bashshur R, Doarn CR, Frenk JM, et al. Telemedicine and the COVID-19 pandemic, lessons for the future. Telemed J E Health 2020;26(5):571–3.

18. Weber DJ, Al-Tawfiq JA, Babcock HM, et al. Multisociety statement on coronavirus disease 2019 (COVID-19) vaccination as a condition of employment for healthcare personnel. Infect Control Hosp Epidemiol 2021;1–9. https://doi.org/10.1017/ice.2021.322.

19. Joint statement in support of COVID-19 vaccine mandates for all workers in health and long-term care. Available at: https://www.acponline.org/acp_policy/statements/joint_statement_covid_vaccine_mandate_2021.pdf. Accessed October 16, 2021.

20. AHA Policy Statement on mandatory COVID-19 vaccination of health care personnel. Available at: https://www.aha.org/public-comments/2021-07-21-aha-policy-statement-mandatory-covid-19-vaccination-health-care. Accessed October 16, 2021.

21. Wendlandt B, Kime M, Carson S. The impact of family visitor restrictions on healthcare workers in the ICU during the COVID-19 pandemic. Intensive Crit Care Nurs 2021;103123. https://doi.org/10.1016/j.iccn.2021.103123.

22. Hindmarch W, McGhan G, Flemons K, et al. COVID-19 and long-term care: the essential role of family caregivers. Can Geriatr J 2021;24(3):195–9.

23. Nassar Junior AP, Besen B, Robinson CC, et al. Flexible versus restrictive visiting policies in ICUs: a systematic review and meta-analysis. Crit Care Med 2018; 46(7):1175–80.

24. Excess deaths associated with COVID-19. Available at: https://www.cdc.gov/nchs/nvss/vsrr/covid19/excess_deaths.htm. Accessed September 17, 2021.

25. Czeisler ME, Marynak K, Clarke KEN, et al. Delay or avoidance of medical care because of COVID-19-related concerns - United States, June 2020. MMWR Morb Mortal Wkly Rep 2020;69(36):1250–7.

26. Woolf SH, Chapman DA, Sabo RT, et al. Excess deaths from COVID-19 and other causes in the US, March 1, 2020, to January 2, 2021. JAMA 2021. https://doi.org/10.1001/jama.2021.5199.

27. Luo J, Tong L, Crotty BH, et al. Telemedicine adoption during the COVID-19 pandemic: gaps and inequalities. Appl Clin Inform Aug 2021;12(4):836–44.

28. Sun R, Blayney DW, Hernandez-Boussard T. Health management via telemedicine: learning from the COVID-19 experience. J Am Med Inform Assoc 2021. https://doi.org/10.1093/jamia/ocab145.

29. Amirav I, Newhouse MT. COVID-19: time to embrace MDI+ valved-holding chambers. J Allergy Clin Immunol 2020;146(2):331.

30. Sethi S, Barjaktarevic IZ, Tashkin DP. The use of nebulized pharmacotherapies during the COVID-19 pandemic. Ther Adv Respir Dis 2020;14. https://doi.org/10.1177/1753466620954366. 1753466620954366.

31. Background E. Environmental services. Available at: https://www.cdc.gov/infectioncontrol/guidelines/environmental/background/services.html. Accessed October 29, 2021.

32. Interim infection prevention and control recommendations for healthcare personnel during the coronavirus disease 2019 (COVID-19) pandemic. Available at: https://www.cdc.gov/coronavirus/2019-ncov/hcp/infection-control-recommendations.html. Accessed October 19, 2021.

33. Heating, ventilation, and air conditioning systems in health-care facilities. Available at: https://www.cdc.gov/infectioncontrol/guidelines/environmental/background/air.html#c3. Accessed October 16, 2021.

34. Filtration/disinfection. Available at: https://www.ashrae.org/technical-resources/filtration-disinfection#mechanical. Accessed October 16, 2021.

35. Keller SC, Pau S, Salinas AB, et al. Barriers to physical distancing among health-care workers on an academic hospital unit during the coronavirus disease 2019 (COVID-19) pandemic. Infect Control Hosp Epidemiol 2021;1–7. https://doi.org/10.1017/ice.2021.154.

36. Romero-Gameros CA, Colin-Martinez T, Waizel-Haiat S, et al. Diagnostic accuracy of symptoms as a diagnostic tool for SARS-CoV 2 infection: a cross-sectional study in a cohort of 2,173 patients. BMC Infect Dis 2021;21(1):255.

37. Vilke GM, Brennan JJ, Cronin AO, et al. Clinical features of patients with COVID-19: is temperature screening useful? J Emerg Med 2020;59(6):952–6.

38. Amer HA, Alowidah IA, Bugtai C, et al. Challenges to infection control team during COVID-19 pandemic in a quaternary medical center in Saudi Arabia. Infect Control Hosp Epidemiol 2021;1–20. https://doi.org/10.1017/ice.2021.72.

39. Zhang H, Dimitrov D, Simpson L, et al. A web-based, mobile-responsive application to screen health care workers for COVID-19 symptoms: rapid design, deployment, and usage. JMIR Form Res 2020;4(10):e19533.

40. Overview of testing for SARS-CoV-2 (COVID-19). Available at: https://www.cdc.gov/coronavirus/2019-ncov/hcp/testing-overview.html. Accessed October 19, 2021.

41. Kobayashi T, Trannel A, Holley SA, et al. COVID-19 serial testing among hospitalized patients in a midwest tertiary medical center, July-September 2020. Clin Infect Dis 2020. https://doi.org/10.1093/cid/ciaa1630.

42. Rhee C, Baker M, Vaidya V, et al. Incidence of nosocomial COVID-19 in patients hospitalized at a large US academic medical center. JAMA Netw Open 2020; 3(9):e2020498.

43. Lichtman A, Greenblatt E, Malenfant J, et al. Universal symptom monitoring to address presenteeism in healthcare workers. Am J Infect Control 2021;49(8): 1021–3.

44. Chow EJ, Schwartz NG, Tobolowsky FA, et al. Symptom screening at illness onset of health care personnel with SARS-CoV-2 infection in King County, Washington. JAMA 2020;323(20):2087–9.

45. Chow A, Htun HL, Kyaw WM, et al. Asymptomatic health-care worker screening during the COVID-19 pandemic. Lancet 2020;396(10260):1393–4.

46. Roberts SC, Peaper DR, Thorne CD, et al. Mass severe acute respiratory coronavirus 2 (SARS-CoV-2) testing of asymptomatic healthcare personnel. Infect Control Hosp Epidemiol 2021;42(5):625–6.

47. Klompas M, Morris CA, Sinclair J, et al. Universal masking in hospitals in the Covid-19 era. N Engl J Med 2020;382(21):e63.

48. Leung NHL, Chu DKW, Shiu EYC, et al. Respiratory virus shedding in exhaled breath and efficacy of face masks. Nat Med 2020;26(5):676–80.

49. Walker J, Fleece ME, Griffin RL, et al. Decreasing high-risk exposures for healthcare workers through universal masking and universal SARS-CoV-2 testing upon entry to a tertiary care facility. Clin Infect Dis 2020. https://doi.org/10.1093/cid/ciaa1358.

50. Wang X, Ferro EG, Zhou G, et al. Association between universal masking in a health care system and SARS-CoV-2 positivity among health care workers. JAMA 2020;324(7):703–4.

51. Seidelman JL, Lewis SS, Advani SD, et al. Universal masking is an effective strategy to flatten the severe acute respiratory coronavirus virus 2 (SARS-CoV-2) healthcare worker epidemiologic curve. Infect Control Hosp Epidemiol 2020; 41(12):1466–7.

52. Chu DK, Akl EA, Duda S, et al. Physical distancing, face masks, and eye protection to prevent person-to-person transmission of SARS-CoV-2 and COVID-19: a systematic review and meta-analysis. Lancet 2020;395(10242):1973–87.

53. Core infection prevention and control practices for safe healthcare delivery in all settings –recommendations of the HICPAC. Available at: https://www.cdc.gov/hicpac/recommendations/core-practices.html. Accessed September 17, 2021.

54. The National Institute for Occupational Safety and Health (NIOSH): eye safety. Available at: https://www.cdc.gov/niosh/topics/eye/eye-infectious.html. Accessed October 10, 2021.

55. Mask use in the context of COVID-19. Available at: https://apps.who.int/iris/bitstream/handle/10665/337199/WHO-2019-nCov-IPC_Masks-2020.5-eng.pdf?sequence=1&isAllowed=y. Accessed October 14, 2021.

56. Tran K, Cimon K, Severn M, et al. Aerosol generating procedures and risk of transmission of acute respiratory infections to healthcare workers: a systematic review. PLoS One 2012;7(4):e35797.

57. Mask use in the context of COVID-19. Available at: https://www.who.int/ publications/i/item/advice-on-the-use-of-masks-in-the-community-during-home-care-and-in-healthcare-settings-in-the-context-of-the-novel-coronavirus-(2019-ncov)-outbreak. Accessed October 22, 2021.

58. Mask use in the context of COVID-19. Available at: https://www.who.int/ publications/i/item/advice-on-the-use-of-masks-in-the-community-during-home-care-and-in-healthcare-settings-in-the-context-of-the-novel-coronavirus-(2019-ncov)-outbreak. Accessed October 29, 2021.

59. Klompas M, Baker M, Rhee C. What is an aerosol-generating procedure? JAMA Surg 2021;156(2):113–4.

60. McCormick WL, Koster MP, Sood GN, et al. Level of respiratory protection for healthcare workers caring for coronavirus disease 2019 (COVID-19) patients: a survey of hospital epidemiologists. Infect Control Hosp Epidemiol 2021;1–2. https://doi.org/10.1017/ice.2021.74.

61. Barycka K, Szarpak L, Filipiak KJ, et al. Comparative effectiveness of N95 respirators and surgical/face masks in preventing airborne infections in the era of SARS-CoV2 pandemic: a meta-analysis of randomized trials. PLoS One 2020; 15(12):e0242901.

62. Implementing Filtering Facepiece Respirator (FFR) reuse, including reuse after decontamination, when there are known shortages of N95 respirators. Available at: https://www.cdc.gov/coronavirus/2019-ncov/hcp/ppe-strategy/ decontamination-reuse-respirators.html. Accessed September 17, 2021.

63. Fisher EM, Shaffer RE. Considerations for recommending extended use and limited reuse of filtering facepiece respirators in health care settings. J Occup Environ Hyg 2014;11(8):D115–28.

64. Peters A, Palomo R, Ney H, et al. The COVID-19 pandemic and N95 masks: reusability and decontamination methods. Antimicrob Resist Infect Control 2021; 10(1):83.

65. Li DF, Alhmidi H, Scott JG, et al. A simulation study to evaluate contamination during reuse of N95 respirators and effectiveness of interventions to reduce contamination. Infect Control Hosp Epidemiol 2021;1–6. https://doi.org/10.1017/ice. 2021.218.

66. FDA recommends transition from use of decontaminated disposable respirators - letter to health care personnel and facilities. Available at: https://www.fda.gov/ medical-devices/letters-health-care-providers/fda-recommends-transition-use-decontaminated-disposable-respirators-letter-health-care-personnel-and. Accessed September 17, 2021.

67. Fabre V, Cosgrove SE, Hsu YJ, et al. N95 filtering face piece respirators remain effective after extensive reuse during the coronavirus disease 2019 (COVID-19) pandemic. Infect Control Hosp Epidemiol 2021;42(7):896–9.

68. Degesys NF, Wang RC, Kwan E, et al. Correlation between N95 extended use and reuse and fit failure in an emergency department. JAMA 2020;324(1):94–6.

69. Bergman MS, Viscusi DJ, Zhuang Z, et al. Impact of multiple consecutive donnings on filtering facepiece respirator fit. Am J Infect Control 2012;40(4):375–80.

70. Cheng VC, Wong SC, Tong DW, et al. Multipronged infection control strategy to achieve zero nosocomial coronavirus disease 2019 (COVID-19) cases among Hong Kong healthcare workers in the first 300 days of the pandemic. Infect Control Hosp Epidemiol 2021;1–10. https://doi.org/10.1017/ice.2021.119.

71. COVID-19 simulation exercises packages. Available at: https://www.who.int/
emergencies/diseases/novel-coronavirus-2019/training. Accessed September
17, 2021.

72. Pan D, Rajwani K. Implementation of simulation training during the COVID-19
pandemic: a New York Hospital experience. Simul Healthc 2021;16(1):46–51.

73. Team CC-R. Characteristics of health care personnel with COVID-19 - United
States, February 12-April 9, 2020. MMWR Morb Mortal Wkly Rep 2020;69(15):
477–81.

74. Interim guidance for managing healthcare personnel with SARS-CoV-2 infection
or exposure to SARS-CoV-2. Available at: https://www.cdc.gov/coronavirus/
2019-ncov/hcp/guidance-risk-assesment-hcp.html. Accessed January 2, 2022.

75. Klompas M, Baker MA, Rhee C, et al. A SARS-CoV-2 cluster in an acute care hospital. Ann Intern Med 2021;174(6):794–802.

76. Shah VP, Breeher LE, Hainy CM, et al. Evaluation of healthcare personnel exposures to patients with severe acute respiratory coronavirus virus 2 (SARS-CoV-2)
associated with personal protective equipment. Infect Control Hosp Epidemiol
2021;1–5. https://doi.org/10.1017/ice.2021.219.

77. Habermann EB, Tande AJ, Pollock BD, et al. Providing safe care for patients in
the coronavirus disease 2019 (COVID-19) era: a case series evaluating risk for
hospital-associated COVID-19. Infect Control Hosp Epidemiol 2021;1–7. https://
doi.org/10.1017/ice.2021.38.

78. Saidel-Odes L, Nesher L, Nativ R, et al. An outbreak of coronavirus disease 2019
(COVID-19) in hematology staff via airborne transmission. Infect Control Hosp
Epidemiol 2021;1–2. https://doi.org/10.1017/ice.2020.1431.

79. Heinzerling A, Stuckey MJ, Scheuer T, et al. Transmission of COVID-19 to health
care personnel during exposures to a hospitalized patient - Solano County, California, February 2020. MMWR Morb Mortal Wkly Rep 2020;69(15):472–6.

80. McGloin JM, Asokaraj N, Feeser B, et al. Coronavirus disease 2019 (COVID-19)
outbreak on an inpatient psychiatry unit: Mitigation and prevention. Infect Control
Hosp Epidemiol 2021;1–2. https://doi.org/10.1017/ice.2021.233.

81. Thompson ER, Williams FS, Giacin PA, et al. Universal masking to control
healthcare-associated transmission of severe acute respiratory coronavirus virus
2 (SARS-CoV-2). Infect Control Hosp Epidemiol 2021;1–7. https://doi.org/10.
1017/ice.2021.127.

82. Ng K, Poon BH, Kiat Puar TH, et al. COVID-19 and the risk to health care workers:
a case report. Ann Intern Med 2020;172(11):766–7.

83. Baker MA, Rhee C, Fiumara K, et al. COVID-19 infections among HCWs exposed
to a patient with a delayed diagnosis of COVID-19. Infect Control Hosp Epidemiol
2020;41(9):1075–6.

84. Howell A, Havens L, Swinford W, et al. PPE effectiveness - yes, the buck and virus
can stop here. Infect Control Hosp Epidemiol 2021;1–3. https://doi.org/10.1017/
ice.2021.75.

85. Karan A, Klompas M, Tucker R, et al. The risk of SARS-CoV-2 transmission from
patients with undiagnosed Covid-19 to roommates in a large academic medical
center. Clin Infect Dis 2021. https://doi.org/10.1093/cid/ciab564.

86. Chow K, Aslam A, McClure T, et al. Risk of healthcare-associated transmission of
SARS-CoV-2 in hospitalized cancer patients. Clin Infect Dis 2021. https://doi.org/
10.1093/cid/ciab670.

87. Lindstrom JC, Engebretsen S, Kristoffersen AB, et al. Increased transmissibility of
the alpha SARS-CoV-2 variant: evidence from contact tracing data in Oslo,

January to February 2021. Infect Dis (Lond) 2021;1–6. https://doi.org/10.1080/23744235.2021.1977382.

88. Chan ER, Jones LD, Redmond SN, et al. Use of whole-genome sequencing to investigate a cluster of severe acute respiratory syndrome coronavirus 2 (SARS-CoV-2) infections in emergency department personnel. Infect Control Hosp Epidemiol 2021;1–3. https://doi.org/10.1017/ice.2021.208.

89. Ariza-Heredia EJ, Frenzel E, Cantu S, et al. Surveillance and identification of clusters of healthcare workers with coronavirus disease 2019 (COVID-19): multidimensional interventions at a comprehensive cancer center. Infect Control Hosp Epidemiol 2021;42(7):797–802.

90. Britton A, Jacobs Slifka KM, Edens C, et al. Effectiveness of the Pfizer-BioNTech COVID-19 vaccine among residents of two skilled nursing facilities experiencing COVID-19 outbreaks - Connecticut, December 2020-February 2021. MMWR Morb Mortal Wkly Rep 2021;70(11):396–401.

91. Teran RA, Walblay KA, Shane EL, et al. Postvaccination SARS-CoV-2 infections among skilled nursing facility residents and staff members - Chicago, Illinois, December 2020-March 2021. MMWR Morb Mortal Wkly Rep 2021;70(17):632–8.

92. Baker MA, Fiumara K, Rhee C, et al. Low risk of COVID-19 among patients exposed to infected healthcare workers. Clin Infect Dis 2020. https://doi.org/10.1093/cid/ciaa1269.

93. Karmarkar EN, Blanco I, Amornkul PN, et al. Timely intervention and control of a novel coronavirus (COVID-19) outbreak at a large skilled nursing facility-San Francisco, California, 2020. Infect Control Hosp Epidemiol 2020;1–8. https://doi.org/10.1017/ice.2020.1375.

94. Lesho EP, Walsh EE, Gutowski J, et al. A cluster-control approach to a coronavirus disease 2019 (COVID-19) outbreak on a stroke ward with infection control considerations for dementia and vascular units. Infect Control Hosp Epidemiol 2021;1–7. https://doi.org/10.1017/ice.2020.1437.

95. McDougal AN, Elhassani D, DeMaet MA, et al. Outbreak of coronavirus disease 2019 (COVID-19) among operating room staff of a tertiary referral center: an epidemiologic and environmental investigation. Infect Control Hosp Epidemiol 2021;1–7. https://doi.org/10.1017/ice.2021.116.

Laboratory Diagnosis for SARS-CoV-2 Infection

Bianca B. Christensen, MD, MPH[a], Marwan M. Azar, MD, FAST, FIDSA[b],
Sarah E. Turbett, MD[a,c,*]

KEYWORDS

- SARS-CoV-2 diagnostics • COVID-19 • Nucleic acid amplification testing • Serology
- Antigen testing

KEY POINTS

- Understanding performance characteristics, advantages, limitations, and best clinical uses of SARS-CoV-2 diagnostic assays is important when interpreting test results for clinical management, infection control purposes, and public health decision making.
- Nucleic acid amplification testing (NAAT) such as reverse-transcriptase polymerase chain reaction remains the gold standard for diagnosis of acute SARS-CoV-2 infection.
- Antigen tests can be used to diagnose acute infection in symptomatic individuals when NAAT is unavailable or not easily accessible; testing should be performed within 3 to 7 days of symptom onset to maximize sensitivity. Antigen tests can be used to screen for COVID-19 infection in high-risk congregate or community settings to identify infected individuals quickly to prevent ongoing transmission.
- Antigen tests have the potential for use as a marker of transmissibility in individuals with COVID-19 infection (especially when positive), but the performance of current assays suffers from significant interassay and interuser variability; more data are needed to establish their use in this regard.
- Serologic testing is best used when identifying individuals with prior or late COVID-19 infection and in the diagnosis of multisystem inflammatory syndrome.

INTRODUCTION

Diagnostic testing for SARS-CoV-2 continues to be a critical component of the pandemic response. Numerous SARS-CoV-2 tests that provide rapid, accurate, and reliable results at various stages of COVID-19 infection are now available. Having a clear understanding of test characteristics, advantages, limitations, and best clinical

[a] Department of Pathology, Massachusetts General Hospital, 55 Fruit Street, Boston, MA 02114, USA; [b] Department of Infectious Diseases, Yale School of Medicine, 135 College Street, New Haven, CT 06510, USA; [c] Department of Medicine, Massachusetts General Hospital, 55 Fruit Street, Boston, MA 02114, USA
* Corresponding author. Department of Medicine, Massachusetts General Hospital, 55 Fruit Street, GRB-526, Boston, MA 02114.
E-mail address: turbett.sarah@MGH.harvard.edu

Infect Dis Clin N Am 36 (2022) 327–347
https://doi.org/10.1016/j.idc.2022.02.002   **id.theclinics.com**
0891-5520/22/© 2022 Elsevier Inc. All rights reserved.

uses is critical when interpreting test results for clinical management, infection control purposes, and public health decision making. Here, we provide an overview of SARS-CoV-2 diagnostic testing with a focus on assay types that are commonly used in the clinical setting. Test characteristics and "best use" scenarios are described.

Virological Biomarkers During the Course of COVID-19 Infection

The natural history of COVID-19 infection consists of an acute phase, which can range from asymptomatic to severe illness, followed by a convalescent period that can range from weeks to months. Throughout these phases, specific virological and immunologic biomarkers appear at different time points; these markers serve as targets for diagnostic testing in infected individuals (**Fig. 1**). SARS-CoV-2 RNA is the first viral marker identified in persons with infection, with detectable levels present in the respiratory tract shortly preceding or around the time of symptom onset.[1] RNA concentrations peak during the first week of symptoms, then decline in levels during the next 2 to 3 weeks.[2] However, viral RNA can persist at detectable levels for months despite clinical infection resolution, particularly in immunosuppressed individuals.[3,4] Similarly, SARS-CoV-2 viral antigens also become detectable in the respiratory tract around the time of symptom onset in those who become symptomatic; however, antigen levels decrease faster compared with viral RNA, with a decline in levels approximately 1 week after symptoms.[5] Viral dynamics are generally similar among asymptomatic persons with SARS-CoV-2 infection, although the time to RNA and antigen clearance tends to be shorter. Due to these characteristics, the detection of viral RNA (via molecular-based testing) and/or antigens in respiratory samples serve as markers of acute infection in symptomatic and asymptomatic individuals.

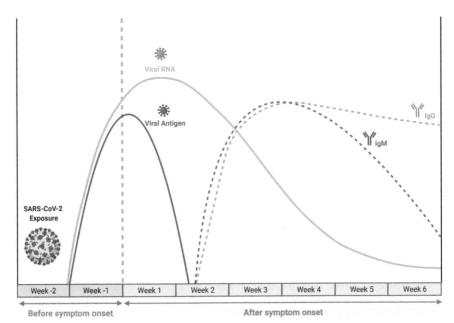

Fig. 1. Timing of virological and immunologic biomarkers during COVID-19 infection. (*Adapted from* "time course of COVID-19 infection and Test positivity", by BioRender.com (2021). Retrieved from https://app.biorender.com/biorender-templates.)

In contrast, SARS-CoV-2 immunoglobulins are not reliably detectable until 2 or more weeks after symptom onset at which time both IgM and IgG isotypes appear at approximately the same time interval.[6] IgM antibodies begin to decline by 2 months postsymptom onset, whereas IgG antibodies persist beyond that time frame.[6] Based on these characteristics, detectable antibodies are indicators of recent or past SARS-COV-2 infection and are of limited value during acute infection.

Common Molecular, Antigen, and Antibody Targets

SARS-CoV-2 is an enveloped single-stranded RNA virus within the *Coronaviridae* family.[76] The genome contains open reading frames (ORFs) that encode both nonstructural and structural proteins (**Fig. 2**). Key structural proteins include spike (S), envelope (E), membrane (M), and nucleocapsid (N), which play roles in viral entry or assembly (**Fig. 3**).[2] Molecular-based tests often target regions of the genome that encode ORF1ab (including RNA-dependent RNA polymerase [RdRp]), S, E, M, and N proteins; common antigen and antibody targets include the N and S proteins.

Molecular-Based Testing

Overview
Molecular diagnostics is the analysis of genetic material and the products they encode in an effort to identify disease-causing sequences or microbes. One type of molecular diagnostic testing, nucleic acid amplification testing (NAAT), is used for the detection of SARS-CoV-2 RNA, most commonly from upper respiratory tract samples and is the reference method for COVID-19 diagnosis in both symptomatic and asymptomatic individuals, particularly during acute infection.

SARS-CoV-2 nucleic acid amplification testing methodologies
The most common NAAT method used for SARS-CoV-2 identification is reverse-transcriptase polymerase chain reaction (RT-PCR). SARS-CoV-2 RNA extracted from an individual sample is reverse transcribed using reverse transcriptase into complementary DNA (cDNA), which is then denatured by heat to create 2 single-stranded pieces of DNA.[7,8] Using the original strands as templates, DNA polymerase synthesizes cDNA, resulting in the duplication of the original DNA. The cycle of denaturing and synthesizing continues for 30 to 45 cycles, depending on the assay, amplifying any target genes present in the sample. The number of cycles necessary to produce the predetermined detectable level of viral genes is called the cycle or crossing threshold (Ct; **Fig. 4**).[7,8] Ct values are semiquantitative and inversely proportional to the level of viral RNA present in a sample.

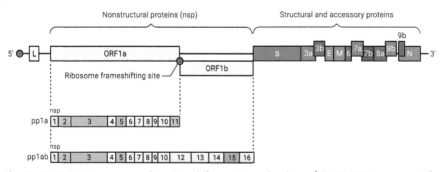

Fig. 2. SARS-CoV-2 genome. (*Reprinted from* "Organization of SARS-COV genome", by BioRender.com (2021). Retrieved from https://app.biorender.com/biorender-templates.)

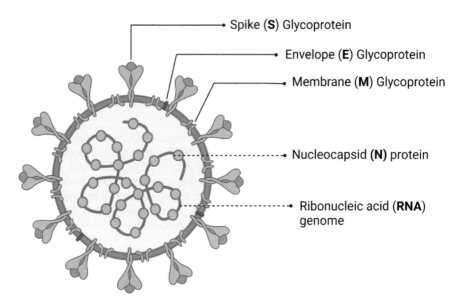

Fig. 3. SARS-CoV-2 structure. (*Adapted from* "human coronavirus Structure", by BioRender. com (2021). Retrieved from https://app.biorender.com/biorender-templates.)

In addition to RT-PCR, isothermal nucleic acid amplification (NAA), including loop-mediated or transcription-mediated amplification, is a common alternative method used by clinical laboratories for SARS-CoV-2 nucleic acid detection. Isothermal NAA achieves enzymatic amplification at a constant temperature, as opposed to PCR where temperature cycling is required. Isothermal NAA therefore eliminates the need for thermal cyclers for high-temperature DNA denaturation, decreasing the device footprint and making technology more amenable to bench-top, point-of-care (POC) testing.

SARS-CoV-2 target genes vary between assays and include the RdRp ORF1ab, E, N, S, and M genes (see **Fig. 2**).[7,9–11] Importantly, the E gene is not specific to SARS-CoV-2 and may result in cross-reactivity with other Sarbecoviruses, including SARS-CoV-1.[10] Because of the potential for cross-reactivity and for genetic reassortment in any individual gene target, most assays use at least two targets to maximize test performance.

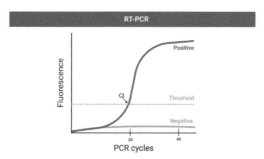

Fig. 4. RT-PCR. (*Adapted from* "COVID-19 diagnostic Test through RT-PCR", by BioRender. com (2021). Retrieved from https://app.biorender.com/biorender-templates.)

An indeterminate result occurs when only one of the two (or more) gene targets detected by NAAT is identified.[9] This scenario may occur when the amount of genetic material in the specimen is low such as in cases of early or late infection, poor specimen collection, or cross-contamination. Repeat testing may be helpful to confirm the result, although these results can be considered presumptively positive.[9] In contrast, an inconclusive result occurs when repeat testing fails to determine the presence or absence of viral RNA.

Molecular testing approaches
Although the mechanism of detecting SARS-CoV-2 viral RNA is the same, RT-PCR and other NAAT-based assays differ in a variety of ways including (1) the testing protocol (one vs two steps), (2) testing prioritization (rapid vs batched), (3) testing strategy (individual vs pooling), (4) testing location (laboratory vs point of care [including home testing]), and (5) the number of detectable viral targets in a given assay (single SARS-CoV-2 target assays vs small multiviral target panels vs extended multiviral target panels). Examples of these options as well as their advantages and limitations are described in **Table 1**.

Molecular test characteristics
In ideal settings, SARS-CoV-2 NAATs are generally highly sensitive and specific for the diagnosis of COVID-19.[7,12,13] However, several factors influence the performance of SARS-CoV-2 RNA detection including (1) specimen handling, (2) specimen type, (3) timing of testing in relation to viral acquisition and symptom onset, and (4) presence of symptoms/disease severity. These factors may negatively affect the sensitivity of testing, resulting in false-negative results. They are discussed below:

Specimen handling. The most common source of errors in laboratory testing is in the preanalytical phase, which encompasses specimen collection, adequacy, storage, and transport and precedes test preparation, analysis, reporting, and interpretation. Poorly collected specimens may not contain sufficient viral RNA to attain the threshold of detection for molecular methods, while prolonged transport time and inadequate storage may accelerate degradation of chemically unstable viral RNA in a specimen, leading to false-negative results. Unfortunately, unlike respiratory cultures and direct/indirect fluorescent antibody testing in which specimen adequacy can be ascertained through assessment of the number of columnar epithelial cells in the specimen, molecular testing does not include a similar step. CDC provides best practice recommendations for specimen collection, which varies across specimen types.[14] For specimen storage, CDC recommends storage at 2 to 8° C for up to 72 hours after specimen collection and at $\leq -70°C$ if transport is not possible within 72 hours of collection.

Specimen type. Testing sensitivity varies substantially across specimen types with lower respiratory tract specimens (LRTS) generally yielding higher sensitivities than upper respiratory tract specimens (URTS; **Table 2**). The use of LRTS for initial testing is impractical because patients cannot often expectorate a sample; additionally, many of the commercially available SARS-CoV-2 NAATs are not authorized for use with LRTS. Because of these factors, the Infectious Diseases Society of America (IDSA) recommends initially obtaining an URTS for NAAT testing.[15] If testing is negative but suspicion for COVID persists, IDSA recommends pursuing LRTS testing. Among URTS, nasopharyngeal (NP) swabs are considered the gold standard specimen type; alternative acceptable specimen types include saliva, midturbinate (MT), and anterior nasal (AN) swabs. Although still considered an accepted sample type for molecular testing, IDSA no longer recommends collecting oropharyngeal (OP) specimens

Table 1
Overview of molecular diagnostics

Testing Protocol	Definition	Advantages	Limitations
One-step RT-PCR	Assay where nucleic acid extraction, amplification, and detection are performed in a single reaction	Relatively fast depending on the assay Relatively automated Reduced laboratory errors Reduced potential for contamination Potential for high-throughput application	Less flexibility related to use of reagents and consumables More difficult to troubleshoot potential errors related to test process
Two-step RT-PCR	Assay where nucleic acid extraction is performed in a separate reaction from amplification and detection	Improved flexibility related to use of reagents and consumables Easier to troubleshoot errors related to test process	More labor intensive than one-step processes Longer result turnaround time

Testing Prioritization	Definition	Advantages	Limitations
Rapid testing	Single use test that can provide results in <60 min	Rapid result turnaround time Relatively easy to perform Can be performed at the POC depending on the assay	Variable sensitivity and specificity depending on the assay Lower throughput
Batched testing	Test where multiple individual specimens can be processed and analyzed simultaneously in parallel, typically with a result time of several hours	Higher throughput Relatively easy to perform depending on the assay	Longer result turnaround time More laboratory technologist training and expertise required depending on the assay

Testing Strategy	Definition	Advantages	Limitations
Individual testing	One specimen is tested individually with a given assay	Higher sensitivity compared with pooled testing (lower risk of false-negative results) Lower risk of laboratory error	Lower throughput compared with pooled testing Higher resource utilization per specimen tested
Pooled testing	Multiple specimens are combined and tested as one specimen with a given assay. If the pooled test is negative all	Higher throughput: increases the number of specimens that can be tested using the same amount of reagents and	Increased risk of false-negative results due to dilution of samples through the pooling process

specimen samples are considered negative. If SARS-CoV-2 RNA is detected with the pooled test, each specimen within the pool is then individually tested to identify the positive sample | supplies / Improved resource utilization when prevalence of SARS-CoV-2 is low and number of negative results is expected to be high / Can estimate the positive rate in a given population | Requires high degree of laboratory organization to prevent errors / supplies

Testing Location	Definition	Advantages	Limitations
Laboratory-based	Tests performed in clinical laboratories that meet specific regulatory requirements for testing	Reference standard for molecular-based diagnosis given high sensitivity and specificity / Higher throughput depending on the assay used	Longer result turnaround time / Requires laboratory technologist training and expertise
Point of Care (POC)	Tests performed at or near specimen collection (eg, outpatient clinics, schools, congregate settings)	Low complexity testing requiring minimal operator experience and training / Rapid result turnaround time	Variable sensitivity and specificity depending on the assay / Lower throughput
Viral Testing Targets	**Definition**	**Advantages**	**Limitations**
Single viral target assay	Assay that detects the presence of only one viral target (SARS-CoV-2)	High sensitivity and specificity	Limited spectrum of pathogen identification
Small multiviral target assay	Assay that detects the presence of a few viral targets (Influenza A, Influenza B, SARS-CoV-2, ± respiratory syncytial virus)	High sensitivity and specificity / Broader spectrum of pathogen identification compared with single viral target assays	Potential reduced sensitivity compared with single viral target assays / Limited spectrum of pathogen identification compared with extended multiviral target assays
Extended multiviral target assay	Assay that detects the presence of man viral (and bacterial) targets	High sensitivity and specificity / Broadest spectrum of pathogen identification	Potential reduced sensitivity compared with single viral target and small multiviral target assays

Data from Refs.[10,69–74]

Table 2
Test characteristics by specimen type

Specimen Type	Sensitivity (95% CI)	Specificity (95% CI)	Advantages	Limitations
NP	N/A (reference method)	N/A (reference method)	Reference method, reducing the potential for false-positive or false-negative results	Requires testing supplies Can only be collected by health-care professionals Higher potential for aerosol generation More invasive compared with other methods Uncomfortable procedure
Anterior nares swab (AN)	89% (83%–94%)	100% (99%–100%)	Potential for self-collection Less invasive compared with NP More comfortable procedure for patients Lower potential for aerosol generation	Reduced sensitivity compared with NP (higher risk of FN results) Requires testing supplies
Saliva (with or without coughing)	90%–99% (85%–100%)	96%–98% (83%–100%)	Potential for self-collection Less invasive compared with all other URT specimen types More comfortable procedure for patients Lower potential for aerosol generation (saliva without coughing only) Requires fewer testing supplies	Reduced sensitivity compared with NP (higher risk of FN results) Often requires formal specimen validation by clinical laboratories as specimen type is not frequently authorized for use on many commercially available NAAT platforms Higher risk of invalid results given complexity of specimen type which can lead to more repeat testing and delayed result turnaround time
MT swab	95% (83%–99%)	100% (89%–100%)	Potential for self-collection Less invasive compared with NP More comfortable procedure for	Reduced sensitivity compared with NP (higher risk of FN results) Requires testing supplies

Specimen	Sensitivity	Sensitivity	Advantages	Disadvantages
			patients Lower potential for aerosol generation	Reduced sensitivity compared with all other URT specimen types (higher risk of FN results) Requires testing supplies Can only be collected by health-care professionals
OP swab	76% (58%–88%)	98% (96%–99%)	Less invasive compared with NP More comfortable procedure for patients Lower potential for aerosol generation	
Combined AN/OP swab	95% (69%–99%)	99% (92%–100%)	Potential for self-collection Less invasive compared with NP More comfortable procedure for patients Lower potential for aerosol generation	Reduced sensitivity compared with NP (higher risk of FN results)Requires testing suppliesRequires formal specimen validation by clinical laboratories as combined specimen type is not authorized for use on commercially available NAAT platforms

Data *from* Refs. [15,19,75]

alone due to low sensitivity but instead to combine them with AN specimens. Studies evaluating the sensitivity of saliva in comparison with NP have yielded mixed results including decreased (compared with combination NP/OP specimens), equivalent, or greater sensitivity.[16] Variability in reference tests, timing of specimen collection relative to symptom onset, specimen collection processes for saliva, patient demographics, comorbidities, and disease severity significantly limit the interpretation of testing performance across specimen types.[15–19] Although perhaps slightly less sensitive than NP specimens, alternative URTS have the advantage of being less invasive and easier to collect which is especially important in frequent/routine testing schemes. Additionally, saliva specimens may be especially amenable to self-collection including in the home setting and reduce the need for swabs and other supplies that are prone to shortages, although specialized saliva collection kits may improve specimen adequacy. Of note, because many commercial NAAT platforms do not have FDA EUA for saliva, individual laboratories would be required to validate this sample type locally.[20]

Testing timing. The sensitivity of SARS-CoV-2 NAAT is highly dependent on the quantity of viral RNA in a clinical specimen. Because the amount of viral RNA in a clinical specimen varies in relation to the time from infection and from symptom onset (in those who go on to develop symptoms), the timing of testing is an important factor when considering testing sensitivity. The SARS-CoV-2 virus becomes detectable in URTS at a median of 4 to 6 days after infection (median of 4 days for the Delta variant; incubation period 2–14 days; slightly shorter incubation period for Omicron) and 2 to 5 days before symptom onset. In symptomatic individuals, viral loads peak between 0.6 days prior and 5 days after symptom onset, then drop precipitously after 7 days of symptom onset but often remain at detectable levels for multiple weeks after infection.[21–24] Therefore, testing done too early (before viral loads increase beyond the threshold of detection) or too late (after viral loads decrease below the threshold of detection) will lead to false-negative results.

Presence of symptoms and disease severity. Although viral loads have been demonstrated to peak early in the disease course and to progressively decline thereafter in most patients (apart from highly immunocompromised patients who may maintain prolonged high viral loads), the presence of symptoms and the severity of illness may also correlate with viral loads in clinical specimens and therefore the clinical sensitivity of molecular testing. Studies comparing viral loads in URTS of symptomatic versus asymptomatic or presymptomatic patients have yielded conflicting results, with most studies showing similar initial viral loads among mildly symptomatic, presymptomatic, and asymptomatic patients.[24–32] The rate of viral clearance seems to be similar or slightly faster in asymptomatic patients compared with presymptomatic and symptomatic patients.[33–35] Notably, assessing the rate of viral clearance is limited by the fact that the onset of viral replication in asymptomatic patients is often unknown leading to asynchronous viral dynamics with matched symptomatic patients. Additionally, multiple studies comparing mild and severe cases of COVID-19 have shown that viral loads tend to be higher at any point in time after symptom onset and persist longer in those with severe disease, suggesting that NAAT sensitivity is potentially higher in this population.[21,36–42]

Cycle threshold values and their role in clinical decision making
Ct values are inversely proportional to the relative amount of viral RNA present in a sample, with lower Ct values representing high RNA titer (fewer PCR cycles needed to reach positive threshold) and higher Ct values representing lower RNA titer (more

PCR cycles needed to reach the positive threshold). Given this relationship, there has been significant interest in using Ct values as surrogate markers of genomic load in the clinical setting. In particular, Ct values have been used as a proxy for transmissibility, to predict illness severity, and to help distinguish active infection, which would require potential treatment and isolation, from persistent RNA detection.[43–45] However, although Ct values do generally correlate well with RNA concentrations, limited data exist to support the use of Ct values in the above-described settings. Additionally, as RT-PCR tests are designed to be qualitative in nature, these assays have not undergone extensive evaluation to optimize the relationship between Ct values and RNA levels, which can lead to lower correlation at low and high RNA concentrations.[46] Finally, significant variability in Ct values has been shown both within and across RT-PCR platforms; Rhoads and colleagues reported intra-assay variability of up to 3 cycles (10-fold viral load difference) and interassay variability of up to 14 cycles (4000-fold viral load difference) for Ct values when reviewing proficiency testing across 700 laboratories in the United States.[47] Due to all of these factors, IDSA does not recommend the use of Ct values for clinical decision making and cautions providers about using these data to predict disease severity or to determine infection status and infectivity.[46] If Ct values are to be used for clinical decision making, consultation with infectious diseases experts should be considered.

Antigen-Based Testing

Overview
Antigen tests are immunoassays that use tagged antibodies to detect specific SARS-CoV-2 antigens within a primary specimen. Many assays are currently authorized by the FDA for the diagnosis of COVID-19, most of which target the N and S proteins (see **Fig. 3**) and can be performed on NP or nasal swab specimens.[7,48,49]

Antigen test characteristics
Overall, antigen tests are sensitive and specific tools for SARS-CoV-2 detection with reported 81% sensitivity (95% CI 72%–88%) and 99% specificity (95% CI: 99–100) compared with NAAT.[50] Sensitivity is improved when used within 7 days of symptom onset, when viral burden in the URT is highest.[50] Additionally, studies comparing antigen testing and NAAT to viral culture have shown higher correlation between positive antigen tests and culture positivity when compared with NAAT, suggesting that antigen tests may be a better marker of infectiousness and transmissibility in certain clinical situations.[51] However, more data are needed to better understand the association between antigen tests and transmissibility; until then, antigen tests should only be used to approximate infectiousness in individuals with COVID-19.[50]

As with other respiratory antigen detection tests and compared with most commercially available NAATs, SARS-CoV-2 antigen tests are relatively inexpensive and easy to perform, require little operator training and experience, and provide rapid results (approximately 15–30 minutes).[10,11,50,52] Given these characteristics, antigen tests are commonly used at the POC where results can be communicated to providers and patients in real time to allow for more informed clinical decision making.

Clinical utility of antigen testing compared with nucleic acid amplification testing
Although NAAT remains the diagnostic test standard for acute COVID-19 infection, antigen tests can be used to diagnose acute infection in both asymptomatic and symptomatic individuals when NAAT is unavailable or results are delayed; testing should be performed within 7 days of symptom onset to maximize sensitivity.[50] Given the reduced sensitivity of antigen detection tests compared with NAAT, negative results must be interpreted in the appropriate clinical context, which includes a

comprehensive evaluation of an individual's pretest probability for COVID-19 infection. Negative antigen tests in symptomatic individuals with high clinical suspicion for COVID-19 should have results confirmed with NAAT given the potential for false-negative antigen test results.[7,11,48,50] In contrast, given their high specificity, positive antigen test results in symptomatic individuals generally do not require confirmatory NAAT and individuals with positive results should be considered infected with COVID-19.[48,50] Confirmatory NAAT can be considered in select situations in antigen-positive, symptomatic individuals with low likelihood of SARS-CoV-2 infection because, although rare, false-positive results have been reported. CDC-designed algorithms using antigen based testing in these population are available at https://www.cdc.gov/coronavirus/2019-ncov/lab/resources/antigen-tests-guidelines.html and provide specific guidance for test interpretation, including indications for additional testing, depending on the antigen test results.[48,53]

Asymptomatic, exposed individuals may also benefit from antigen testing when NAAT is unavailable because positive tests do reliably indicate SARS-CoV-2 infection. As with NAAT, negative antigen results do not preclude COVID-19 infection in asymptomatic individuals with high risk for infection (close contact or suspected exposure) and do not obviate the need for quarantine. Per CDC guidance, both NAAT and antigen tests can be used to shorten the duration of quarantine in exposed unvaccinated asymptomatic individuals if performed at least 5 days after last exposure.[54]

Finally, the rapid turnaround time and relatively low cost of antigen detection tests compared with NAATs make these tests appealing serial screening tools for SARS-CoV-2 detection in high-risk congregate and community settings, where identifying infected individuals quickly is paramount to preventing transmission.[48]

Serologic Testing

Overview
Serologic testing detects the presence of SARS-CoV-2 specific antibodies in clinical specimens from individuals with prior SARS-CoV-2 infection, vaccination, and/or recent receipt of anti-SARS-Cov-2 monoclonal antibody therapy. Currently, nearly 100 assays have received FDA EUA for clinical use; common antibody targets include the nucleocapsid (anti-N) protein, which is produced in response to natural infection and the spike (anti-S) protein, which is produced in response to either natural infection or vaccination (**Table 3** for guidance on the interpretation of SARS-CoV-2 serologic assays by vaccination status). Common specimen types include serum and/or plasma . Depending on the assay, different classes of antibodies may be detected, ranging

Table 3			
Interpretation of SARS-CoV-2 serologic assays by vaccination status			
Vaccination Status	Anti-N Antibody	Anti-S Antibody	Interpretation
Unvaccinated	Positive	Positive	Previously infected
Unvaccinated	Negative	Negative	Not previously vaccinated or infected
Vaccinated	Positive	Positive	Vaccinated and previously infected
Vaccinated	Negative	Positive	Vaccinated and not previously infected[a]

[a]Immunocompromised patients may have negative serology postvaccination.
Adapted from Centers for Disease Control and Prevention. Interim Guidelines for COVID-19 Antibody Testing. *Cent Dis Control Prev.* 2020:1-8. https://www.cdc.gov/coronavirus/2019-ncov/lab/resources/antibody-tests-guidelines.html. Accessed October 20, 2021.

from IgM, IgG, IgA, or total antibody, the latter of which does not discern between specific class types. Assays are qualitative or semiquantitative in nature and, generally, do not distinguish between neutralizing (protective) and nonneutralizing antibodies.

Serologic testing characteristics
In general, SARS-CoV-2 serologic assays are reasonably sensitive and specific; however, several factors, including (1) test method, (2) test timing in relation to symptom onset, (3) type of antibodies measured, and (4) host type, can affect test performance.[55] These factors are discussed below:

Test method. There are several available SARS-CoV-2 serologic testing methods including lateral flow assays (LFA), enzyme-linked immunosorbent assay (ELISA), and chemiluminescent immunoassays (CIA).[56,57] LFA are generally low complexity tests that can be performed at the POC, whereas ELISA and CIA are laboratory-based tests with the potential for high-throughput testing.[57] In general, LFA are less sensitive than ELISA and CIA, with a recent-meta-analysis showing a pooled sensitivity of only 66% for LFA compared with 84.3% and 97.8% for ELISA and CIA, respectively.[9,10,55] Pooled specificity ranged from 99.6% to 99.7%.[55] Given this observed variability across assay methodologies, clinicians should be aware of the test characteristics of the specific platforms used by their institutions so as to interpret negative test results in the appropriate context.

Test timing. Due to the kinetics of antibody production in response to infection, sensitivity for all serologic assays is low within the first 2 weeks following infection, with reported pooled sensitivities of 23% to 63% at week 1 and 68% to 96% at week 2.[57] Sensitivity significantly improves by 3 weeks after infection with pooled sensitivity of 84% to 95%.[57] Due to this reduced sensitivity early in infection, serologic testing should be avoided during this time frame to prevent potential false-negative results. Levels of S-specific, RBD-specific, and N-specific IgM and IgG antibodies seem to develop concurrently after infection and follow similar dynamic changes during convalescence.[58]

Types of antibodies measured. Because small differences in specificity can have disproportionate effects on false-positive rates when SARS-CoV-2 prevalence is low, IDSA recommends using serologic tests with high specificity ($\geq$99.5%).[57] Generally, serologic assays that detect IgG or total antibodies (IgM, IgA, and IgG) have higher specificities ($\geq$99%) compared with assays that detect IgM or IgA only or combined IgM and IgG; these assays should be prioritized for use if serologic testing is indicated.[57] When a false-positive test is suspected based on low pretest probability and/or low prevalence, orthogonal testing using two sequential serologic assays that target different protein targets can be done to increase the positive predictive value of an initial positive result.

Host type. Patients with immune deficiencies limiting their host immune response to SARS-CoV-2 antigens, especially those on lymphocyte depleting or suppressing agents, may fail to seroconvert after exposure to SARS-CoV-2. As a result, serologic methods may not reliably identify immunosuppressed individuals with prior infection.

Clinical utility of serologic testing
A detailed description of "best use" scenarios for SARS-CoV-2 serologic testing can be found in **Table 4**. In general, serologic testing plays a limited role in the diagnosis of acute infection and is more commonly used for surveillance purposes. Currently authorized antibody tests provide a qualitative result (positive/negative). Although

Table 4		
Best uses of SARS-CoV-2 diagnostic testing		
NAAT[15]	**Antigen-Based**[50]	**Serology**[57]
Symptomatic individuals suspected of having COVID-19	Screening in high-risk congregate or community settings	Confirmation of past SARS-CoV-2 infection, 3–4 wk after symptom onset
Asymptomatic individuals with possible or known exposure to COVID-19	Symptomatic individuals suspected of having COVID-19, when NAAT is not easily available	Diagnose COVID-19 infection in symptomatic patients with high clinical suspicion and negative NAAT testing
Asymptomatic individuals being admitted to the hospital, regardless of exposure history to COVID-19	Prior to an event or travel to identify asymptomatic or presmptomatic COVID-19 infection	Diagnose current or past COVID-19 infection in patients with MIS
Asymptomatic patients undergoing procedures when PPE or other resources are limited	Congregate settings experiencing an outbreak in need of rapid turnaround	

some tests additionally provide a numerical result, these tests are classified as semi-quantitative rather than quantitative by the FDA; hence, the utility of numerical values is not known at this time. One exception is their use to support the diagnosis of multi-system inflammatory syndrome (MIS) in children and adults as NAAT can be negative because most cases present 2 to 6 weeks after initial infection. Additionally, recent data have suggested that knowing SARS-CoV-2 serostatus in hospitalized individuals suffering from COVID-19 may be helpful for making treatment decisions related to anti-SARS CoV-2 monoclonal antibody therapy, particularly in immunosuppressed patients unlikely to mount any immune response; however, more data are needed to support the routine use of these assays in this setting.[59] Importantly, although good correlation between some serologic assays (anti-S) and neutralizing antibodies has been reported, full correlates of immunity have not been established and may differ across viral variants, antibody types, assays, and patient populations. Thus, serologic testing should not routinely be used to determine immunity in previously infected or vaccinated individuals.[57,60,61]

Effects of SARS-CoV-2 Variants on Diagnostic Testing Performance

Because the SARS-CoV-2 pandemic has continued, many SARS-CoV-2 variants, with various mutations in the viral genome, have emerged. In addition to affecting the over-all clinical characteristics of this virus, the presence of these mutations has also affected the test performance of certain diagnostics tests, leading to false-negative results.[62] For example, specific spike protein mutations identified in Alpha (B.1.1.7) and Omicron (B.1.1.529) variants can cause false-negative NAAT results ("S gene target failure" [SGTF]) if the S gene is the predominant gene target for a given NAAT. Importantly, most NAATs detect more than one viral target, minimizing the likelihood of a false-negative result even if one target is affected by a specific mutation present in a circulating variant. In fact, in some instances, failure of a specific gene target to amplify in the setting of other amplified SARS-CoV-2 gene targets (such as SGTF) can even be advantageous because these patterns can serve as proxies for detection of certain variants. For example, the identification of the SGTF pattern has been used as a proxy for detection of Alpha and Omicron variants both in the United States and abroad (ECDC).[7,63,64] In contrast, S gene mutations in the Delta variant (B.1.617.2) typically do not lead to S gene drop out. Currently, the FDA monitors the potential impact of novel mutations on test performance; up-to-date information can be found at: https://www.fda.gov/medical-devices/coronavirus-covid-19-and-medical-devices/sars-cov-2-viral-mutations-impact-covid-19-tests. Additionally, in February of 2021, the FDA published guidance for test developers and manufacturers for the evaluation of novel viral mutations on COVID-19 test performance in an effort to identify issues with commercial testing in real-time.[65]

Compared with NAAT, most antigen tests detect the viral nucleocapsid protein and would be unaffected by mutations in the spike protein, although rare mutations in the N gene that may affect the sensitivity of diagnostic tests have been reported.[49] More recently, reports of reduced antigen-testing sensitivity have been reported for the rapidly emerging Omicron variant.[62] Reasons for this reduced sensitivity are as of yet unclear but include mutations in target antigens, variations in viral burden, or tropism to an anatomic site/specimen other than the one being tested (such as for saliva when nasal swab being performed). Evaluation of these reports related to Omicron is an area of ongoing investigation.

Testing in Specific Patient Populations/Clinical Settings

Reinfected individuals
Genotypically confirmed reinfection with SARS-CoV-2 has been documented in both immunocompetent and immunocompromised individuals with most cases occurring ≥90 days after the primary infection, presumably because of the development of short-term protective immunity. Considering this and the potential for prolonged shedding of viral particles without true infectiousness for weeks to months after initial infection, retesting should generally be avoided within 90 days of primary infection. In symptomatic or asymptomatic individuals presenting ≥90 days after initial infection/illness, standard testing criteria should be applied. For individuals presenting 45 to 89 days after initial infection and with high suspicion for reinfection based on clinical criteria without or without additional predisposing host factors and no alternate cause of symptoms, testing should be considered because some cases of reinfection have occurred as early as 48 days after initial infection.[66,67] In these circumstances, a repeat positive NAAT test with a low Ct value (lower than 33 per CDC investigative reinfection criteria) would be suggestive of reinfection.[68] Ultimately, however, reinfection can only be confirmed with genomic sequencing of both the initial and subsequent infecting viruses to determine if the patient was reinfected with a different virus.

SUMMARY

The diagnosis of SARS-CoV-2 infection relies on several considerations including the presence and duration of COVID-19 symptoms and the diagnostic testing methods used. Molecular testing, most often RT-PCR, offers the highest sensitivity and specificity during acute infection, with URTS being the preferred initial specimen type for testing. Antigen testing can also be used for acute diagnosis when RT-PCR is unavailable or not easily accessible and is of particular use for serial screening in high-risk asymptomatic populations and congregate settings due to its low cost and ease of performance. Finally, antigen testing may have the potential to approximate infectiousness in individuals with COVID-19 infection but the current data are inconclusive and more studies are needed to establish their use in this setting. In contrast, serologic testing is more useful for diagnosing recent or past infection and MIS, with improved sensitivity when performed after more than 14 days of symptoms. In keeping with current guidelines, COVID-19 serologic assays should not be used during the acute phase of infection.

DISCLOSURE

S.E. Turbett receives grant support from the Centers for Disease Control and Prevention for COVID-19-related work. She also receives royalties from UpToDate. The remaining authors have nothing to disclose.

REFERENCES

1. van den Borst B, Peters JB, Brink M, et al. comprehensive health assessment 3 months after recovery from acute coronavirus disease 2019 (COVID-19). Clin Infect Dis 2021;73(5):e1089.
2. Wang QJ, Yao YZ, Song JS, et al. Kinetic changes in virology, specific antibody response and imaging during the clinical course of COVID-19: a descriptive study. BMC Infect Dis 2020;20(1):818.
3. Nussenblatt V, Roder AE, Das S, et al. Year-long COVID-19 infection reveals within-host evolution of SARS-CoV-2 in a patient with B cell depletion. medRxiv 2021. https://doi.org/10.1101/2021.10.02.21264267. Published online October 5, 2021.
4. Choi B, Choudhary MC, Regan J, et al. Persistence and evolution of SARS-CoV-2 in an immunocompromised host. N Engl J Med 2020;383(23):2291–3.
5. Greninger AL, Dien Bard J, Colgrove RC, et al. Clinical and infection prevention applications of SARS-CoV-2 genotyping: an IDSA/ASM consensus review document. Clin Infect Dis. Published online November 3, 2021. doi:10.1093/cid/ciab761
6. Iyer AS, Jones FK, Nodoushani A, et al. Persistence and decay of human antibody responses to the receptor binding domain of SARS-CoV-2 spike protein in COVID-19 patients. Sci Immunol 2020;5(52). https://doi.org/10.1126/SCIIMMUNOL.ABE0367.
7. Gitman MR, Shaban Mv, Paniz-Mondolfi AE, et al. Laboratory diagnosis of sars-cov-2 pneumonia. Diagnostics 2021;11(7). https://doi.org/10.3390/diagnostics11071270.
8. Jayamohan H, Lambert CJ, Sant HJ, et al. SARS-CoV-2 pandemic: a review of molecular diagnostic tools including sample collection and commercial response with associated advantages and limitations. doi:10.1007/s00216-020-02958-1/Published
9. Mardian Y, Kosasih H, Karyana M, et al. Review of current COVID-19 diagnostics and opportunities for further development. Front Med 2021;8. https://doi.org/10.3389/fmed.2021.615099.
10. Gulholm T, Basile K, Kok J, et al. Laboratory diagnosis of severe acute respiratory syndrome coronavirus 2. Pathology 2020;52(7):745–53.
11. la Marca A, Capuzzo M, Paglia T, et al. Testing for SARS-CoV-2 (COVID-19): a systematic review and clinical guide to molecular and serological in-vitro diagnostic assays. Reprod Biomed Online 2020;41(3):483–99.
12. Lieberman JA, Pepper G, Naccache SN, et al. Comparison of commercially available and laboratory-developed assays for in vitro detection of SARS-CoV-2 in clinical laboratories. J Clin Microbiol 2020;58(8). https://doi.org/10.1128/JCM.00821-20.

13. Nalla AK, Casto AM, Casto AM, et al. Comparative performance of SARS-CoV-2 detection assays using seven different primer-probe sets and one assay kit. J Clin Microbiol 2020;58(6). https://doi.org/10.1128/JCM.00557-20.

14. Centers for Disease Control and Prevention. Interim guidelines for clinical specimens for COVID-19 | CDC, 2019. Centers for Disease Control and Prevention; 2020. p. 1–5. Accessed October 18, 2021. https://www.cdc.gov/coronavirus/2019-ncov/lab/guidelines-clinical-specimens.html. Available at.

15. Hanson KE, Caliendo AM, Arias CA, et al. The infectious diseases society of america guidelines on the diagnosis of COVID-19: molecular diagnostic testing. Published online December 23, 2020. Accessed November 27, 2021. https://www.idsociety.org/practice-guideline/covid-19-guideline-diagnostics/.   Available at.

16. Butler-Laporte G, Lawandi A, Schiller I, et al. Comparison of saliva and nasopharyngeal swab nucleic acid amplification testing for detection of SARS-CoV-2: a systematic review and meta-analysis. JAMA Intern Med 2021;181(3):353–60.

17. Bastos ML, Perlman-Arrow S, Menzies D, et al. The sensitivity and costs of testing for SARS-CoV-2 infection with saliva versus nasopharyngeal swabs : a systematic review and meta-analysis. Ann Intern Med 2021;174(4):501–10.

18. Tsang NNY, So HC, Ng KY, et al. Diagnostic performance of different sampling approaches for SARS-CoV-2 RT-PCR testing: a systematic review and meta-analysis. Lancet Infect Dis 2021;21(9):1233–45.

19. Lee RA, Herigon JC, Benedetti A, et al. Performance of saliva, oropharyngeal swabs, and nasal swabs for SARS-CoV-2 molecular detection: a systematic review and meta-analysis. J Clin Microbiol 2021;59(5). https://doi.org/10.1128/JCM.02881-20.

20. Williams E, Bond K, Zhang B, et al. Saliva as a noninvasive specimen for detection of sars-cov-2. J Clin Microbiol 2020;58(8). https://doi.org/10.1128/JCM.00776-20/ASSET/344BF6A9-26C9-44D7-9114-392784B80298/ASSETS/GRAPHIC/JCM.00776-20-F0001.

21. He X, Lau EHY, Wu P, et al. Temporal dynamics in viral shedding and transmissibility of COVID-19. Nat Med 2020;26(5):672–5.

22. Zou L, Ruan F, Huang M, et al. SARS-CoV-2 viral load in upper respiratory specimens of infected patients. N Engl J Med 2020;382(12):1177–9.

23. Azar MM, Shin JJ, Kang I, et al. Diagnosis of SARS-CoV-2 infection in the setting of the cytokine release syndrome. Expert Rev Mol Diagn 2020;20(11):1087–97.

24. Lee S, Kim T, Lee E, et al. Clinical course and molecular viral shedding among asymptomatic and symptomatic patients with SARS-CoV-2 infection in a community treatment center in the republic of korea. JAMA Intern Med 2020;180(11):1447–52.

25. Ra SH, Lim JS, Kim GU, et al. Upper respiratory viral load in asymptomatic individuals and mildly symptomatic patients with SARS-CoV-2 infection. Thorax 2021;76(1):61–3.

26. Arons MM, Hatfield KM, Reddy SC, et al. Presymptomatic SARS-CoV-2 infections and transmission in a skilled nursing facility. N Engl J Med 2020;382(22):2081–90.

27. Chau NVV, Lam VT, Dung NT, et al. The natural history and transmission potential of asymptomatic severe acute respiratory syndrome coronavirus 2 infection. Clin Infect Dis 2020;71(10):2679–87.

28. Lavezzo E, Franchin E, Ciavarella C, et al. Suppression of a SARS-CoV-2 outbreak in the Italian municipality of Vo. Nature 2020;584(7821):425–9.

29. Han MS, Seong MW, Kim N, et al. Viral RNA load in mildly symptomatic and asymptomatic children with COVID-19, Seoul, South Korea. Emerg Infect Dis 2020;26(10):2497–9.

30. Zhou R, Li F, Chen F, et al. Viral dynamics in asymptomatic patients with COVID-19. Int J Infect Dis 2020;96:288–90.

31. Kociolek LK, Muller WJ, Yee R, et al. Comparison of upper respiratory viral load distributions in asymptomatic and symptomatic children diagnosed with SARS-CoV-2 infection in pediatric hospital testing programs. J Clin Microbiol 2020; 59(1). https://doi.org/10.1128/JCM.02593-20.

32. Hasanoglu I, Korukluoglu G, Asilturk D, et al. Higher viral loads in asymptomatic COVID-19 patients might be the invisible part of the iceberg. Infection 2021; 49(1):117–26.

33. Hu Z, Song C, Xu C, et al. Clinical characteristics of 24 asymptomatic infections with COVID-19 screened among close contacts in Nanjing, China. Sci China Life Sci 2020;63(5):706–11.

34. Yang R, Gui X, Xiong Y. Comparison of clinical characteristics of patients with asymptomatic vs symptomatic coronavirus disease 2019 in Wuhan, China. JAMA Netw open 2020;3(5). https://doi.org/10.1001/JAMANETWORKOPEN. 2020.10182.

35. Yongchen Z, Shen H, Wang X, et al. Different longitudinal patterns of nucleic acid and serology testing results based on disease severity of COVID-19 patients. Emerg Microbes Infect 2020;9(1):833–6.

36. Zheng S, Fan J, Yu F, et al. Viral load dynamics and disease severity in patients infected with SARS-CoV-2 in Zhejiang province, China, January-March 2020: retrospective cohort study 2020;369. https://doi.org/10.1136/BMJ.M1443.

37. Guo X, Jie Y, Ye Y, et al. Upper respiratory tract viral ribonucleic acid load at hospital admission is associated with coronavirus disease 2019 disease severity. Open Forum Infect Dis 2020;7(7). https://doi.org/10.1093/OFID/OFAA282.

38. To KKW, Tsang OTY, Leung WS, et al. Temporal profiles of viral load in posterior oropharyngeal saliva samples and serum antibody responses during infection by SARS-CoV-2: an observational cohort study. Lancet Infect Dis 2020;20(5): 565–74.

39. Chen X, Zhu B, Hong W, et al. Associations of clinical characteristics and treatment regimens with the duration of viral RNA shedding in patients with COVID-19. Int J Infect Dis 2020;98:252–60.

40. Chen J, Qi T, Liu L, et al. Clinical progression of patients with COVID-19 in Shanghai, China. J Infect 2020;80(5):e1–6.

41. Yan D, Liu XY, Zhu YN, et al. Factors associated with prolonged viral shedding and impact of lopinavir/ritonavir treatment in hospitalised non-critically ill patients with SARS-CoV-2 infection. Eur Respir J 2020;56(1). https://doi.org/10.1183/13993003.00799-2020.

42. Liu Y, Yan LM, Wan L, et al. Viral dynamics in mild and severe cases of COVID-19. Lancet Infect Dis 2020;20(6):656–7.

43. Peltan ID, Beesley SJ, Webb BJ, et al. Evaluation of potential COVID-19 recurrence in patients with late repeat positive SARS-CoV-2 testing. PLoS One 2021; 16(5). https://doi.org/10.1371/JOURNAL.PONE.0251214.

44. Bullard J, Dust K, Funk D, et al. predicting infectious severe acute respiratory syndrome coronavirus 2 from diagnostic samples. Clin Infect Dis 2020;71(10): 2663–6.

45. Zacharioudakis IM, Prasad PJ, Zervou FN, et al. Association of SARS-CoV-2 genomic load with outcomes in patients with COVID-19. Ann Am Thorac Soc 2021;18(5):900–3.
46. IDSA and AMP joint statement on the use of SARS-CoV-2 PCR cycle threshold (Ct) values for clinical decision-making.
47. Rhoads D, Peaper DR, She RC, et al. college of american pathologists (CAP) microbiology committee perspective: caution must be used in interpreting the cycle threshold (Ct) value. Clin Infect Dis 2021;72(10):e685–6.
48. Centers for Disease Control and Prevention. Interim guidance for antigen testing for sars-cov-2. centers for disease control and prevention. 2020. Available at. https://www.cdc.gov/coronavirus/2019-ncov/lab/resources/antigen-tests-guidelines.html. Accessed October 19, 2021.
49. Bourassa L, Perchetti GA, Phung Q, et al. A SARS-CoV-2 nucleocapsid variant that affects antigen test performance. J Clin Virol 2021;141. https://doi.org/10.1016/j.jcv.2021.104900.
50. Hanson KE, Caliendo AM, Arias CA, et al. IDSA guidelines on the diagnosis of COVID-19: antigen testing. 2021. Available at. https://www.idsociety.org/practice-guideline/covid-19-guideline-antigen-testing/. Accessed November 27, 2021.
51. Pekosz A, Parvu V, Li M, et al. Antigen-based testing but not real-time polymerase chain reaction correlates with severe acute respiratory syndrome coronavirus 2 viral culture. Clin Infect Dis 2021;73(9):e2861–6.
52. Dinnes J, Deeks JJ, Berhane S, et al. Rapid, point-of-care antigen and molecular-based tests for diagnosis of SARS-CoV-2 infection. Cochrane Database Syst Rev 2021;(3):2021.
53. Humphries RM, Azar MM, Caliendo AM, et al. To test, perchance to diagnose: Practical strategies for severe acute respiratory syndrome coronavirus 2 testing. Open Forum Infect Dis 2021;8(4). https://doi.org/10.1093/ofid/ofab095.
54. Centers for Disease Control and Prevention. science brief: options to reduce quarantine for contacts of persons with SARS-CoV-2 infection using symptom monitoring and diagnostic testing | CDC. Available at. https://www.cdc.gov/coronavirus/2019-ncov/science/science-briefs/scientific-brief-options-to-reduce-quarantine.html?CDC_AA_refVal=https%3A%2F%2Fwww.cdc.gov%2Fcoronavirus%2F2019-ncov%2Fmore%2Fscientific-brief-options-to-reduce-quarantine.html. Accessed November 27, 2021.
55. Lisboa Bastos M, Tavaziva G, Abidi SK, et al. Diagnostic accuracy of serological tests for covid-19: systematic review and meta-analysis. BMJ 2020;370. https://doi.org/10.1136/BMJ.M2516.
56. U.S. Food and Drug Administration. In vitro diagnostics EUAs - Serology and other adaptive immune response tests for SARS-CoV-2. Available at. https://www.fda.gov/medical-devices/coronavirus-disease-2019-covid-19-emergency-use-authorizations-medical-devices/in-vitro-diagnostics-euas-serology-and-other-adaptive-immune-response-tests-sars-cov-2#individual-serological. Accessed November 27, 2021.
57. Hanson KE, Caliendo AM, Arias CA, et al. IDSA guidelines on the diagnosis of COVID-19: serologic testing. Available at. https://www.idsociety.org/practice-guideline/covid-19-guideline-serology/. Accessed November 27, 2021.
58. Li K, Huang B, Wu M, et al. Dynamic changes in anti-SARS-CoV-2 antibodies during SARS-CoV-2 infection and recovery from COVID-19. Nat Commun 2020;11(1):1–11.

59. Horby PW, Mafham M, Peto L, et al, RECOVERY Collaborative Group. Casirivi-
    mab and imdevimab in patients admitted to hospital with COVID-19 (RECOV-
    ERY): a randomised, controlled, open-label, platform trial. medRxiv 2021;16.
    https://doi.org/10.1101/2021.06.15.21258542. Published online June.

60. Khoury DS, Cromer D, Reynaldi A, et al. Neutralizing antibody levels are highly
    predictive of immune protection from symptomatic SARS-CoV-2 infection. Nat
    Med 2021;27(7):1205–11. https://doi.org/10.1038/S41591-021-01377-8.

61. Centers for Disease Control and Prevention. Interim guidelines for COVID-19 anti-
    body testing. Center for Disease Control and Prevention; 2020. p. 1–8. Available
    at. https://www.cdc.gov/coronavirus/2019-ncov/lab/resources/antibody-tests-
    guidelines.html. Accessed October 19, 2021.

62. U.S. Food and Drug Administration. SARS-CoV-2 Viral Mutations: Impact on
    COVID-19 Tests | FDA. Available at. https://www.fda.gov/medical-devices/
    coronavirus-covid-19-and-medical-devices/sars-cov-2-viral-mutations-impact-
    covid-19-tests. Accessed January 5, 2022.

63. ECDC. Methods for the detection and characterisation of SARS-CoV-2 variants -
    first update 20 Dec 2021. Published online 2021.

64. Centers for Disease Control and Prevention. Genetic variants of SARS-CoV-2 may
    lead to false negative results with molecular tests for detection of SARS-CoV-2 -
    letter to clinical laboratory staff and health care providers | FDA. Cdc. Published
    online 2021:1-5. Available at. https://www.fda.gov/medical-devices/letters-health-
    care-providers/genetic-variants-sars-cov-2-may-lead-false-negative-results-
    molecular-tests-detection-sars-cov-2. Accessed November 25, 2021.

65. U.S. Food and Drug Administration. Contains nonbinding recommendations pol-
    icy for evaluating impact of viral mutations on COVID-19 tests guidance for test
    developers and food and drug administration staff preface public comment.
    2021. Available at. https://www.fda.gov/regulatory-. Accessed January 5, 2022.

66. Klein J, Brito AF, Trubin P, et al. Longitudinal immune profiling of a SARS-CoV-2
    reinfection in a solid organ transplant recipient. J Infect Dis 2021. https://doi.
    org/10.1093/INFDIS/JIAB553. Published online October 29.

67. Tillett RL, Sevinsky JR, Hartley PD, et al. Genomic evidence for reinfection with
    SARS-CoV-2: a case study. Lancet Infect Dis 2021;21(1):52–8.

68. Centers for Disease Control and Prevention. Investigative criteria for suspected
    cases of SARS-CoV-2 reinfection (ICR). *Centers for Disease Control and Preven-
    tion* 2020. p. 1–3. Available at. https://www.cdc.gov/coronavirus/2019-ncov/php/
    invest-criteria.html. Accessed November 25, 2021.

69. U.S. Food and Drug Administration. FAQs on testing for SARS-CoV-2 | FDA. Avail-
    able at. https://www.fda.gov/medical-devices/coronavirus-covid-19-and-
    medical-devices/faqs-testing-sars-cov-2. Accessed December 22, 2021.

70. Peaper DR, Landry ML. Laboratory diagnosis of viral infection. Handb Clin Neurol
    2014;123:123.

71. Daniel EA, Esakialraj LBH, S A, et al. Pooled testing strategies for SARS-CoV-2
    diagnosis: a comprehensive review. Diagn Microbiol Infect Dis 2021;101(2):
    115432.

72. U.S. Food and Drug Administration. Pooled sample testing and screening testing
    for COVID-19 | FDA. Available at. https://www.fda.gov/medical-devices/
    coronavirus-covid-19-and-medical-devices/pooled-sample-testing-and-
    screening-testing-covid-19. Accessed December 22, 2021.

73. Wacker MJ, Godard MP. Analysis of one-step and two-step real-time RT-PCR us-
    ing superscript III. J Biomol Tech 2005;16(3):266. Available at:/pmc/arti-
    cles/PMC2291734/. Accessed December 22, 2021.

74. Centers for Disease Control and Prevention. Information on rapid molecular assays, RT-PCR, and other molecular assays for diagnosis of influenza virus infection | CDC. Available at. https://www.cdc.gov/flu/professionals/diagnosis/molecular-assays.htm. Accessed December 22, 2021.

75. U.S. Food and Drug Administration. COVID-19 Testing Supplies: FAQs on Testing for SARS-CoV-2 | FDA. Published online 2020:1-18. Available at. https://www.fda.gov/medical-devices/coronavirus-covid-19-and-medical-devices/covid-19-testing-supplies-faqs-testing-sars-cov-2. Accessed November 27, 2021.

76. Lu R, Zhao X, Niu P, et al. Genomic characterisation and epidemiology of 2019 novel coronavirus: implications for virus origins and receptor binding. Lancet 2020;395:565–74.

Pharmacologic Treatment and Management of Coronavirus Disease 2019

Amy Hirsch Shumaker, PharmD, BCPS, AAHIVP[a,b,]*,
Adarsh Bhimraj, MD[c]

KEYWORDS

- COVID-19 • SARS CoV-2 • Monoclonal antibodies • Corticosteroids • Tocilizumab
- Baricitinib • Antivirals

KEY POINTS

- Most patients with mild or moderate COVID-19 recover without treatments, but patients with high risk of progression or patients with severe or critical COVID-19 can benefit from pharmacotherapy.
- Treatments like glucocorticoids, interleukin (IL)-6 inhibitors, and Janus kinase (JAK) inhibitors have shown a mortality benefit in severe or critical COVID-19.
- Treatments like anti-SARS CoV-2 antibodies and direct-acting antivirals have been shown to decrease the need for medically attended visits, hospitalizations or length of hospital stay.
- Assessing severity of COVID-19 and duration of illness is necessary to identify patients who will benefit most from specific therapies.

INTRODUCTION

At the outset of the pandemic, efficacy data for potential treatments were sparse and of low quality. Despite the dynamic demands of the pandemic, it is remarkable how much our understanding of the efficacy and harms of coronavirus disease 2019 (COVID-19) treatment options has evolved in less than 2 years. During these months, pivotal adaptive COVID-19 treatment trials like SOLIDARITY[1] and RECOVERY[2,3] were successfully completed and have been instrumental in guiding treatment recommendations for the management of patients with COVID-19.

[a] Clinical Pharmacy Specialist-Infectious Disease, Department of Pharmacy, VA Northeast Ohio Healthcare System, 10701 East Boulevard, Pharmacy 119 (W), Cleveland, OH 44106, USA; [b] Senior Clinical Instructor, School of Medicine, Case Western Reserve University, 10900 Euclid Ave, Cleveland, OH 44106-7341; [c] Section Head Neurologic Infectious Diseases, Department of Infectious Diseases, Cleveland Clinic, 9500 Euclid Avenue/g21, Cleveland, OH 44195, USA
* Corresponding author. Infectious Disease, 10701 East Boulevard, Pharmacy 119 (W), Cleveland, OH 44106.
E-mail address: amy.hirsch@va.gov

Infect Dis Clin N Am 36 (2022) 349–364
https://doi.org/10.1016/j.idc.2022.02.001
0891-5520/22/Published by Elsevier Inc.
id.theclinics.com

The Infectious Disease Society of America (IDSA) and the National Institutes of Health have produced comprehensive guidelines for the treatment and management of patients with COVID-19.[4,5] The IDSA Guideline has used the GRADE Methodology[58] in the development of their treatment guideline. GRADE (Grading of Recommendations Assessment, Development and Evaluation) provides a framework that allows for frontline clinicians to appreciate the confidence in an estimate of treatment effect in a given patient population and for a particular outcome. The IDSA guidelines use 4 categories of ratings for the quality of evidence: high, moderate, low, and very low; these ratings are based on the certainty of the treatment effect, as well as any methodological concerns or risk of bias within the supporting evidence base. The word "recommend" in the IDSA COVID guideline indicates a strong recommendation, and the word "suggest" indicates a conditional recommendation.

Treatment recommendations are developed around PICO (population, intervention, comparator, outcome) questions. For example, "in hospitalized patients with COVID-19 (population), should hydroxychloroquine (intervention) versus no hydroxychloroquine (comparator) be used"? This question can be applied for various outcomes of COVID-19, like mortality, hospitalization, progression to mechanical ventilation, and serious adverse events.

As a clinician applying treatment recommendations to patients with COVID-19, it is vital to classify the patient's current disease severity (population) because subtle differences in the known benefits and harms (outcomes) of various treatments exist (interventions/comparators). **Fig. 1** displays the spectrum of disease for patients with COVID-19, and certain types of treatments may be more advantageous or harmful at a particular stage of disease. From a mechanistic perspective, early in the infection, when viral burden is high and the host's adaptive immune system has not mounted an

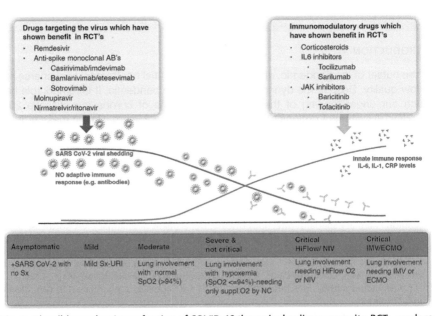

Fig. 1. Plausible mechanisms of action of COVID-19 therapies by disease severity. RCTs, randomized controlled trials; ABs, antibodies; Sx, symptoms; URI, upper respiratory infection; Spo2, oxygen saturation as measured by pulse oximetry; NC, nasal cannula; NIV, noninvasive ventilation; IMV, invasive mechanical ventilation; ECMO, extracorporeal membrane oxygenation.

adequate response, treatments targeting viral replication can be more effective. Examples would be antiviral therapies like remdesivir, molnupiravir, nirmatrelvir/ritonavir, and neutralizing antibody therapies. Like influenza, the earlier the antiviral therapies are administered the more efficacious they likely would be. There may be subsets of patients like immunocompromised patients or patients who have not had an adaptive immune response, with high viral burden even later in the disease process, who may still benefit from antiviral treatments. Treatments like glucocorticoids may also be harmful early in mild or moderate disease.

OTHER CLINICAL CONSIDERATIONS WHEN CHOOSING CORONAVIRUS DISEASE 2019 PHARMACOTHERAPIES

As a treating clinician it is also important to appreciate the contraindications and relative contraindications for COVID-19 treatments as well as the specific criteria in the US Food and Drug Administration (FDA) Emergency Use Authorizations (EUAs). For example, many trials of immunomodulatory agents such as interleukin (IL)-6 or Janus kinase (JAK) inhibitors for autoimmune or hematologic processes excluded patients with active infections, but these are not absolute contraindications to their use except in certain types of infections. Patients with a hypercoagulable state or a history of clots were often excluded from the studies of JAK inhibitors due to the risk of clots; however, many patients with COVID-19 who are severely or critically ill are on prophylactic anticoagulation. It is also important to identify if the patients have other acute diseases that either mimic COVID-19 or present concomitantly with COVID-19. Patients can have a positive result of severe acute respiratory syndrome coronavirus 2 (SARS CoV-2) polymerase chain reaction (PCR) from a nasopharyngeal sample, and present with pulmonary diseases caused by a bacterial pneumonia or pulmonary edema. Patients with COVID-19 can also have pulmonary embolism contributing to their symptoms and hypoxemia. It is important to avoid anchoring bias to COVID-19 and consider other causes. Many of the COVID-19 therapies have an EUA from the US FDA, rather than a full approval, so it is necessary to follow the scope of the authorization for these agents.

Here we provide a review of treatment options by class based on a patient's current clinical stage of disease with a focus on agents that have efficacy demonstrated through well-designed randomized controlled trials (RCTs). In this review, we focus on a few important therapeutic options for the management of patients with COVID-19, and pooled estimates of treatment effect are derived from the IDSA guidelines. **Table 1** is a summary table of treatments available in the United States. Preexposure and postexposure prophylaxis, as well as anticoagulation, are outside the scope of this review and are discussed. Because the evidence behind the guidelines and the guidelines themselves are rapidly being updated, we encourage readers to refer to the continuously updated IDSA and National Institutes of Health guidelines.

MANAGEMENT OF AMBULATORY PATIENTS WITH MILD OR MODERATE CORONAVIRUS DISEASE 2019 WHO ARE AT RISK FOR SEVERE DISEASE

The disease severity for ambulatory patients with COVID-19 can range from asymptomatic to severe disease. Recommendations for ambulatory patients who are asymptomatic or have mild to moderate disease and have risk factors for severe disease should be promptly identified and treated. Mild COVID-19 is when there are clinical features suggestive of upper respiratory tract involvement without features of lung or other end organ involvement. Moderate COVID-19 includes pulmonary involvement without hypoxia. Most patients improve with supportive care at this stage, but patients

Table 1
Currently available coronavirus disease 2019 therapies by disease severity and care location

Care Location and COVID-19 Severity	Pharmacologic Treatments Available in the United States
Ambulatory mild to moderate disease (not hypoxic)	• Casirivimab/imdevimab, bamlanivimab/etesevimab, sotrovimab, or bebtelovimabfor high-risk patients. • Systemic glucocorticoids have no demonstrated benefit and may harm. • No clear benefit for convalescent plasma, hydroxychloroquine, azithromycin, lopinavir/ritonavir, or ivermectin.
Hospitalized for mild to moderate COVID-19 (not hypoxic)	• Systemic glucocorticoids have no demonstrated benefit and may harm. • Casirivimab/imdevimab, bamlanivimab/etesevimab, sotrovimab, bebtelovimab: no FDA approval or emergency use authorization for inpatient use. • No clear benefit for convalescent plasma, hydroxychloroquine, azithromycin, lopinavir/ritonavir, or ivermectin.
Hospitalized for severe, but not critical, COVID-19 (hypoxic needing low-flow supplemental oxygen)	• Glucocorticoids (dexamethasone 6 mg daily for 10 days or until discharge or an equivalent dose of hydrocortisone). • May consider remdesivir. • Tocilizumab or sarilumab in progressive disease & elevated inflammatory makers. • Baricitinib or tofacitinib in patients with elevated inflammatory markers. • No clear benefit for convalescent plasma, hydroxychloroquine, azithromycin, lopinavir/ritonavir, or ivermectin.
Hospitalized for critically ill COVID-19, needing noninvasive ventilation or high-flow oxygen	• Glucocorticoids (dexamethasone 6 mg daily for 10 days or until discharge or an equivalent dose of hydrocortisone). • Tocilizumab or sarilumab in progressive disease & elevated inflammatory makers. • Baricitinib or tofacitinib in patients with elevated inflammatory markers • No clear benefit for convalescent plasma, hydroxychloroquine, azithromycin, lopinavir/ritonavir, or ivermectin.
Hospitalized for critically ill COVID-19, needing invasive mechanical ventilation or ECMO	• Glucocorticoids (dexamethasone6 mg daily for 10 days or until discharge or an equivalent dose of hydrocortisone. • Tocilizumab or sarilumab in progressive disease & elevated inflammatory makers. • Baricitinib or tofacitinib in patients with elevated inflammatory markers. • No clear benefit for hydroxychloroquine, azithromycin, Lopinavir/ritonavir and remdesivir. • No clear benefit for convalescent plasma, hydroxychloroquine, azithromycin, lopinavir/ritonavir, or ivermectin.

Abbreviation: ECMO, extracorporeal membrane oxygenation.

with risk factors can progress to more severe or critical disease or death and may benefit from pharmacotherapies. There are no universally accepted clinical prediction rules or risk calculators, but the US FDA EUAs mention a few of these risk factors to consider for treatment with anti-SARS CoV-2 antibodies. More research is needed to identify precise prediction instruments and determinants that both increase and decrease the risk of severe disease and how potentially protective factors like prior infection or vaccination influence risk stratification. Other potential benefits include use of antiviral and antibody therapies in early disease to reduce symptom duration, period of infectivity, and the risk of postacute sequelae of COVID-19, although impact on these outcomes has not been established and is an area of active inquiry.

Certain interventions may provide more benefit and less harm, depending on the patient's severity of disease.

NEUTRALIZING MONOCLONAL ANTIBODY TREATMENTS

These agents interact with the receptor-binding domain of the spike glycoprotein of SARS CoV-2. Neutralizing antibodies directed at SARS-CoV-2 have been derived from convalescent plasma, recombinant approaches using humanized mice, or a combination of the approaches. Modifications to various portions of the antibody can provide advantages that can alter the pharmacokinetics of the various compounds and may be more or less active against potential variants. Bamlanivimab was the first available neutralizing antibody, and it was given FDA EUA status as monotherapy for COVID-19 treatment of those at high risk for severe disease in November 2020. Issuance of the EUA was based on data from the phase 2 BLAZE-1 trial in which bamlanivimab was compared with placebo.[6] Owing to the emergence of viral variants and availability of combination neutralizing antibodies, the US FDA revoked the EUA for bamlanivimab monotherapy on April 16, 2021.

Combining 2 antibodies such as bamlanivimab/etesevimab or casirivimab/imdevimab or developing antibodies that target the highly conserved regions of SARS CoV-2 may help to overcome any decrease in activity due to circulating variants.[7] Similarly, neutralizing antibodies like sotrovimab, which target the highly conserved region of the spike receptor-binding domain, may offer an advantage against circulating variants. Sotrovimab has been shown to neutralize SARS CoV-2 in vitro, including variants of concern.[8]

In ambulatory patients with mild to moderate COVID-19 who are at high risk for progression to severe disease, early intervention with neutralizing monoclonal antibody treatments has been shown to reduce mortality,[9] progression to hospitalization,[9–11] and severe disease.[11] Three neutralizing monoclonal antibody treatments, bamlanivimab/etesevimab, casirivimab/imdevimab, and sotrovimab have been granted EUA for the treatment of COVID-19 in those patients who are at high risk for severe disease. The IDSA treatment guidelines suggest using these agents rather than no neutralizing monoclonal antibody treatment in ambulatory patients with mild to moderate COVID-19 at high risk for progression to severe disease[4]; however, it is important to ensure that the neutralizing antibodies are active against the locally circulating variants. **Fig. 2** lists the risk factors for the progression to severe COVID-19 or hospitalization per US FDA EUA.

Neutralizing monoclonal antibody treatments are well tolerated; however, these agents require an intravenous infusion or other parenteral route of injection, and monitoring for 1 hour postadministration. The Centers for Disease Control and Prevention recommends that those receiving neutralizing monoclonal antibodies should wait to receive a COVID vaccine for at least 90 days after administration.[12]

The following medical conditions or other factors may place adults and pediatric patients (age 12–17 y and weighing at least 40 kg) at higher risk for progression to severe COVID-19:

- Older age (for example ≥65 y of age)
- Obesity or being overweight (for example, adults with BMI >25 kg/m², or if age 12–17, have BMI ≥85th percentile for their age and gender based on CDC growth charts
- Pregnancy
- Chronic kidney disease
- Diabetes
- Immunosuppressive disease or immunosuppressive treatment
- Cardiovascular disease (including congenital heart disease) or hypertension
- Chronic lung diseases (for example, chronic obstructive pulmonary disease, asthma [moderate-to-severe], interstitial lung disease, cystic fibrosis and pulmonary hypertension)
- Sickle cell disease
- Neurodevelopmental disorders (for example, cerebral palsy) or other conditions that confer medical complexity (for example, genetic or metabolic syndromes and severe congenital anomalies)
- Having a medical-related technological dependence (for example, tracheostomy, gastrostomy, or positive pressure ventilation [not related to COVID-19])

Fig. 2. Risk factors and conditions placing adults and pediatric patients at higher risk for progression to severe COVID-19 per FDA EUA.

ANTIVIRAL AGENTS FOR AMBULATORY PATIENTS WITH MILD OR MODERATE CORONAVIRUS DISEASE 2019

In late 2021, several oral antiviral agents were authorized by the US FDA. Logistical challenges associated with infusion of neutralizing antibody treatments may be lessened with the availability of easier-to-administer oral antiviral agents.

Molnupiravir

Molnupiravir is an oral antiviral that targets the genetic machinery that is responsible for SARS COV-2 viral replication. Molnupiravir is an oral prodrug that is converted to its active form and acts as a substrate for RNA-dependent RNA polymerase. After it is incorporated into the viral RNA, serial mutations develop, resulting in a virus that is less fit for ongoing viral replication.[13] In the MOVe-OUT trial, patients at risk for severe COVID-19 were randomized to molnupiravir or placebo. In an interim analysis, patients receiving molnupiravir had a lower risk of hospitalization or death through day 29, compared with placebo (relative risk, 0.52; 95% confidence interval [CI], 0.33, 0.80)[14]; however, in the final results, the benefits of molnupiravir were diminished. Mortality was lower in patients receiving molnupiravir (RR, 0.11; 95% CI, 0.01, 0.86); however, mortality events were sparse.[15] Molnupiravir was granted US FDA EUA on December 23, 2021, for the treatment of patients with mild to moderate COVID-19 who are at high risk for progression to severe disease when there are no other alternative COVID-19 treatments available.[16] Molnupiravir should not be used in pregnant individuals due to evidence of fetal harm in animal studies.[17] Molnupiravir must be initiated within 5 days of symptom onset.

Nirmatrelvir/Ritonavir

Nirmatrelvir/ritonavir (Paxlovid), a combination of a novel SARS CoV-2 protease inhibitor, nirmatrelvir, and low dose of the human immunodeficiency virus protease ritonavir, used as a pharmacokinetic booster, was granted US FDA EUA on December 22, 2021.[18] Data for authorization are based on results from the EPIC-HR study, which was a randomized trial of nirmatrelvir/ritonavir compared with placebo in nonhospitalized adult patients with COVID-19 at high risk for severe disease. Nirmatrelvir/ritonavir reduced COVID-19-related hospitalization compared with placebo (RR, 0.12; 95% CI, 0.06, 0.26). Similarly, there were no deaths in those who received nirmatrelvir/ritonavir, whereas there were 12 deaths in the placebo group.[19] Given the use of ritonavir as a boosting agent, there are significant drug interactions even with short-course therapy that need careful management, specifically with drugs that are metabolized by CYP3A4. Nirmatrelvir also requires renal dose adjustment in those with moderate renal impairment and is not recommended in those with severe renal impairment.

Remdesivir

Remdesivir may be considered in ambulatory patients with mild to moderate COVID-19 who are at risk for progression to severe disease or death, but it should be initiated within 7 days of symptom onset. In the PINETREE trial, treatment with remdesivir for 3 days, compared with placebo in ambulatory patients showed a reduction in hospitalizations (hazard ratio [HR], 0.28; 95% CI, 0.1, 0.75) and COVID-19-related medically attended visits though day 28 (HR, 0.19; 95% CI, 0.07, 0.56).[20] Administering 3 consecutive days of infusions has significant resource and access challenges but should be considered for high-risk populations if more accessible alternatives are not available.

REPURPOSED TREATMENTS
Fluvoxamine

Selective serotonin reuptake inhibitors (SSRIs) may play a role in systemic inflammation given their affinity for the sigma-1 receptor. Fluvoxamine has been shown to have the highest affinity for these receptors compared with other SSRIs,[21] and inhibition of sigma-1 receptors by fluvoxamine resulted in cytokine release in preclinical models of bacterial infection.[22] SSRIs also have been shown to decrease platelet aggregation and neutrophil activation,[23,24] which may mitigate inflammatory and thrombotic events related to COVID-19. In vitro models suggest that fluvoxamine has also demonstrated enhanced viral endocytosis of the SARS CoV-2 spike protein.[25]

Two RCTs have evaluated the SSRI fluvoxamine in the management of COVID-19 in ambulatory patients with a diagnostic test positive for SARS CoV-2 infection.[26,27] The 2 trials compared fluvoxamine 100 mg either 2 or 3 times per day with placebo. Both trials reported on mortality by day 28 (IDSA guidelines pooled relative risk [2 studies]; RR, 0.69; 95% CI, 0.38, 1.27; low certainty of evidence) and hospitalization by day 28 (IDSA guidelines pooled relative risk [2 studies]; RR, 0.75; 95% CI. 0.57, 0.99; low certainty of evidence). The primary outcome of the TOGETHER trial was a composite outcome of a prolonged emergency room visit or hospitalization through day 28. In the composite outcome, patients who received fluvoxamine had a lower relative risk of emergency room visit/hospitalization compared with placebo (RR, 0.68; 95% CI, 0.52, 0.88); however, the difference in the composite outcome was largely driven by emergency room visits lasting greater than 6 hours. Given the resource constraints in Brazil during the time of the TOGETHER study, it is unclear if these results would be generalizable to other settings. STOP-COVID 2 was a contactless, randomized trial in outpatients with SARS CoV-2 that compared fluvoxamine with placebo that was stopped prematurely for futility when fluvoxamine was no different from placebo in the outcome of clinical deterioration. In addition, it became difficult to enroll in this study with the widespread availability of vaccines and outpatient monoclonal antibodies.[28]

WHAT NOT TO USE IN AMBULATORY PATIENTS WITH MILD OR MODERATE CORONAVIRUS DISEASE 2019

Hydroxychloroquine, azithromycin, and lopinavir/ritonavir have not shown evidence of benefit in RCTs.[4,29] Although there are several reported studies evaluating ivermectin in ambulatory patients with COVID-19, there does not seem to be any meaningful benefit on mortality or progression to severe disease.[4] There is a need for well-done clinical trials to evaluate ivermectin's utility for the treatment of COVID-19, and some of the early reports showing benefit have since been retracted.[30] Use of systemic glucocorticoids in mild to moderate COVID-19 may be harmful. Although the RECOVERY trial was not done in ambulatory patients, and was conducted in hospitalized patients, it demonstrated a trend to increase mortality when used in patients with mild to moderate COVID-19 (RR, 1.19; 95% CI, 0.92, 1.55).[3]

PHARMACOLOGIC TREATMENT OF PATIENTS HOSPITALIZED FOR MILD OR MODERATE CORONAVIRUS DISEASE 2019
Neutralizing Monoclonal Antibody Treatments

The US FDA has not authorized the neutralizing monoclonal antibody treatments for patients admitted to the hospital for COVID-19. The ACTIV-3 study was an early trial of bamlanivimab for the management of hospitalized patients with COVID-19.[31] In this trial, a single dose of bamlanivimab 7000 mg was compared with placebo in hospitalized patients who were positive for SARS CoV-2 who had a duration of illness less than or equal to 12 days. In this trial, more than 50% of patients in each group were on supplemental oxygen at baseline. Enrollment of this trial was stopped prematurely when the prespecified futility criteria were met and data were censored on October 26, 2020. Patients receiving bamlanivimab had a higher risk of mortality compared with those who did not receive bamlanivimab (HR, 2.00; 95% CI, 0.67, 5.99). The IDSA guideline panel has strongly recommended against the use of bamlanivimab in hospitalized patients based on the lack of clinical benefit demonstrated.[4] To date, EUAs for all neutralizing antibodies have excluded patients who are hospitalized due to COVID-19, who require oxygen therapy, or who require an increase in baseline oxygen flow due to COVID-19.

In the RECOVERY trial, hospitalized patients with COVID-19 were randomized to a single dose of casirivimab/imdevimab or usual care. In the overall population, there was no mortality benefit at 28 days; however, a prespecified analysis done before unblinding tested the hypothesis that casirivimab/imdevimab would be more beneficial in patients who tested negative for SARS CoV-2 antibodies. In this analysis, in seronegative patients, casirivimab/imdevimab conferred a mortality benefit compared with standard of care (RR, 0.80; 95% CI, 0.70, 0.91).[32] Two subsequent arms of the ACTIV-3 study, including sotrovimab or Brii-196 and Brii-198 were also stopped when futility criteria were met, and there was no clear signal toward benefit for patients in either of these arms who tested negative for SARS-CoV-2 antibodies at the time of randomization.[31] At present, no neutralizing monoclonal antibodies have EUA or US FDA approval for patients hospitalized due to COVID or with severe COVID.

Convalescent Plasma

Convalescent plasma has been used as a treatment of COVID-19 since the early days of the pandemic; it works similar to neutralizing antibodies as a passive immunotherapy, where naturally derived antibodies from the convalescent donor infused into an infected patient may inhibit viral entry into cells or assist in viral phagocytosis or antibody-dependent cellular cytotoxicity.

RCTs in hospitalized patients have demonstrated that convalescent plasma has no effect on mortality compared with no treatment (IDSA guidelines pooled relative risk [18 studies]: RR, 0.98; 95% CI, 0.93, 1.03; moderate certainty of evidence). In hospitalized patients who receive convalescent plasma compared with those who do not, data suggest a worrying trend toward an increase in the need for mechanical ventilation ([4 studies]; RR, 1.10; 95% CI, 0.94, 1.29; low certainty of evidence) and an increase in the risk of adverse events ([11 studies], RR, 1.08; 95% CI, 0.94, 1.26).

PHARMACOLOGIC TREATMENT OF SEVERE CORONAVIRUS DISEASE 2019

Patients with severe COVID-19 are those who have pulmonary disease with hypoxia on room air needing treatment with low-flow oxygen. Most existing criteria for trials consider an oxygen saturation as measured by pulse oximetry level less than 94% or 90% and tachypnea (respiratory rate >30) as severe COVID-19. Such criteria help standardize classification in trials, but by no means do they capture the complexity of COVID-19 severity, so clinical judgment should supplement such criteria.

Certain patients develop proinflammatory state characterized by a clinical worsening approximately 7 to 10 days after onset of symptoms. This worsening can be characterized by increasing oxygen requirements and the development of acute respiratory distress syndrome as well as symptoms of hypoperfusion, which may result in progressive organ failure, and complications may involve multiple organ systems (see Winkler and colleagues' article, "Infection Prevention and Control of SARS-CoV-2 In Healthcare Settings," in this issue). Typically, this syndrome is marked by increasing systemic markers of inflammation like C-reactive protein (CRP), D-dimer, ferritin, as well as proinflammatory cytokines.[33,34]

Antivirals

Remdesivir may be considered in patients hospitalized with severe COVID-19, because in the trial ACCT-1 it showed early recovery or time to discharge. However, it did not show a mortality benefit based on a pooled analysis of 3 studies by the IDSA guideline panel (RR, 0.92; 95% CI, 0.77, 1.10).[35–37] Unfortunately, given the varied outcomes of these trials pooling of nonmortal events like clinical improvement was not possible; however, there was a trend toward greater clinical improvement at day 28[37] and reduced need for mechanical ventilation[36] in patients receiving remdesivir.

Remdesivir is solubilized in a vehicle that is renally eliminated, and remdesivir is not recommended for patients with an estimated glomerular filtration rate of less than 30 mL/min. Case series are available to support the use in creatinine clearance less than 30 mL/min[38–40]; however, pharmacovigilance reports provide evidence for adverse renal outcomes,[41,42] so providers must assess the risk versus benefit of remdesivir use and consultation with pharmacy colleagues is recommended. Transaminase elevations may occur with remdesivir, and clinicians should consider discontinuing use if alanine aminotransferase levels increase to greater than 10 times the upper limit of normal.

Glucocorticoids

Glucocorticoids, especially dexamethasone, have demonstrated a mortality benefit, and their use is recommended by the IDSA guidelines for severe or critical illness. In the RECOVERY trial,[3] patients were randomized with dexamethasone 6 mg daily for 10 days or usual care. Patients receiving dexamethasone had a lower risk of death (RR, 0.83; 95% CI, 0.74, 0.92) and were more likely to be discharged from the hospital through day 28 (RR, 1.11; 95% CI, 1.04, 1.19). Glucocorticoids are generally well tolerated; however, patients may experience significant hyperglycemia.

Interleukin-6 antagonists

Several agents have been studied to attempt to reduce the impact of the inflammatory cascade on disease course. Tocilizumab is the most frequently studied IL-6 antagonist in RCTs. To date there are 8 RCTs evaluating tocilizumab compared with no tocilizumab in the management of COVID-19. Although enrollment criteria for these studies varied, studies included hospitalized patients with evidence of pneumonia or severe disease. In the 8 randomized trials, there is a trend toward reduced mortality at day 28 in those who receive tocilizumab compared with no tocilizumab (IDSA guidelines pooled relative risk [8 studies] RR, 0.91, 95% CI, 0.79, 1.04; moderate certainty of evidence). Two studies that seem to show the largest effect on the reduction of mortality included patients who received tocilizumab around the time of an escalation in their oxygen requirements[43,44]; this may indicate that the timing of tocilizumab therapy is an important factor; however, this needs to be evaluated a priori in clinical trials. After pooling of all the RCTs, patients receiving tocilizumab are less likely to develop clinical deterioration, which was characterized by progression to mechanical ventilation or death in most of the trials (IDSA guidelines pooled relative risk [7 studies]; RR, 0.83, 95% CI, 0.77, 0.89; moderate certainty of evidence).

Unfortunately, there have been shortages of tocilizumab, leading frontline clinicians to look for alternative agents. Sarilumab is another IL-6 inhibitor that is being evaluated for the management of severe COVID-19. The IDSA guidelines suggest the use of sarilumab in those who would otherwise qualify for tocilizumab in addition to standard of care, rather than standard of care alone, when tocilizumab is not available. Data from 3 RCTs and network meta-analysis support this recommendation.[43,45–47]

Janus Kinase Inhibitors

JAK are a group of kinases expressed on many cell surfaces that mediate cytokine signaling. JAK1 and JAK2 inhibitors have been developed and used in inflammatory conditions such as rheumatoid arthritis and ulcerative colitis. The most studied JAK inhibitor in the management of COVID-19 is baricitinib. In the ACTT-2 trial,[48] baricitinib combined with remdesivir was compared with remdesivir with placebo. Notably, study participants were prohibited from receiving glucocorticoids for COVID-19. These data have limited applicability given the widespread use of glucocorticoids in the management of severe COVID-19; however, this study provides guidance into treatment options for those in whom glucocorticoids are contraindicated.

In a large RCT, the COV-BARRIER trial,[49] patients with severe COVID-19 and elevated inflammatory markers were randomized to receive renally dosed baricitinib or no baricitinib. Mortality at day 60 was lower in those receiving baricitinib compared with no baricitinib (HR, 0.62; 95% CI, 0.47–0.83; moderate certainty of evidence). Of note, more than two-thirds of study participants received glucocorticoids.

Tofacitinib has also been evaluated in the STOP-COVID trial in which it was compared with placebo in recently hospitalized patients with PCR-confirmed COVID-19 pneumonia.[50] In this trial, patients receiving tofacitinib had a lower risk of a composite end point of death or respiratory failure at 28 days, compared with participants who did not receive tofacitinib (RR, 0.63; 95% CI, 0.41, 0.97). Owing to the limited number of mortal events, one cannot exclude a beneficial or harmful effect on mortality (RR, 0.49; 95% CI, 0.15, 1.63). Similarly, the study was not able to exclude a beneficial or harmful effect on progression to mechanical ventilation or extracorporeal membrane oxygenation (ECMO) (RR, 0.25; 95% CI, 0.03, 2.20). Participants receiving tofacitinib experienced numerically more serious adverse events by day 28. Unfortunately, this study excluded patients with an immunosuppressive condition so the results should not be generalized to that population which is at risk for severe COVID-19. In addition, the results from the COV-BARRIER and STOP-COVID trials should not be generalized to other JAK inhibitors, such as ruxolitinib, because currently available data do not suggest a clinical benefit.[51,52]

The US FDA has issued a drug safety communication for tofacitinib after the review of a large, randomized safety trial. Their results indicated an increased risk of serious heart-related events such as heart attack or stroke, cancer, blood clots, and death when tofacitinib is used for ulcerative colitis or arthritis. Given the shared mechanism of action, the US FDA broadened its warnings to include other agents used for rheumatoid arthritis and include baricitinib and upadacitinib.[53]

Baricitinib requires renal dose adjustment; see **Table 2** for dosing.

PHARMACOLOGIC TREATMENT OF PATIENTS WITH CORONAVIRUS DISEASE 2019 NEEDING NONINVASIVE VENTILATION OR HIGH-FLOW OXYGEN

This severity of critically ill patients requires more ventilator or oxygenation support, with either high-flow oxygen or noninvasive ventilation. High-flow oxygen therapy involves delivery of oxygen via special devices at rates up to 10 to 15 L/min.

We strongly recommend systemic glucocorticoids in critically ill patients with COVID-19 because they have shown the highest 28-day mortality benefit when used in this subpopulation (odds ratio [OR], 0.66; 95% CI, 0.54; 0.82).[54] In critically ill patients, dexamethasone 6 mg daily for 10 days is preferred, but doses up to 20 mg daily can be used if indicated for other reasons. Hydrocortisone 50 mg administered intravenously every 6 hours is an alternative that can also be considered. Safety data in critically ill patients is reassuring.[47]

In addition to glucocorticoids, we recommend using either IL-6 inhibitors (tocilizumab preferred over sarilumab) or JAK inhibitors (baricitinib preferred over tofacitinib) in those patients who have elevated levels of inflammatory markers like CRP. The trials done so far have not identified specific subpopulations of critically ill patients already being treated with corticosteroids that would benefit with additional treatment with IL-6 or JAK inhibitors.

PHARMACOLOGIC TREATMENT OF PATIENTS WITH CORONAVIRUS DISEASE 2019 NEEDING INVASIVE MECHANICAL VENTILATION OR EXTRACORPOREAL MEMBRANE OXYGENATION
Glucocorticoids

The IDSA guidelines recommend dexamethasone rather than no dexamethasone in critically ill patients with COVID-19. Data supporting this recommendation is based on a systematic review of 7 RCTs that demonstrated a reduction in the odds of mortality in patients treated with glucocorticoids compared with those not treated with glucocorticoids (OR, 0.66; 95% CI, 0.54, 0.82). In addition, patients who received glucocorticoids were more likely to be discharged from the hospital through day 28, compared with those who did not receive glucocorticoids (RR, 1.11; 95% CI: 1.04, 1.19).

Interleukin-6 Inhibitors

To date, there are no randomized trials specifically comparing IL-6 inhibitors with not using IL-6 inhibitors in those on mechanical ventilation and/or ECMO; however,

Table 2 Renal dosing baricitinib		
eGFR Range	Adults and Pediatric Patients 9 y and Older	Pediatric Patients 2–9 y
eGFR ≥ 60 mL/	4 mg once daily	2 mg once daily
eGFR 30 to < 60 mL/min	2 mg once daily	1 mg once daily
eGFR 15 to < 30 mL/min	1 mg once daily	Not recommended
eGFR < 15	Not recommended	Not recommended

Several trials included patients on mechanical ventilation at baseline[43,44,55,56] and many studies allowed for patients to receive glucocorticoids for COVID-19. The IDSA guidelines suggest the use of tocilizumab in addition to the standard of care, rather than standard of care alone. Systemic inflammatory markers are often elevated in critically ill patients with COVID-19; however, there is no randomized trial data to demonstrate a specific cutoff for CRP that would indicate the appropriate patient for tocilizumab. In RECOVERY, patients were required to have a CRP of 75 mg/L or greater to be included in the IL-6 arm.

Janus Kinase Inhibitors

The role of baricitinib in critically ill patients on invasive mechanical ventilation or ECMO was evaluated in an addendum to the COV-Barrier study.[57] In this small trial with about 50 patients per arm, participants who were on invasive mechanical ventilation or ECMO and at least 1 elevated inflammatory marker were randomized 1:1 to receive baricitinib or standard of care. In this study, there was a reduction in the 60-day mortality rate in those who received baricitinib compared with no baricitinib (RR, 0.56; 95% CI, 0.47, 0.97).

Antivirals

The IDSA guideline does not suggest the use of remdesivir in patients with COVID-19 who are critically ill because the subgroup analysis of ACCT-1 failed to demonstrate a reduction in mortality (RR, 1.23; 95% CI, 0.99, 1.53) in mechanically ventilated patients.[36] Results also failed to demonstrate a beneficial effect of remdesivir on time to clinical recovery (HR, 0.98; 95% CI, 0.70, 1.36).

SUMMARY

It is important for frontline clinicians managing patients with COVID-19 to evaluate the setting as well as the severity of illness for each patient. Agile clinical guidelines are available to inform clinicians about place in therapy for various treatment options. Rigorous guideline methodologies, like GRADE, can be applied in the setting of rapidly emerging and evolving literature to support clinicians and guide decision making.

CLINICS CARE POINTS

- Treating providers must assess each patient's severity of COVID-19 and apply the treatment guidelines based on the clinical severity. Treatments directed at ambulatory patients with COVID-19 are generally recommended for those who are at high risk for progression to severe disease, death, or hospitalization.

- Most patients with mild to moderate disease without risk factors for progression to severe disease will improve without COVID-19 pharmacotherapy.
- The efficacy of neutralizing monoclonal antibodies demonstrated in clinical trials may not be equivalent to the overall effectiveness in real-life settings due to the emergence of circulating variants with reduced susceptibility.
- The ease of use of the oral antivirals may be limited by clinically significant drug interactions with nirmatrelvir/ritonavir and due to reproductive health concerns with molnupiravir.
- Patients with severe COVID-19 appear to benefit from glucocorticoids, baricitinib, interleukin-6 inhibitors, and remdesivir; however additional studies are needed to determine the optimal timing and combination of these agents.

DISCLOSURE

A. H. Shumaker and A. Bhimraj: The authors have nothing to disclose.

REFERENCES

1. Consortium WST. Repurposed Antiviral Drugs for Covid-19 — Interim WHO Solidarity Trial Results. N Engl J Med 2020. https://doi.org/10.1056/NEJMoa2023184.
2. Group TRC. Effect of Hydroxychloroquine in Hospitalized Patients with Covid-19. N Engl J Med 2020. https://doi.org/10.1056/NEJMoa2022926.
3. Dexamethasone in Hospitalized Patients with Covid-19. N Engl J Med 2021; 384(8):693–704.
4. idsa-covid-19-gl-tx-and-mgmt-v5.6.0.pdf. Available at: https://www.idsociety.org/globalassets/idsa/practice-guidelines/covid-19/treatment/idsa-covid-19-gl-tx-and-mgmt-v5.6.0.pdf. Accessed November 21, 2021.
5. National Institutes of Health COVID-19 Treatment Guidelines. National Institutes of Health COVID-19 Treatment Guidelines. Available at: https://www.covid19treatmentguidelines.nih.gov/. Accessed November 21, 2021.
6. SARS-CoV-2 Neutralizing Antibody LY-CoV555 in Outpatients with Covid-19 | NEJM. Available at: https://www.nejm.org/doi/10.1056/NEJMoa2029849. Accessed November 21, 2021.
7. Hurt AC, Wheatley AK. Neutralizing Antibody Therapeutics for COVID-19. Viruses 2021;13(4):628.
8. Pinto D, Park YJ, Beltramello M, et al. Cross-neutralization of SARS-CoV-2 by a human monoclonal SARS-CoV antibody. Nature 2020;583(7815):290–5.
9. Dougan M, Nirula A, Azizad M, et al. Bamlanivimab plus Etesevimab in Mild or Moderate Covid-19. N Engl J Med 2021;385(15):1382–92.
10. Weinreich DM, Sivapalasingam S, Norton T, et al. REGN-COV2, a Neutralizing Antibody Cocktail, in Outpatients with Covid-19. N Engl J Med 2021;384(3): 238–51.
11. Gupta A, Gonzalez-Rojas Y, Juarez E, et al. Early Treatment for Covid-19 with SARS-CoV-2 Neutralizing Antibody Sotrovimab. N Engl J Med 2021;385(21): 1941–50.
12. COVID-19 Vaccine FAQs for Healthcare Professionals | CDC. 2021. Available at: https://www.cdc.gov/vaccines/covid-19/hcp/faq.html. Accessed November 22, 2021.
13. Kabinger F, Stiller C, Schmitzová J, et al. Mechanism of molnupiravir-induced SARS-CoV-2 mutagenesis. Nat Struct Mol Biol 2021;28(9):740–6.

14. Merck and Ridgeback's Investigational Oral Antiviral Molnupiravir Reduced the Risk of Hospitalization or Death by Approximately 50 Percent Compared to Placebo for Patients with Mild or Moderate COVID-19 in Positive Interim Analysis of Phase 3 Study.. Available at: Merck.com https://www.merck.com/news/merck-and-ridgebacks-investigational-oral-antiviral-molnupiravir-reduced-the-risk-of-hospitalization-or-death-by-approximately-50-percent-compared-to-placebo-for-patients-with-mild-or-moderat/. Accessed November 21, 2021.
15. Jayk Bernal A, Gomes da Silva MM, Musungaie DB, et al. Molnupiravir for Oral Treatment of Covid-19 in Nonhospitalized Patients. N Engl J Med 2021. https://doi.org/10.1056/NEJMoa2116044. NEJMoa2116044.
16. Available at: https://www.fda.gov/media/155053/download. Accessed January 17, 2022.
17. Zhou S, Hill CS, Sarkar S, et al. β-d-N4-hydroxycytidine Inhibits SARS-CoV-2 Through Lethal Mutagenesis But Is Also Mutagenic To Mammalian Cells. J Infect Dis 2021;224(3):415–9.
18. Available at: https://www.fda.gov/media/155049/download. Accessed January 17, 2022.
19. Available at: https://www.fda.gov/media/155194/download. Accessed January 17, 2022.
20. Gottlieb RL, Vaca CE, Paredes R, et al. Early Remdesivir to Prevent Progression to Severe Covid-19 in Outpatients. N Engl J Med 2021. https://doi.org/10.1056/NEJMoa2116846.
21. Narita N, Hashimoto K, Tomitaka S, et al. Interactions of selective serotonin reuptake inhibitors with subtypes of sigma receptors in rat brain. Eur J Pharmacol 1996;307(1):117–9.
22. Rosen DA, Seki SM, Fernández-Castañeda A, et al. Modulation of the sigma-1 receptor–IRE1 pathway is beneficial in preclinical models of inflammation and sepsis. Sci Transl Med 2019;11(478). https://doi.org/10.1126/scitranslmed.aau5266. eaau5266.
23. McCloskey DJ, Postolache TT, Vittone BJ, et al. Selective serotonin reuptake inhibitors: measurement of effect on platelet function. Transl Res 2008;151(3):168–72.
24. Duerschmied D, Suidan GL, Demers M, et al. Platelet serotonin promotes the recruitment of neutrophils to sites of acute inflammation in mice. Blood 2013;121(6):1008–15.
25. Glebov OO. Low-Dose Fluvoxamine Modulates Endocytic Trafficking of SARS-CoV-2 Spike Protein: A Potential Mechanism for Anti-COVID-19 Protection by Antidepressants. Front Pharmacol 2021;12:787261. https://doi.org/10.3389/fphar.2021.787261.
26. Reis G, Moreira-Silva EA, dos S, et al. Effect of early treatment with fluvoxamine on risk of emergency care and hospitalisation among patients with COVID-19: the TOGETHER randomised, platform clinical trial. Lancet Glob Health 2021;0(0). https://doi.org/10.1016/S2214-109X(21)00448-4.
27. Lenze EJ, Mattar C, Zorumski CF, et al. Fluvoxamine vs Placebo and Clinical Deterioration in Outpatients With Symptomatic COVID-19: A Randomized Clinical Trial. JAMA 2020;324(22):2292–300.
28. Available at: https://dcricollab.dcri.duke.edu/sites/NIHKR/KR/GR-Slides-08-20-21.pdf. Accessed January 25, 2022.
29. Ayerbe L, Risco-Risco C, Forgnone I, et al. Azithromycin in patients with COVID-19: a systematic review and meta-analysis. J Antimicrob Chemother 2021. https://doi.org/10.1093/jac/dkab404. dkab404.

30. Available at: https://www.researchsquare.com/article/rs-100956/v3. Accessed January 20, 2022.
31. Lundgren JD, Grund B, Barkauskas CE, et al, ACTIV-3/TICO LY-CoV555 Study Group. A Neutralizing Monoclonal Antibody for Hospitalized Patients with Covid-19. N Engl J Med 2021;384(10):905–14.
32. Group RC, Horby PW, Mafham M, et al. Casirivimab and imdevimab in patients admitted to hospital with COVID-19 (recovery): a Randomised, controlled, Open-Label. Platform Trial; 2021. https://doi.org/10.1101/2021.06.15.21258542.
33. Mehta P, McAuley DF, Brown M, et al. COVID-19: consider cytokine storm syndromes and immunosuppression. Lancet Lond Engl 2020;395(10229):1033–4.
34. Wang C, Kang K, Gao Y, et al. Cytokine Levels in the Body Fluids of a Patient With COVID-19 and Acute Respiratory Distress Syndrome: A Case Report. Ann Intern Med 2020;173(6):499–501.
35. Pan H, Peto R, Henao-Restrepo AM, et al, WHO Solidarity Trial Consortium. Repurposed Antiviral Drugs for Covid-19 - Interim WHO Solidarity Trial Results. N Engl J Med 2021;384(6):497–511.
36. Beigel JH, Tomashek KM, Dodd LE, et al. Remdesivir for the Treatment of Covid-19 - Final Report. N Engl J Med 2020;383(19):1813–26.
37. Wang Y, Zhang D, Du G, et al. Remdesivir in adults with severe COVID-19: a randomised, double-blind, placebo-controlled, multicentre trial. Lancet 2020; 395(10236):1569–78.
38. Wang S, Huynh C, Islam S, et al. Assessment of Safety of Remdesivir in Covid -19 Patients with Estimated Glomerular Filtration Rate (eGFR) < 30 ml/min per 1.73 m^2. J Intensive Care Med 2021. https://doi.org/10.1177/08850666211070521. 8850666211070521.
39. Biancalana E, Chiriacò M, Sciarrone P, et al. Remdesivir, Renal Function and Short-Term Clinical Outcomes in Elderly COVID-19 Pneumonia Patients: A Single-Centre Study. Clin Interv Aging 2021;16:1037–46.
40. Aiswarya D, Arumugam V, Dineshkumar T, et al. Use of Remdesivir in Patients With COVID-19 on Hemodialysis: A Study of Safety and Tolerance. Kidney Int Rep 2021;6(3):586–93.
41. Rocca E, Gauffin O, Savage R, et al. Remdesivir in the COVID-19 Pandemic: An Analysis of Spontaneous Reports in VigiBase During 2020. Drug Saf 2021;44(9): 987–98.
42. de O Silva NA, de SA Zara AL, Figueras A, et al. Potential kidney damage associated with the use of remdesivir for COVID-19: analysis of a pharmacovigilance database. Cad Saude Publica 2021;37(10):e00077721.
43. REMAP-CAP Investigators, Gordon AC, Mouncey PR, et al. Interleukin-6 Receptor Antagonists in Critically Ill Patients with Covid-19. N Engl J Med 2021;384(16): 1491–502.
44. RECOVERY Collaborative Group. Tocilizumab in patients admitted to hospital with COVID-19 (RECOVERY): a randomised, controlled, open-label, platform trial. Lancet Lond Engl 2021;397(10285):1637–45.
45. Lescure FX, Honda H, Fowler RA, et al. Sarilumab in patients admitted to hospital with severe or critical COVID-19: a randomised, double-blind, placebo-controlled, phase 3 trial. Lancet Respir Med 2021;9(5):522–32.
46. Sivapalasingam S, Lederer DJ, Bhore R, et al. A randomized placebo-controlled trial of sarilumab in hospitalized patients with Covid-19. J Infect Dis 2021. https://doi.org/10.1101/2021.05.13.21256973.
47. Shankar-Hari M, Vale CL, Godolphin PJ, et al, WHO Rapid Evidence Appraisal for COVID-19 Therapies (REACT) Working Group. Association Between

Administration of IL-6 Antagonists and Mortality Among Patients Hospitalized for COVID-19: A Meta-analysis. JAMA 2021;326(6):499–518.

48. Kalil AC, Patterson TF, Mehta AK, et al. Baricitinib plus Remdesivir for Hospitalized Adults with Covid-19. N Engl J Med 2021;384(9):795–807.

49. Marconi VC, Ramanan AV, de Bono S, et al. Efficacy and safety of baricitinib for the treatment of hospitalised adults with COVID-19 (COV-BARRIER): a randomised, double-blind, parallel-group, placebo-controlled phase 3 trial. Lancet Respir Med 2021. https://doi.org/10.1016/S2213-2600(21)00331-3. S2213-2600(21)00331-3.

50. Guimarães PO, Quirk D, Furtado RH, et al. Tofacitinib in Patients Hospitalized with Covid-19 Pneumonia. N Engl J Med 2021;385(5):406–15.

51. Cao Y, Wei J, Zou L, et al. Ruxolitinib in treatment of severe coronavirus disease 2019 (COVID-19): A multicenter, single-blind, randomized controlled trial. J Allergy Clin Immunol 2020;146(1):137–46.e3.

52. Available at: https://clinicaltrials.gov/ct2/show/results/NCT04362137. Accessed January 20, 2022.

53. Commissioner O of the. Janus Kinase (JAK) inhibitors: Drug Safety Communication - FDA Requires Warnings about Increased Risk of Serious Heart-related Events, Cancer, Blood Clots, and Death. FDA 2021. Available at: https://www.fda.gov/safety/medical-product-safety-information/janus-kinase-jak-inhibitors-drug-safety-communication-fda-requires-warnings-about-increased-risk. Accessed November 22, 2021.

54. The WHO Rapid Evidence Appraisal for COVID-19 Therapies (REACT) Working Group. Association Between Administration of Systemic Corticosteroids and Mortality Among Critically Ill Patients With COVID-19: A Meta-analysis. JAMA 2020; 324(13):1330–41.

55. Rosas IO, Bräu N, Waters M, et al. Tocilizumab in Hospitalized Patients with Severe Covid-19 Pneumonia. N Engl J Med 2021;384(16):1503–16.

56. Veiga VC, Prats JAGG, Farias DLC, et al. Effect of tocilizumab on clinical outcomes at 15 days in patients with severe or critical coronavirus disease 2019: randomised controlled trial. BMJ 2021;372:n84. https://doi.org/10.1136/bmj.n84.

57. Ely EW, Ramanan AV, Kartman CE, et al. Baricitinib plus standard of care for Hospitalised adults with COVID-19 on invasive mechanical ventilation or extracorporeal membrane oxygenation: results of a Randomised. Placebo-Controlled Trial; 2021. https://doi.org/10.1101/2021.10.11.21263897.

58. Guyatt GH, Oxman AD, Vist GE, et al. GRADE: an emerging consensus on rating quality of evidence and strength of recommendations. BMJ 2008;336(7650): 924–6. https://doi.org/10.1136/bmj.39489.470347.AD.

COVID-19 in the Critically Ill Patient

Taison D. Bell, MD, MBA[a,b,*]

KEYWORDS

- COVID-19 • COVID • SARS-CoV-2 • Critically ill • Critical care • ARDS
- Acute respiratory distress syndrome • Coronavirus

KEY POINTS

- Severe COVID-19 is characterized by dyspnea, tachypnea, hypoxemia, and bilateral pulmonary infiltrates. The proportion of patients with COVID who develop severe disease has been decreasing over time.
- Age greater than or equal to 65 years is the strongest risk factor for developing severe COVID-19. Additional risk factors include obesity, anxiety disorders and depression, chronic diseases, and complicated diabetes.
- Although the primary driver of critical illness from COVID-19 is the acute respiratory disease syndrome, many other organ systems may be involved due to direct viral injury, hyperinflammatory responses, or complications of critical illness.
- Therapeutic agents generally attempt to target the earlier stage of illness mediated by viral replication or the later inflammatory stages with immunomodulatory agents.

INTRODUCTION

COVID-19 has become the fourth leading cause of mortality worldwide since the beginning of 2020, accounting for just less than 1 in every 20 deaths in the United States. However, when accounting for excess deaths, the estimates could be as high as 1 in every 10 deaths.[1] In the United States, the pandemic caused approximately 375,000 deaths in 2020, which was surpassed in 2021 with more than 450,000 deaths.[2] However, with vaccination, the rate of critical illness and death is dramatically reduced.[3] The epidemiology, pathogenesis, and treatment of severe and critical COVID-19 are discussed in this chapter.

[a] Internal Medicine, Division of Pulmonary/Critical Care, University of Virginia School of Medicine, 310 Maroon Creek Court, Charlottesville, VA 22903, USA; [b] Division of Infectious Diseases and International Health, University of Virginia School of Medicine, 310 Maroon Creek Court, Charlottesville, VA 22903, USA
* Division of Infectious Diseases and International Health, University of Virginia School of Medicine, 310 Maroon Creek Court, Charlottesville, VA 22903.
E-mail address: TDB4C@hscmail.mcc.virginia.edu

Infect Dis Clin N Am 36 (2022) 365–377
https://doi.org/10.1016/j.idc.2022.02.005   **id.theclinics.com**
0891-5520/22/© 2022 Elsevier Inc. All rights reserved.

EPIDEMIOLOGY

For epidemiologic purposes, severe COVID-19 is defined as subjective dyspnea, a respiratory rate of 30 or more breaths per minute, a blood oxygen saturation of 93% or less, a ratio of the partial pressure of arterial oxygen to the fraction of inspired oxygen (Pao_2:Fio_2 or P/F ratio) of less than 300 mm Hg, or infiltrates in more than 50% of the lung field.[4] Studies demonstrate that the proportion of patients infected with SARS-CoV-2 who develop severe COVID-19 requiring hospitalization varies widely and depend on several factors—including geographic differences in admission patterns and population characteristics. Early reports from Wuhan, China suggested admission rates as high as 20% with around 25% of admitted patients needing intensive care (around 5% of all cases).[5,6] Reports from the Lombard region of Italy showed the proportion of intensive care unit (ICU) admissions ranged from to 5% to 16%.[7,8]

The proportion of cases admitted to the ICU seems to be decreasing over time. In Germany the proportion of hospitalized patients requiring ICU care dropped from 30% at the beginning of the year to 14% in December 2020, corresponding to a relative drop of more than 50%.[9] There are several underlying reasons for this trend—including increasing experience managing patient with high oxygen needs outside of the ICU, improvements in therapeutic options, and growing population immunity.

Risk Factors for Severe Disease

Several risk factors have been linked to worse outcomes from COVID-19 (**Table 1**). Age is the strongest risk factor, with those aged 65 years and older representing 81% of US COVID-19–related deaths despite making up around 17% of the population.[2] In an analysis of 540,667 adults hospitalized for COVID-19, 94.9% of admissions were in patients with at least one underlying medical condition. Essential hypertension (50.4%), disorders of lipid metabolism (49.4%), and obesity (33.0%) were the most common conditions.[10(p667)] The strongest risk factors for death were obesity (absolute risk reduction [aRR] = 1.30), anxiety disorders (aRR = 1.28), and diabetes with complication (aRR = 1.26). In addition, the total number of conditions was linked with increased risk for mortality, with aRRs of death ranging from 1.53 for patients with 1 condition to 3.82 for patients with more than 10 conditions (compared with patients with no underlying conditions).

Table 1 Risk factors for severe COVID-19	
Age ≥65 y	Cancer
Cerebrovascular disease	Chronic kidney disease
Chronic lung diseases	Chronic liver disease
Diabetes type 1 and 2	Chronic heart diseases
Immunosuppression	Mental health disorders (schizophrenia, depression, and other mood disorders)
Obesity (BMI≥30 kg/m^2)	Pregnancy and recent pregnancy
Smoking or history of smoking	Tuberculosis

Abbreviation: BMI, body mass index.
Adapted from CDC COVID-19 Response Team. Severe Outcomes Among Patients with Coronavirus Disease 2019 (COVID-19) - United States, February 12-March 16, 2020. MMWR Morb Mortal Wkly Rep. 2020;69(12):343-346. Published 2020 Mar 27. https://doi.org/10.15585/mmwr.mm6912e2.

Racial and Ethnic Disparities

When compared with White populations, higher rates of infection, hospitalization, and death have been observed in Black, Hispanic, and Asian Americans and Pacific Islander (AAPI) populations.[11] According to a Kaiser Family Foundation and the Epic Health Research Network analysis, hospitalization and deaths rates were between 2 and 3 times higher for Black, Hispanic, and AAPI patients.[12] The disparity has been linked with higher rates of chronic conditions and poorer access to health care in marginalized communities.[13] In a study that compared mortality rates due to SARS-CoV-2 infection by race among 11,210 hospitalized adults, there was no difference in all-cause, in-hospital mortality between White and Black patients after adjusting for age, sex, insurance status, comorbidity, neighborhood deprivation, and site of care[14]; this argues against an independent predisposition to severe disease driven by genetics, but rather the impacts of structural racism on health and access to health care in communities of color (see Chapter 4 for further discussion of racial and ethnic disparities in COVID-19).

Protection from Vaccination

The risk of severe COVID is substantially reduced with vaccination. In an observational study of more than 6.5 million individuals in Israel, the BNT162b2 (Pfizer-BioNTech) vaccine demonstrated 97% efficacy for both COVID-19–related hospitalization and COVID-19–related death before the spread of the Delta variant.[15(p2)] Among adults aged 65 years and older, an evaluation of 417 COVID-19–related hospitalizations demonstrated an adjusted vaccine effectiveness of 94% against COVID-19–associated hospitalization for full vaccination and 64% for partial vaccination with either Pfizer-BioNTech or the mRNA-1273 (Moderna) vaccines.[16] In comparison to the mRNA vaccines, a single dose of the Ad26.COV2.S (Johnson and Johnson) vaccine has shown lower efficacy in preventing moderate-to-severe COVID-19. In a phase III efficacy trial, a single dose had 66.9% efficacy in preventing moderate-to-severe/critical COVID-19 beginning at or after 14 days postvaccination.[17] Vaccination against COVID-19 is covered in detail in Chapter 13.

Although vaccination has consistently shown protection from severe outcomes from COVID-19, protection from infection has been shown to wane with the emergence of the Delta and Omicron variants. In a cohort of health care workers, vaccine effectiveness during the Delta predominant period was 66% compared with 91% during the months preceding Delta predominance.[18] Further erosion in vaccine effectiveness have been observed with the Omicron variant,[19] although protection from severe illness remains robust for most vaccine recipients. In an analysis of more than 1 million people who had completed primary vaccination, the risk for severe outcomes was higher among persons who were aged 65 years and older, were immunosuppressed, or had at least 1 of 6 underlying chronic conditions—including pulmonary, liver, kidney, cardiac, neurologic disease, and diabetes mellitus.[20] Further, 78% of those who died had 4 or more risk factors.

PATHOGENESIS AND CLINICAL FEATURES

Although the primary driver of critical illness from COVID-19 is respiratory disease, critical illness can manifest in several ways and affect several organ systems. For critically ill patients there may be multiple mechanisms involved, although a common link to complications stem from hyperinflammatory responses.

Viral-Mediated Phase Versus the Immune-Mediated Phase

COVID-19 is characterized by 3 stages. In the first stage mild symptoms typical of other viral respiratory tract infections predominate. As viral replication continues and the immune response develops, ongoing infection can lead to complications from stage 2 disease, characterized by moderate respiratory symptoms. In the case of mild disease, viral replication decreases during this stage as well as the immune response during convalescence. For patients who subsequently develop worsening disease, a hyperinflammatory state leads to stage 3 disease with acute respiratory distress syndrome (ARDS), which may be complicated by circulatory failure/cardiac failure and multiorgan dysfunction syndrome.[21] Therapeutic agents for COVID generally target the earlier stage of viral replication with antiviral agents or the later stage with immunomodulatory agents.[22]

Pulmonary Manifestations

Viral pneumonia is the most frequent serious manifestation of infection, characterized by fever, cough, dyspnea, and bilateral infiltrates on chest imaging characteristic of ARDS.[5,6] Viral replication in the upper and lower respiratory tract induces cellular death and injury in airway epithelial cells, causing the release of various damage-associated molecular patterns and pathogen-associated molecular patterns. These mediators lead to the induction of proinflammatory cytokines and subsequent filling of the alveolar space, impairing gas exchange and respiratory mechanics.[23] For patients who require mechanical ventilation complications from alveolar stretch injury can occur—such as barotrauma and ventilator induced lung injury, pneumothorax, and pneumomediastinum.[24] Hypercapnia is rare unless there is concomitant chronic obstructive pulmonary disease or a history of narcotic overdose.

Cardiovascular Manifestations

Cardiac injury is a common complication in critically ill patients, especially in those with concomitant severe pulmonary disease. Several mechanisms may be involved, including myocarditis, hypoxia-induced injury, physiologic stress (Takotsubo) cardiomyopathy, vasculopathy, pulmonary embolism, ARDS, shock, and cytokine storm. In one New York City cohort of patients on mechanical ventilation, multiple cardiac complications were described—including arrhythmias (18%), myocardial infarction (8%), and heart failure (2%).[25]

Neurologic Manifestations

Delirium, encephalopathy, and other neurologic manifestations are common findings in critically ill patients with COVID-19. In one review of 214 hospitalized patients in Wuhan, 36.4% had neurologic manifestations. In comparison to patients with nonsevere disease, those with severe infection had a higher chance of neurologic manifestations, such as acute cerebrovascular diseases (5.7% vs 1%), impaired consciousness (14.8% vs 2.4%), and skeletal muscle injury (19.3% vs 4.8%).[26] In a review of critically ill patients in France 13 patients underwent MRI for unexplained encephalopathy without a localizing neurologic examination. Leptomeningeal enhancement was noted in 8 patients (61.5%) and bilateral frontotemporal hypoperfusion was noted in all 11 patients who underwent perfusion imaging. In addition, 2 patients (15.4%) were noted to have acute or subacute ischemic strokes.[27]

Renal Manifestations

Acute kidney injury (AKI) commonly occurrence in patients with critical illness from COVID-19. In a meta-analysis of around 13,000 hospitalized patients the overall prevalence of AKI was 17%, with 5% of overall patients requiring renal replacement therapy. In addition, AKI was associated with an increased odds of death (pooled odds ratio 15.27; 95% confidence interval [CI] 4.82–48.36).[28] The cause of AKI is likely multifactorial and includes virus-mediated injury, cytokine storm, angiotensin II pathway activation, complement activation, hypercoagulation, and microangiopathy interacting with known risk factors for AKI in critically ill patients (**Fig. 1**).[29] In an autopsy series of 42 patients who died from COVID-19, the most common finding on kidney histopathology was acute tubular necrosis.[30]

Gastrointestinal Manifestations

Patients with severe COVID-19 are at high risk for developing a range of gastrointestinal complications, including bowel ischemia, transaminase elevation, acalculous cholecystitis, gastrointestinal bleeding, pancreatitis, Ogilvie syndrome, and severe ileus.[31] In one evaluation of propensity-matched patients of critically ill patients with or without COVID-19, those with COVID-19 were more likely to develop gastrointestinal complications (74% vs 37%). Specifically, patients with COVID-19 developed more transaminase elevation (55% vs 27%), severe ileus (48% vs 22%), and bowel ischemia (4% vs 0%).[32]

Thrombosis and Vasculopathy

Estimates of venous thromboembolism (VTE) in critically ill patients with COVID-19 have varied widely but seem to have declined from 20% to 25% in the earlier phase of the pandemic to around 7% to 15%.[33–36] Rates of deep venous thrombosis have generally been higher in studies that routinely perform surveillance. The mechanism of hypercoagulability is likely related to endothelial injury, microvascular inflammation, immobilization in critically ill patients, and microangiopathy.[37] In many instances, VTE has been noted despite the routine use of prophylactic anticoagulation. The American Society of Hematology recommends routine prophylactic intensity pharmacologic prophylaxis over intermediate or therapeutic anticoagulation, as trials demonstrated an increased risk of bleeding without mortality benefit among critically ill patients.[38] Select patients may benefit from therapeutic dose anticoagulation.[39]

Secondary Infection

Prolonged ICU admissions place critically ill COVID-19 patients at risk for hospital-acquired infections. Common complications include secondary pneumonia, central line–associated bloodstream infection, and urinary tract infections. In endemic areas, strongyloidiasis reactivation is also of concern, particularly in those who receive immunosuppressive agents, such as dexamethasone. Several reports have described

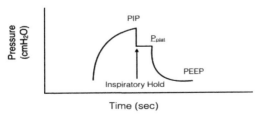

Time (sec)

Fig. 1. Measuring plateau pressure for mechanical ventilation. (*From* Pacheco GS, Mendelson J, Gaspers M. Pediatric Ventilator Management in the Emergency Department. Emerg Med Clin North Am. 2018;36(2):401-413. https://doi.org/10.1016/j.emc.2017.12.008; with permission.)

invasive aspergillus in immunocompetent hosts, although the true prevalence is uncertain.[40,41]

Secondary bacterial infections have been noted in COVID-19 patients, and patients are frequently treated with empirical antimicrobial agents. However, secondary bacterial infections do not seem to be common. A meta-analysis found that 71.9% of patients hospitalized with COVID-19 before mid-April 2020 received antibiotics despite the fact that only 6.9% of these admissions were associated with bacterial infections.[42] The Infectious Disease Society of America and National Institutes of Health COVID-19 treatment guidelines do not recommend either for or against empirical broad spectrum antimicrobial therapy.[39,43] However, if broad spectrum antimicrobials are used, effort should be made to obtain culture data and there should be regular reassessment of the appropriateness of ongoing use.

DIAGNOSIS
Laboratory Findings

Laboratory findings in critically ill patients with COVID-19 are varied and include leukopenia or leukocytosis, lymphopenia, thrombocytopenia, and elevated D-dimer, aminotransferases, lactate dehydrogenase, and ferritin levels.[44] Many patients with severe COVID-19 also display evidence of a pronounced inflammatory response that is similar to the cytokine release syndrome with elevated serum levels of C-reactive protein, ferritin, and interleukin-6. Patients with evidence of a hyperinflammatory response have a higher risk of progression to mechanical ventilation and death.[45]

Imaging

Chest imaging findings can be nonspecific but frequent findings in critically ill patients include multifocal consolidation and ground-glass opacities.[46] Peak severity in lung findings usually occurs after the first week of symptom onset. In one systemic review of computed tomography findings in more than 2700 patients with COVID-19, the following pulmonary manifestations were noted (**Table 2**):[47]

TREATMENT

The key principles in treatment of patients with severe COVID-19 include high-quality supportive care, antiviral therapies, immunomodulatory therapies, prevention of hospital-acquired conditions, and rigorous infection control procedures to limit nosocomial spread. In addition, managing surges of critically ill patients requires proactive

Table 2	
Computed tomographic manifestations of COVID-19	
CT Finding	**Proportion**
Ground glass opacities(GGO)	83.3%
GGO mixed with consolidation	58.4%
Adjacent pleural thickening	52.5%
Consolidation	44%
Interlobular septal thickening	48.5%
Air bronchogram	46.5%

Modified from Bao C, Liu X, Zhang H, Li Y, Liu J. Coronavirus Disease 2019 (COVID-19) CT Findings: A Systematic Review and Meta-analysis. J Am Coll Radiol. 2020;17(6):701-709. https://doi.org/10.1016/j.jacr.2020.03.006; with permission.

management of hospital staff, bed allocation, and equipment resources to adequately meet the needs of the pool of critically ill patients. In extreme circumstances, crisis of care standard may need to be implemented.[48]

Basic Management

Patients admitted with severe COVID-19 should be monitored closely for disease progression with close observation and pulse oximetry. Oxygen support should be titrated to achieve a saturation between 90% and 96%. For patients with hypotension or shock, fluid resuscitation should be conservative and norepinephrine should be used as the first-line vasoactive agent to achieve a mean arterial pressure of 60 to 65 mm Hg.[49]

Advanced Noninvasive Respiratory Support

In patients unable to achieve adequate oxygen saturation with supplemental nasal cannula, either high-flow nasal cannula or noninvasive ventilation (continuous positive airway pressure/bilevel positive airway pressure) should be used. Deciding if and when to intubate is a critical decision that should be considered for patients on advanced respiratory support. Clinicians should consider the anticipated clinical course and weigh both the risk of premature intubation against the risk of respiratory arrest and emergency intubation.[4] Signs of labored breathing, refractory hypoxemia, and encephalopathy indicate impending respiratory arrest and should prompt urgent endotracheal intubation and mechanical ventilation.

Mechanical Ventilation

The primary lung pathology from severe COVID-19 is ARDS. Therefore, patients on mechanical ventilation should be managed according to established principles of managing ARDS to avoid alveolar collapse, overdistension, and hyperoxia-induced injury.

Sufficient positive end-expiratory pressure (PEEP) should be used to prevent end-expiratory alveolar collapse, and tidal volumes should be limited to between 4 and 8 mL/kg of predicted body weight to achieve an end-inspiratory pressure (plateau pressure [Pplat]) of less than 30 cm H_2O (**Fig. 2**).[50] To achieve low tidal volume lung protective ventilation, permissive hypercapnia should be tolerated to maintain arterial pH less than 7.20. Clinicians should be mindful that excessive PEEP may cause alveolar overdistension and hemodynamic instability from decreased venous filling to the heart. Achieving the lowest driving pressure possible (Pplat–PEEP) is associated with improved mortality and indicates the ideal balance between alveolar collapse and overdistension.[51] Sedation and pain control agents should be used to achieve comfort and synchrony with mechanical ventilation.

In the case of severe hypoxia (P/F < 150 mm Hg) despite conventional lung protective ventilation, paralysis and prone ventilation should be considered (**Fig. 3**). In a pre-COVID randomized trial of intubated patients with ARDS, prone ventilation for 16 hours per day improved oxygenation and mortality.[52] If severe hypoxia persists despite these efforts, rescue therapies, such as inhaled pulmonary vasodilators and extracorporeal membrane oxygenation (ECMO), should be considered.[4]

Antiviral Therapies

Remdesivir is a nucleoside analogue the inhibits the RNA-dependent RNA polymerase of coronaviruses and is recommended for use in combination with dexamethasone for patients admitted and requiring supplemental oxygen.[39] A randomized trial demonstrated an improved time to recovery for hospitalized patients, although benefit was greatest in patients earlier in disease course who were receiving supplemental oxygen

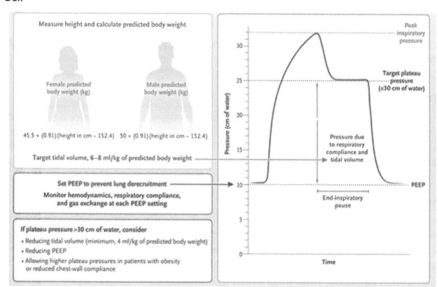

Fig. 2. Goals of mechanical ventilation. (*Adapted from* Berlin DA, Gulick RM, Martinez FJ. Severe Covid-19. N Engl J Med. 2020;383(25):2451-2460. https://doi.org/10.1056/NEJMcp2009575; with permission.)

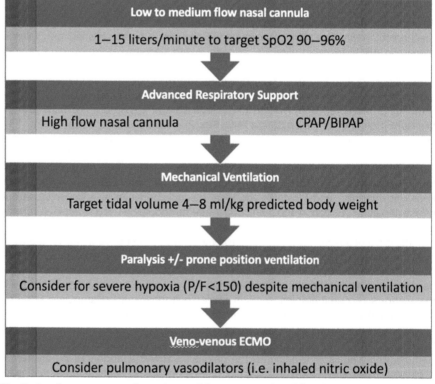

Fig. 3. Respiratory support in patients with COVID-19. (*Modified from* Farkas J. Management of COVID-19 patients admitted to stepdown or ICU. EMCrit Project. Available at https://emcrit.org/ibcc/covid19/. Accessed; with permission.)

but not intubated.[53] A large open-label trial did not demonstrate an in-hospital mortality benefit.[54]

Monoclonal antibodies are generally recommended for outpatients with COVID-19 who are at high risk of progression to severe disease. However, they may be considered for immunocompromised patients on supplemental oxygen therapy through expanded access programs but is otherwise generally not authorized nor recommended for patients with severe or critical COVID-19, based on negative results from several randomized controlled studies.[55,56] Convalescent plasma has not been demonstrated to improve outcomes in hospitalized patients and is not recommended.

Immunomodulatory Therapies

Dexamethasone is considered standard of care for patients with severe COVID-19. A randomized trial of more than 6400 hospitalized patients with COVID-19 showed a reduction in 30-day mortality (22.9% vs 25.7%) with the benefit most pronounced in patients requiring mechanical ventilation (29.3% vs 41.4%).[57]

A second immunomodulatory agent—such as tocilizumab, sarilumab, or baricitinib—should be considered for patients with rapidly escalating oxygen needs or those requiring advanced respiratory support, mechanical ventilation, or ECMO. Tocilizumab and sarilumab are monoclonal antibodies that competitively inhibit interleukin-6 (IL-6) receptor binding. In a meta-analysis of more than 10,000 hospitalized patients receiving anti-IL-6 inhibitors the odd ratios for the association with mortality compared with usual care or placebo were 0.77 (95% CI, 0.68–0.87) for tocilizumab and 0.92 (95% CI, 0.61–1.38) for sarilumab.[58] Anti-IL-6 inhibitors should not be used in patients with a concurrent active infection other than the SARS-CoV-2 infection (including localized infection) or with elevated alanine aminotransferase or aspartate transaminase (AST) greater than 10 times the upper limit of the reference range.

Baricitinib is a selective Janus kinase 1 and 2 inhibitor and can be used as an alternative to the anti-IL-6 inhibitors. In a randomized trial of 1525 hospitalized adults with COVID-19 and elevated inflammatory markers but not receiving invasive mechanical ventilation, adding baricitinib to standard of care reduced 28-day mortality compared with standard of care (8.1% vs 13.1%).[59] It should not be administered if estimated glomerular filtration rate is less than 15 mL/min, the absolute lymphocyte count is less than 200 cells/uL, or if the absolute neutrophil count is less than 500 cells/uL.

CLINICS CARE POINTS

- Patients with severe COVID-19 should be hospitalized and monitored closely for signs of deterioration.

- When to intubate is a critical decision that should depend on the anticipated clinical course and weigh both the risk of premature intubation against the risk of respiratory arrest and emergency intubation.

- Remdesivir and dexamethasone are standard of care for most patients with severe COVID-19. Additional immunomodulatory agents (baricitinib, anti-IL-6 inhibitors) should be considered for patients on high-flow nasal cannula, noninvasive ventilation, or mechanical ventilation.

- The evidenced-based principles for ARDS should be used in patients on mechanical ventilation: low tidal volume ventilation, permissive hypercapnia, and adequate PEEP.

DISCLOSURE

The author has nothing to disclose.

REFERENCES

1. Causes of death (COD) visualization. institute for health metrics and evaluation. 2014. Available at: https://www.healthdata.org/data-visualization/causes-death-cod-visualization. Accessed December 26, 2021.
2. Ahmad FB. Provisional mortality data — United States, 2020. MMWR Morb Mortal Wkly Rep 2021;70. https://doi.org/10.15585/mmwr.mm7014e1.
3. Xu S. COVID-19 vaccination and non–COVID-19 mortality risk — seven integrated health care organizations, United States, December 14, 2020–July 31, 2021. MMWR Morb Mortal Wkly Rep 2021;70. https://doi.org/10.15585/mmwr.mm7043e2.
4. Berlin DA, Gulick RM, Martinez FJ. Severe Covid-19. N Engl J Med 2020;383(25): 2451–60.
5. Huang C, Wang Y, Li X, et al. Clinical features of patients infected with 2019 novel coronavirus in Wuhan, China. Lancet 2020;395(10223):497–506.
6. Zhou F, Yu T, Du R, et al. Clinical course and risk factors for mortality of adult inpatients with COVID-19 in Wuhan, China: a retrospective cohort study. Lancet 2020;395(10229):1054–62.
7. Grasselli G, Pesenti A, Cecconi M. Critical care utilization for the COVID-19 outbreak in lombardy, italy: early experience and forecast during an emergency response. JAMA 2020;323(16):1545–6.
8. Livingston E, Bucher K. Coronavirus disease 2019 (COVID-19) in Italy. JAMA 2020;323(14):1335.
9. Karagiannidis C, Windisch W, McAuley DF, et al. Major differences in ICU admissions during the first and second COVID-19 wave in Germany. Lancet Respir Med 2021;9(5):e47–8.
10. Kompaniyets L. Underlying medical conditions and severe illness among 540,667 adults hospitalized with COVID-19, March 2020–March 2021. Prev Chronic Dis 2021;18. https://doi.org/10.5888/pcd18.210123.
11. Lopez L III, Hart LH III, Katz MH. Racial and ethnic health disparities related to COVID-19. JAMA 2021;325(8):719–20.
12. Rubin-Miller L, Alban C, Sep 16 SSP. COVID-19 racial disparities in testing, infection, hospitalization, and death: analysis of epic patient data. KFF. 2020. Published September 16, 2020. Accessed January 24, 2022. https://www.kff.org/coronavirus-covid-19/issue-brief/covid-19-racial-disparities-testing-infection-hospitalization-death-analysis-epic-patient-data/. Available at.
13. Price JH, Khubchandani J, McKinney M, et al. Racial/Ethnic Disparities in Chronic Diseases of Youths and Access to Health Care in the United States. Biomed Res Int 2013;2013:787616.
14. Yehia BR, Winegar A, Fogel R, et al. Association of race with mortality among patients hospitalized with coronavirus disease 2019 (COVID-19) at 92 US hospitals. JAMA Netw Open 2020;3(8):e2018039.
15. Haas EJ, Angulo FJ, McLaughlin JM, et al. Impact and effectiveness of mRNA BNT162b2 vaccine against SARS-CoV-2 infections and COVID-19 cases, hospitalisations, and deaths following a nationwide vaccination campaign in Israel: an observational study using national surveillance data. Lancet 2021;397(10287): 1819–29. Lond Engl.
16. Tenforde MW, Olson SM, Self WH, et al. Effectiveness of Pfizer-biontech and moderna vaccines against COVID-19 among hospitalized adults aged $\geq$65 years - United States, January-March 2021. MMWR Morb Mortal Wkly Rep 2021; 70(18):674–9.

17. Sadoff J, Gray G, Vandebosch A, et al. Safety and efficacy of single-dose Ad26.-COV2.S vaccine against covid-19. N Engl J Med 2021;384(23):2187–201.

18. Fowlkes A, Gaglani M, Groover K, et al. Effectiveness of COVID-19 vaccines in preventing SARS-CoV-2 infection among frontline workers before and during B.1.617.2 (Delta) variant predominance — eight U.S. locations, December 2020–August 2021. MMWR Morb Mortal Wkly Rep 2021;70(34):1167–9.

19. Enhancing response to Omicron SARS-CoV-2 variant. Available at: https://www.who.int/publications/m/item/enhancing-readiness-for-omicron-(b.1.1.529)-technical-brief-and-priority-actions-for-member-states. Accessed January 24, 2022.

20. Yek C. Risk factors for severe COVID-19 outcomes among persons aged ≥18 years who completed a primary COVID-19 vaccination series — 465 health care facilities, United States, December 2020–October 2021. MMWR Morb Mortal Wkly Rep 2022;71. https://doi.org/10.15585/mmwr.mm7101a4.

21. Siddiqi HK, Mehra MR. COVID-19 illness in native and immunosuppressed states: a clinical–therapeutic staging proposal. J Heart Lung Transpl 2020; 39(5):405–7.

22. Gandhi RT, Lynch JB, del Rio C. Mild or moderate Covid-19. N Engl J Med 2020; 383(18):1757–66.

23. Bohn MK, Hall A, Sepiashvili L, et al. Pathophysiology of COVID-19: mechanisms underlying disease severity and progression. Physiology 2020;35(5):288–301.

24. Ibrahim GS, Alkandari BM, Shady IAA, et al. Invasive mechanical ventilation complications in COVID-19 patients. Egypt J Radiol Nucl Med 2021;52(1):226.

25. Goyal P, Choi JJ, Pinheiro LC, et al. Clinical characteristics of Covid-19 in New York city. N Engl J Med 2020;382(24):2372–4.

26. Mao L, Jin H, Wang M, et al. Neurologic manifestations of hospitalized patients with coronavirus disease 2019 in Wuhan, China. JAMA Neurol 2020;77(6): 683–90.

27. Helms J, Kremer S, Merdji H, et al. Neurologic features in severe SARS-CoV-2 infection. N Engl J Med 2020. https://doi.org/10.1056/NEJMc2008597.

28. Robbins-Juarez SY, Qian L, King KL, et al. Outcomes for patients with COVID-19 and Acute kidney injury: a systematic review and meta-analysis. Kidney Int Rep 2020;5(8):1149–60.

29. Batlle D, Soler MJ, Sparks MA, et al. Acute kidney injury in COVID-19: emerging evidence of a distinct pathophysiology. J Am Soc Nephrol 2020;31(7):1380–3.

30. Santoriello D, Khairallah P, Bomback AS, et al. Postmortem kidney pathology findings in patients with COVID-19. J Am Soc Nephrol 2020;31(9):2158–67.

31. Kaafarani HMA, El Moheb M, Hwabejire JO, et al. Gastrointestinal complications in critically ill patients with COVID-19. Ann Surg 2020;272(2):e61–2.

32. El Moheb M, Naar L, Christensen MA, et al. Gastrointestinal complications in critically ill patients with and without COVID-19. JAMA 2020;324(18):1899–901.

33. Cui S, Chen S, Li X, et al. Prevalence of venous thromboembolism in patients with severe novel coronavirus pneumonia. J Thromb Haemost 2020;18(6):1421–4.

34. Middeldorp S, Coppens M, van Haaps TF, et al. Incidence of venous thromboembolism in hospitalized patients with COVID-19. J Thromb Haemost 2020;18(8): 1995–2002.

35. Hill JB, Garcia D, Crowther M, et al. Frequency of venous thromboembolism in 6513 patients with COVID-19: a retrospective study. Blood Adv 2020;4(21): 5373–7.

36. Bilaloglu S, Aphinyanaphongs Y, Jones S, et al. Thrombosis in hospitalized patients with COVID-19 in a New York city health system. JAMA 2020;324(8): 799–801.

37. Connors JM, Levy JH. COVID-19 and its implications for thrombosis and antico-agulation. Blood 2020;135(23):2033–40.
38. Cuker A, Tseng EK, Nieuwlaat R, et al. American society of hematology 2021 guidelines on the use of anticoagulation for thromboprophylaxis in patients with COVID-19. Blood Adv 2021;5(3):872–88.
39. NIH COVID-19 Treatment Guidelines. COVID-19 treatment guidelines. Available at: https://www.covid19treatmentguidelines.nih.gov/management/clinical-management/hospitalized-adults–therapeutic-management/. Accessed January 26, 2022.
40. Bartoletti M, Pascale R, Cricca M, et al. Epidemiology of invasive pulmonary aspergillosis among intubated patients with COVID-19: a prospective study. Clin Infect 2021;73(11):e3606–14.
41. Koehler P, Cornely OA, Böttiger BW, et al. COVID-19 associated pulmonary aspergillosis. Mycoses 2020;63(6):528–34.
42. Langford BJ, So M, Raybardhan S, et al. Bacterial co-infection and secondary infection in patients with COVID-19: a living rapid review and meta-analysis. Clin Microbiol Infect 2020;26(12):1622–9.
43. Bhimraj A, Morgan RL, Shumaker AH, et al. Infectious diseases society of america guidelines on the treatment and management of patients with COVID-19. Clin Infect 2020;27:ciaa478. Published online April.
44. Wang D, Hu B, Hu C, et al. Clinical characteristics of 138 hospitalized patients with 2019 novel coronavirus-infected pneumonia in Wuhan, China. JAMA 2020; 323(11):1061–9.
45. Webb BJ, Peltan ID, Jensen P, et al. Clinical criteria for COVID-19-associated hy-perinflammatory syndrome: a cohort study. Lancet Rheumatol 2020;2(12): e754–63.
46. Wong HYF, Lam HYS, Fong AHT, et al. Frequency and distribution of chest radio-graphic findings in patients positive for COVID-19. Radiology 2020;296(2):E72–8.
47. Bao C, Liu X, Zhang H, et al. Coronavirus disease 2019 (COVID-19) CT findings: a systematic review and meta-analysis. J Am Coll Radiol 2020;17(6):701–9.
48. Read "Rapid Expert Consultation on Crisis Standards of Care for the COVID-19 Pandemic (March 28, 2020)" at NAP.Edu. doi:10.17226/25765.
49. Alhazzani W, Møller MH, Arabi YM, et al. Surviving sepsis campaign: guidelines on the management of critically ill adults with coronavirus disease 2019 (COVID-19). Intensive Care Med 2020;46(5):854–87.
50. Acute Respiratory Distress Syndrome Network, Brower RG, Matthay MA, Morris A, et al. Ventilation with lower tidal volumes as compared with traditional tidal volumes for acute lung injury and the acute respiratory distress syndrome. N Engl J Med 2000;342(18):1301–8.
51. Guérin C, Papazian L, Reignier J, et al. Effect of driving pressure on mortality in ARDS patients during lung protective mechanical ventilation in two randomized controlled trials. Crit Care Lond Engl 2016;20(1):384.
52. Guérin C, Reignier J, Richard JC, et al. Prone positioning in severe acute respi-ratory distress syndrome. N Engl J Med 2013;368(23):2159–68.
53. Beigel JH, Tomashek KM, Dodd LE, et al. Remdesivir for the treatment of Covid-19 - preliminary report. N Engl J Med 2020. https://doi.org/10.1056/NEJMoa2007764.
54. Repurposed antiviral drugs for COVID-19 –interim WHO SOLIDARITY trial results | medRxiv. Available at: https://www.medrxiv.org/content/10.1101/2020.10.15.20209817v1. Accessed January 26, 2022.

55. Self WH, Sandkovsky U, Reilly CS, et al. Efficacy and safety of two neutralising monoclonal antibody therapies, sotrovimab and BRII-196 plus BRII-198, for adults hospitalised with COVID-19 (TICO): a randomised controlled trial. Lancet Infect Dis 2021;0(0).
56. ACTIV-3/TICO LY-CoV555 Study Group, et al. A neutralizing monoclonal antibody for hospitalized patients with Covid-19. N Engl J Med 2021;384(10):905–14.
57. RECOVERY Collaborative Group, Horby P, Lim WS, et al. Dexamethasone in hospitalized patients with Covid-19. N Engl J Med 2021;384(8):693–704.
58. Shankar-Hari M, Vale CL, Godolphin PJ, et al, WHO Rapid Evidence Appraisal for COVID-19 Therapies (REACT) Working Group. Association between administration of IL-6 antagonists and mortality among patients hospitalized for COVID-19: a meta-analysis. JAMA 2021;326(6):499–518.
59. Marconi VC, Ramanan AV, de Bono S, et al. Efficacy and safety of baricitinib for the treatment of hospitalised adults with COVID-19 (COV-BARRIER): a randomised, double-blind, parallel-group, placebo-controlled phase 3 trial. Lancet Respir Med 2021;9(12):1407–18.

Postacute Sequelae of Severe Acute Respiratory Syndrome Coronavirus 2 Infection

Aluko A. Hope, MD, MSCE[a],*, Teresa H. Evering, MD, MS[b],*

KEYWORDS

- COVID-19 • SARS-CoV-2 • Postacute sequelae of SARS-CoV-2 infection (PASC)
- Long COVID • Long-haul COVID • Postacute COVID-19

KEY POINTS

- Postacute sequelae of SARS-CoV-2 (PASC) infection or long COVID is a heterogeneous, multisystem, relapsing and remitting illness that can affect patients infected with SARS-CoV-2 regardless of the severity of the acute infection.
- Estimates of the incidence and prevalence of long COVID symptoms vary widely across published studies.
- The diagnosis of long COVID is currently primarily based on history and physical examination and may require a multidisciplinary approach to care.
- The overall approach to the treatment of long COVID is to focus on symptom management, functional goals, and improvements in the quality of life.

INTRODUCTION

The clinical spectrum of severe acute respiratory syndrome coronavirus 2 (SARS-CoV-2) infection ranges from asymptomatic to critical illness, which may include severe sepsis and acute respiratory failure.[1] When symptomatic, acute coronavirus disease 2019 (COVID-19) illness will typically last days to weeks, and most of the symptoms are thought to be mediated by the replication of the virus and the initial immune response to the infection.[2] As the COVID-19 pandemic continues, it has become increasingly clear that clinical sequelae and symptoms may persist for weeks to months beyond the acute stage of SARS-CoV-2 infection for a significant proportion of patients. This chronic illness has been termed postacute sequelae of SARS-CoV-2 (PASC) infection, post-COVID syndrome, or long COVID. A less common postacute hyperinflammatory illness (multisystem inflammatory syndrome in children [MIS-C] and multisystem

[a] Division of Pulmonary, Allergy, and Critical Care Medicine, School of Medicine, Oregon Health & Science University (OHSU), 3181 SW Sam Jackson Park Road, Portland, Oregon, 97239, USA; [b] Department of Medicine, Division of Infectious Diseases, Weill Cornell Medicine, 413 East 69th Street, Belfer Research Building, BB-512, New York, NY 10021, USA
* Corresponding authors.
E-mail addresses: hopeal@ohsu.edu (A.A.H.); evering@med.cornell.edu (T.H.E.)

Infect Dis Clin N Am 36 (2022) 379–395
https://doi.org/10.1016/j.idc.2022.02.004   **id.theclinics.com**
0891-5520/22/© 2022 Elsevier Inc. All rights reserved.

inflammatory syndrome in adults [MIS-A]) has also been characterized. MIS-C and MIS-A will typically occur 2 to 5 weeks after the initial SARS-CoV-2 infection and are thought to be mediated by a dysregulated immune response.[1] Patients with these syndromes may suffer from cardiovascular, gastrointestinal, neurologic, dermatologic, and mucocutaneous manifestations like Kawasaki disease,[3,4] and this is discussed further in Chapter 12. This review highlights what is known about the epidemiology, clinical features, pathophysiology, and risk factors of long COVID and summarizes current rational approaches for the diagnosis, prevention, and treatment of this new syndrome based on emerging literature and expert opinion.

Definitions and Epidemiology

As of this writing, there is no universally accepted case definition for long COVID.[5] The Centers for Disease Control and Prevention defines post-COVID conditions as a range of health problems or symptoms experienced 4 or more weeks after initial infection with SARS-CoV-2.[6] The United Kingdom National Institute for Health and Care Excellence (NICE) guidance classifies acute infection as lasting up to 4 weeks, classifies ongoing symptomatic COVID-19 as lasting up to 12 weeks, and then defines post-COVID syndrome as a cluster of overlapping signs and symptoms across multiple systems that has developed during or after the initial infection and continues for more than 12 weeks after SARS-CoV-2 infection.[7] Using a time frame similar to NICE, the World Health Organization (WHO) proposes a clinical case definition in which long COVID begins 3 months from the onset of probable or confirmed SARS-CoV-2 infection.[8] All current case definitions do, however, acknowledge that long COVID encompasses a wide range of symptoms and can persist, fluctuate, or relapse following the initial SARS-COV-2 infection or can newly appear after initial symptom resolution.

Estimates of the incidence and prevalence of long COVID symptoms vary widely across published studies. The reasons for this variability include the overall severity and spectrum of SARS-CoV-2 infection in the study population, participant sociodemographics and geographic location, the health system, and the public health infrastructure within which the study is completed, the follow-up period from the initial SARS-CoV-2 infection, the spectrum of symptoms on which the reports are based, the methods and tools for data collection, and the chosen study outcome measure.[9] In addition, most studies describing the prevalence and clinical manifestations of long COVID are cross-sectional or observational and are subject to various types of selection or reporter bias that make it difficult to generalize the results beyond the population studied.[10] As an example, participation in app-based self-report surveys requires motivated participants with adequate computer literacy to download the app and track their COVID-19 symptom, thus influencing the responding cohort.[11,12]

Acknowledging the heterogeneity of these studies, in general, for those patients evaluated or treated for acute COVID-19 in the outpatient setting, the reported incidence of long COVID ranges from 10% to 35%[13–15] and can exceed 80% for those treated in the hospital with more severe initial illness.[16,17] In one of the earliest attempts to define the clinical course of COVID-19, a cross-sectional study of symptomatic adults tested in outpatient settings reported that 34% had not returned to their usual state of health 14 to 21 days after SARS-CoV-2 infection.[14] In light of the prolonged course of long COVID, multiple studies have since followed participants for longer durations in a variety of settings. An illustrative selection of those studies is summarized in **Table 1**. Taken together, these studies reveal the global scope of the syndrome and suggest the potential for a significant proportion of patients who are infected with SARS-CoV-2 regardless of severity of the initial infection to develop long COVID.

Table 1
Select publications highlighting long coronavirus disease prevalence

Authors	Population	Participants (n)	Severity of Initial Illness	Evaluation Time Point	Outcome Measure	Prevalence
Carvalho-Schneider et al,[18] 2021	Patients at Tours University Hospital (France)	150	Mild-moderate COVID-19 (n = 116); severe COVID-19 (n = 34)	30 d and 60 d after initial infection	≥ 1 persistent symptom	69% and 66%, respectively
Carfi et al,[19] 2020	Postacute outpatient service in Italy	143	Hospitalized; ICU admission (13%)	60 d since symptom onset (mean)	≥1 persistent symptom	87%
Huang et al,[20] 2021	Hospitalized adults in Wuhan, China	1733	Hospitalized	186 d after symptom onset (median)	≥1 symptom	76%
Goertz et al,[21] 2020	Members of Facebook groups for patients with COVID-19 with persistent complaints in the Netherlands and Belgium, and a panel of individuals registered on a Web site of the Lung Foundation Netherlands	2113	Hospitalized (n = 112); nonhospitalized adults (n = 2001)	79 d after symptom onset (mean)	≥1 symptom from a 29-symptom list	87% fatigue and 71% dyspnea
Sudre et al,[11] 2021	Respondents from United Kingdom, United States and Sweden, self-reporting symptoms in the COVID Symptom Study app	558	Mild to moderate COVID-19 illness based on the low rates of hospitalizations in the cohort	≥28 d, ≥8 wk, and ≥12 wk	≥ 1 symptom	13.3%, 4.5%, and 2.3% had persistent symptoms ≥28, ≥56 and ≥ 84 d, respectively
Blomberg et al,[22] 2021	Prospective cohort of patients testing positive for SARS-CoV-2 in Norway	312	Home-isolated (n = 247); hospitalized (n = 65)	6 mo	Any persistent symptom	61% (189/312)

Abbreviation: ICU, intensive care unit.

Clinical Manifestations

Current literature suggests that long COVID is a heterogeneous, multisystem, relapsing and remitting illness that can affect patients infected with SARS-CoV-2 regardless of the severity of the acute infection.[23]

Although not universal, most patients presenting with long COVID will report a prior history of a viral syndrome with symptoms consistent with an acute COVID-19 infection such as fever, shortness of breath, cough, or change in taste or smell. Several recent review papers or meta-analyses describe the ability of long COVID to manifest across multiple body systems including constitutional,[24] cardiovascular,[25–27] pulmonary,[28] neurologic,[29] neuropsychiatric,[30] musculoskeletal,[31] and gastrointestinal.[32] A recent meta-analysis that included international studies that defined long COVID as ranging from 14 to 110 days postviral infection and included hospitalized and ambulatory treated infections found that the most common symptoms were fatigue (58%), headache (44%), attention disorder (27%), hair loss (25%), difficulty breathing (24%), and loss of taste (23%) or smell (21%).[33] Incidence of gastrointestinal symptoms (eg, diarrhea, nausea, pain) ranged from 3% to 79%.[33] Another recent systematic review and meta-analysis comprising 81 studies of individuals reporting fatigue and cognitive impairment 12 or more weeks after COVID-19 infection revealed the proportion of affected individuals to be 32% and 22%, respectively.[24] Other reported symptoms include cardiac impairments, muscle weakness, and poor exercise tolerance.[34] **Table 2** summarizes common clinical signs and symptoms reported in the long COVID literature, as well as associated differential diagnoses for consideration in patients presenting for evaluation.

Beyond signs and symptoms, long COVID may also be associated with new or worsening difficulties completing activities of daily living and difficulty returning to work. In an observational cohort study of 448 individuals contacted via telephone approximately 60 days after discharge from hospitals across Michigan, persistent symptoms related to the acute COVID-19 illness were present in 159 of 448 (35.5%) and 58 of 488 (11.8%) reported new or worsening difficulties completing activities of daily living.[35] Furthermore, among 195 patients who were employed before hospitalization, 117 had returned to work, whereas 78 could not return because of ongoing health issues or job loss.[35] Similarly, in a large multicenter cohort study of 253 adults previously hospitalized in the United States for COVID-19 who completed 1-month telephone follow-up after hospital discharge, a majority (139 [53.8%]) reported at least 1 new or worsened cardiopulmonary symptom, 130 (52.8%) reported new limitations in activities of daily living or instrumental activities of daily living, and 213 (84.2%) reported that they were not fully back to their pre-COVID level of health and well-being. Importantly, this study suggests a complex relationship between the level of symptoms, degree of disability, and degree of perceived recovery.[36]

Although long COVID is a newly emerging illness, it is worth noting that postinfectious syndromes that share a similarly diffuse degree and constellation of symptoms have been previously described. For example, postinfectious fatigue syndromes have been reported following infections with *Giardia lamblia, Coxiella burnetii,* and *Borrelia burgdorferi,* the causative agent of Lyme disease. Postviral fatigue syndromes have also been described after other viral infections such as Epstein-Barr virus.[50] In a classic paper on the identification and management of postviral fatigue syndromes, a postviral fatigue syndrome was characterized by (1) generalized, relapsing fatigue exacerbated by minor exercise that was associated with disruption of usual daily activities for at least 3 months and (2) subjective cognitive complaints including

Table 2
Postacute sequelae of severe acute respiratory syndrome coronavirus 2 clinical signs and symptoms

Systems	Symptom or Sign	Differential Diagnosis for Consideration
Constitutional[37,38]	Fatigue, fevers, malaise, exercise intolerance	Postviral fatigue, deconditioning, electrolyte imbalance
Cardiovascular[25,27]	Tachycardia, chest pain, chest tightness, palpitations, exercise intolerance	Anemia, heart failure, myocarditis, pericarditis, thromboembolic disease, hypoxemia, pulmonary fibrosis, pulmonary vascular disease, chest wall pain, gastrointestinal source, coronary artery disease, small fiber neuropathy, autonomic impairment
Respiratory[19,20,37,39,40]	Shortness of breath, cough, exercise intolerance	Residual lung disease, reactive airway disease, cryptogenic organizing pneumonia, myocardial involvement, pulmonary embolism, angina variant
Neurologic[29,41]	Headache, dizziness, ataxia, vertigo, nerve pain, smell and taste impairment, seizure like activity	Cerebrovascular disease, migraines, traumatic brain injury, concussion, allergic rhinitis, functional neurologic disorder
Gastrointestinal[32,42]	Abdominal pain, nausea, vomiting, diarrhea, constipation, bloating	Irritable bowel syndrome, inflammatory bowel disease, gluten sensitivity, dysautonomia, parasitic infection
Musculoskeletal and skin[42–44]	Joint pain, myalgia, increased pain and tenderness, numbness and tingling in upper or lower extremities, COVID toes, balance problems, upper back pain	Small fiber neuropathy, ICU-acquired neuromuscular weakness, dysautonomia, reactive arthritis, chronic fatigue syndrome, autoimmune disorders, central desensitization syndromes[41,42]
Neuropsychiatric[30,45]	Anxiety, depression, posttraumatic stress symptoms	Premorbid mood or anxiety disorder, secondary impact from neurologic injury from acute illness (eg, stroke), dysautonomia

(continued on next page)

Table 2 (continued)		
Systems	Symptom or Sign	Differential Diagnosis for Consideration
Sleep[46]	Insomnia, hypersomnia	Premorbid sleep disorder, polypharmacy, mood disorder, hypersomnolence disorders includding narcolepsy, obstructive sleep apnea, restless leg syndrome, circadian rhythm sleep-wake disorders, substance/medication-induced sleep disorder
Autonomic nervous system[26,27,47]	Disequilibrium, dizziness, pre-syncope, blurred vision, chest pain palpitations, positive tilt table, hypotension, difficult-to-control hypertension, breathlessness	Dehydration, autonomic failure, POTS, autoimmune disorders, mast cell activation syndrome, orthostatic hypotension, myocarditis, pulmonary embolism
Neurocognitive[24,37,48,49]	Cognitive changes, light sensitivity, personality changes, change in taste or smell, balance change, gait changes	Premorbid mild cognitive impairment, delirium, depression, anxiety, psychosis, traumatic brain injury, post-ICU syndrome[47]

Abbreviations: ICU, intensive care unit; POTS, postural tachycardia syndrome.

disturbances in concentration and/or short-term memory impairment, with no other "obvious, organic causes for a similar syndrome."[51] In this proposed definition, other supporting criteria could include (1) symptoms such as "myalgias, gastrointestinal disturbances, headache, depression, tinnitus, paresthesias, tinnitus, sleep disturbance, cardiovascular complaints, adverse effects of alcohol, adverse effect of heat"; (2) clinical signs of lymphadenopathy, localized muscle tenderness, or pharyngitis; and (3) laboratory evidence of viral infection and abnormalities in immune function.[51] Myalgic encephalomyelitis or chronic fatigue syndrome (ME/CFS) is a chronic complex disease that has often been described as beginning after a viral infection, although the cause remains unknown. ME/CFS is estimated to affect between 836,000 and 2.5 million people in the United States alone[52] and is characterized by fatigue, postexertional malaise, sleep problems, cognitive impairment, pain, autonomic dysfunction, and neuroendocrine symptoms.[52] These examples demonstrate the ubiquity of postinfectious syndromes that share some similarities with the clinical presentations we now see with long COVID.

Risk Factors for Long Coronavirus Disease

Although the pathophysiology is still to be elucidated and likely includes multiple phenotypes, studies thus far suggest that long COVID may be a syndrome with predisposing, precipitating, and perpetuating factors.[53]

Nonmodifiable and modifiable characteristics such as older age and female sex, obesity, and the presence of multiple preexisting medical comorbidities including immunosuppressive and psychiatric conditions may all be factors associated with an increased risk of protracted symptoms after COVID-19 infection.[11,14] In their neuro-cognitive evaluation of 106 patients (mean age 64.9 years, 26.7% female) 6 months after discharge from a pulmonary COVID-19 unit, Cristillo and colleagues[54] found that more severe pulmonary disease during the acute COVID-19 illness and a measure of prehospital vulnerability captured by the National Health System COVID-19 Decision Support Tool were associated with abnormal levels of cognitive function as determined by age- and education-adjusted Montreal Cognitive Assessment scores. These findings support the hypothesis that premorbid vulnerability and older age play an important role in predicting long-term cognitive sequalae of SARS-CoV-2 infection.[54]

In multiple cross-sectional studies[11,37] as well as in multiple observational studies of long COVID in treatment settings,[55,56] women appear more likely to develop long COVID symptoms than men.[57] In addition, the largest cross-sectional studies of long COVID symptoms in adults have typically shown a predominance of female participants[11,37]; however, it remains unclear if this reflects a true biologic predisposition to long COVID, because reporter bias may also play a role.

In terms of precipitating factors, perhaps not surprisingly, several studies report that the severity of the initial COVID-19 infection seems to be associated with an increased risk of developing long COVID.[11] Similarly, the length of hospitalization and intensive care unit (ICU) admission have also been identified as independent predictors of long COVID at 6 months of follow-up.[58] In a large, prospective cross-sectional study of 558 adults who self-reported their symptoms in the COVID Symptom Study app[59] adults with more than 5 symptoms during the first week of their COVID-19 illness were more likely to experience symptoms beyond 28 days (odds ratio [OR] 3.95 [95% confidence interval (CI) 3.10–5.04]).[11] In this study, in adults older than 70 years, loss of smell, fever, and hoarse voice were symptoms most predictive of developing long COVID, with odd ratios ranging from 4.03 to 7.35.[11] In a prospective multicenter study of 991 patients with COVID-19 requiring ICU admission, persistent post-COVID-19 symptoms were reported in more than two-thirds of patients at 3 months. Among this cohort, independent risk factors for persistent poor health post-COVID-19 included female sex, development of ICU-acquired pneumonia, duration of ICU stay, and acute respiratory distress syndrome.[60] Taken together, the severity of the acute COVID-19 infection whether classified by the number of symptoms, the duration of the hospital stay, or the need for ICU care have all been associated with an increased risk of long COVID.

Few studies have looked at perpetuating factors in protracted recovery in patients diagnosed with long COVID.

Pathophysiology

Both viral direct and indirect mechanisms have been hypothesized to play a role in the pathogenesis of long COVID symptoms, although the pathophysiology is still largely unknown. SARS-CoV-2 uses angiotensin-converting enzyme 2 (ACE2) for cellular entry,[61] and ACE2 is widely expressed on pulmonary and extrapulmonary tissues throughout the body, allowing for the potential of widespread direct virally mediated issue damage.[42] The possibility that there may be persistent viral replication in localized sites has not been excluded. In one recent study that analyzed intestinal biopsies obtained from asymptomatic persons 4 months after COVID-19 onset, there was persistence of SARS-CoV-2 nucleic acids and immunoreactivity in the small bowel of 7 of 14 participants.[62] In addition, in a small meta-analysis of patients with

COVID-19 in Hong Kong, the stool appeared to have a high prevalence of viral RNA, even though 70% of these samples were collected after the respiratory specimens were no longer positive for the virus.[63] Other pathophysiologic mechanisms of COVID-19 that may have lasting adverse effects beyond the acute phase of infection phase include endothelial damage and hypercoagulability/thrombosis and maladaptation of ACE2-related pathways.[2,42] Endothelial dysfunction, small vessel microangiopathy, and fibrin clotting within small capillaries may also contribute to decreased effective oxygen carrying capacity and contribute to shortness of breath and exercise intolerance.[64] A hyperinflammatory syndrome with persistent immune activation and dysregulation of the immune response has also been suggested as a possible mechanism for some of the symptoms.[65,66] The histopathological detection of autoreactive T cells in autopsy samples from individuals infected with COVID-19 supports this latter mechanism.[67,68] Similarly, measures of overt and latent autoimmunity have been demonstrated to persist in some individuals with long COVID.[69]

Impairment in mitochondrial function could be an important contributor to the exercise intolerance and fatigue symptoms in patients with long COVID. A study in which patients with long COVID were tested with Cardio pulmonary exercise testing (CPET) found a lower level of impaired fatty acid oxidation and increased levels of lactate accumulation during exercise regardless of their baseline comorbidities.[70] These results are consistent with impaired energy utilization contributing to the fatigue and functional impairment reported in patients with long COVID.

CONSIDERED APPROACH TO THE EVALUATION OF PATIENTS WITH LONG CORONAVIRUS DISEASE
History

An important part of the evaluation for long COVID is a review the patient's acute COVID-19 illness history, including the effect of the illness and the pandemic on their interpersonal relationships and their social and financial vulnerability. A thorough history should review the main symptoms including fatigue and postexertional malaise.[71] Patients may describe severe exhaustion after minimal exertion, a lack of stamina, or feeling "weighted down." Postexertional malaise may be described as "crashing" after several good days, or several days of worsening symptoms after stressors or triggers. Cognitive difficulties or "brain fog" can include impaired attention, concentration, reduced ability to multitask, difficulty with short-term memory, and word-finding difficulties.[72] Some patients may describe increased irritability or emotionally vulnerable. Reports of unrestful or nonrestorative sleep, often with delayed sleep onset or frequent awakening, are common. Orthostatic intolerance has been reported in long COVID[39,45] and may manifest as syncope, dizziness, lightheadedness, blurred vision, weakness, fatigue, gastrointestinal symptoms (nausea, abdominal pain, bloating, constipation, diarrhea), palpitations, headache, dyspnea, chest pain, temperature intolerance, labile blood pressure, new-onset hypertension, and neck and shoulder pain. Typically, symptoms are triggered or worsened by upright posture. As with other respiratory infections, some patients may experience a persistent breathing discomfort and other respiratory sequelae including chronic cough.[73] Some patients will describe generalized pain in joints, muscle, and soft tissues. Exercise intolerance, burning chest pain, numbness and tingling in the hands or feet, and muscle cramps are also reported.

Clinical Examination

Most patients with long COVID may present with a normal physical examination. Some patients may show signs of fatigue or being generally unwell. Signs of weight loss may be evident in some patients with months of gastrointestinal symptoms. Others may show signs of slow thinking, poor attention, short memory, and impaired word finding. In patients in whom some degree of autonomic dysfunction is suspected, screening patients using the 10-minute NASA Lean Test (NSL) or active stand test may be reasonable.[24,45] The active stand test measures blood pressure and heart rate after 5 minutes of lying supine and then 3 minutes after standing. Orthostatic hypotension is defined as a decrease of greater than 20 mm Hg systolic and greater than 10 mm Hg diastolic after standing for 3 minutes, or during or after a head up tilt to at least 60°.[74] Ten-minute orthostatic vital signs may show a heart rate increase greater than 30 beats per minute (bpm) after standing (or in those aged 12–19 year, more than 40 bpm).[75] Patients with cognitive complaints may benefit from a thorough neurologic examination to identify focal neurologic deficits. Balance and gait may be assessed and compared with age-based norms. For patients with changes in visual acuity or eye pain, a low threshold for a post-COVID-19 retinal examination seems reasonable given that the eyes are known to have ACE2, and such examinations can be a window into microvascular alterations affecting the whole body.[76,77]

Laboratory Testing

Laboratory testing should focus on ruling out comorbid conditions, contributory factors, and common conditions that may explain reported symptoms. It may help to prepare the patient for the fact that most of these test results will be normal. Examples of useful screening tests for initial investigations include complete blood cell count with differential, iron and ferritin levels, comprehensive metabolic panel, urinalysis, thyroid function, vitamin B12 and 25-hydroxy vitamin D levels, and high-sensitivity C-reactive protein, erythrocyte sedimentation rate, and antinuclear antibodies (ANA). More extensive laboratory evaluation may be ordered to identify less common alternative diagnoses and comorbidities, including newly emergent autoimmune conditions.[69,78] Pulmonary function testing and chest imaging are reasonable in patients with chronic breathlessness and/or evidence of oxygen desaturation on exertion.[73] Brain imaging in most cases may be best reserved for patients with focal neurologic deficits or a history of head trauma. Transthoracic echocardiography, cardiac stress testing, and cardiopulmonary exercise testing should be considered on an individual basis based on the patient's associated symptoms and treatment plan.

PREVENTION

Prevention of long COVID can best be achieved through consistent use of established tools for the prevention of COVID-19, including vaccination, the appropriate use of personal protective equipment, hand hygiene, and social distancing. Studies are underway to understand if early use of effective antiviral therapies (eg, monoclonal antibodies or other antiviral therapies) can mitigate or prevent long COVID in patients infected with COVID-19. Reports of the mitigating effects of vaccination on long COVID are intriguing. This includes a large UK prospective, community-based, nested, case-control study using self-reported data that found that when compared with unvaccinated participants, vaccination before SARS-CoV-2 infection was associated with reduced likelihood of symptomatic acute COVID-19, and reduced odds of long-duration (≥28 days) symptoms following the second vaccine dose.[79] Intriguing results from a prospective, single-center study of 449 discharged hospital patients suggest a significant, 35.9% reduction in long COVID at 6 months in those treated with the antiviral remdesivir during the acute period, with multivariate analysis identifying the drug as an independent predictor of the syndrome (OR = 0.641; 95%

CI = 0.413–0.782; P < .001).[58] Although confirmatory, randomized, placebo-controlled trails are needed, these studies support the possibility that a host of interventions, including early effective antiviral interventions and vaccination, may have a substantial mitigating effect on long COVID.

Treatment

Although there are few studies of treatment in long COVID that have shown efficacy or effectiveness, consensus guidance on best approaches to treat these patients based on the lived experience of patient and clinicians are emerging.[71–73,80] The overall approach to treatment of long COVID is to focus on managing symptoms, improving function, and working with the patient to settle on reasonable treatment targets that have the potential to improve their quality of life. Given the wide array and varying magnitude of presentation of long COVID symptoms, multiprong approaches may be needed. Providing patients with the tools for self-management is crucial early in the disease course because patients are often dealing with isolation and uncertainty. The goal of self-management is to help the patient be in control of their disease and healing process. The primary care providers or generalists should remain integrated in the care of these patients to facilitate access to local physiotherapy, occupational therapy, dieticians, or home care. In addition, the primary care provider has an important role in searching for alternative diagnoses, so that not all the patient's symptoms are automatically attributed to this syndrome.

Titrating physical activity: The evaluation may first focus on the patient's medical history, diagnostic tests, pre-COVID-19 level of physical activity, and social determinants of health. Patients should be screened for postexertional symptom exacerbation through careful monitoring of their symptoms both during physical activity and in the days following the activity. Signs of exertional oxygen desaturation, orthostatic intolerance, or autonomic dysfunction may also be important to titrate the appropriate level and type of physical activity during the recovery process. Importantly, telling patients to push through their pain or discomfort during the early periods may lead to worsening postexertional malaise and may prolong recovery. It is important to individualize the patient-reported outcome measure to each patient and to consider the reality of postexertional malaise and energy conservation in the educational interventions. NICE guidelines do not recommend graded exercise therapy or any physical activity program that uses a fixed incremental increase in physical activity. Rather, more recent guidelines recommend a symptom-titrated physical activity approach in which physical activity is continuously monitored an adjusted according to symptoms.[7,71] Educational materials can focus on teaching patients how to recognize when they are crossing their anaerobic threshold, which is often much lower than their pre-COVID-19 baseline. In patients who are limited by dizziness, imbalance, and headache symptoms, adjusting mode of exercise to be recumbent may be beneficial along with compression stockings and use of isometric exercises. Vestibular rehabilitation or balance programs may be appropriate in patients demonstrating vestibular impairment or poor balance.

Accommodating cognitive symptoms: For patients with significant impairments in their well-being due to cognitive symptoms, a referral to a specialist who can complete a thorough assessment of the domains of impairment (eg, speech language pathologist, occupational therapist, neuropsychologist) seems a reasonable treatment approach.[72] The evaluation may focus on the assessment of memory, attention, language, energy and cognitive endurance, sleep, and other symptoms. Patients should be asked about their living situation, their work or school status, and what cognitive symptoms are most troubling them. Educational materials may focus on memory, attention, communication strategies, helping patients understand what types of cognitive activities use up the most cognitive energy, and helping patients to assess factors that may be affecting their cognitive energy such as mood, stress, sleep, pain, or medication changes.

Dysautonomia: For patients with dysautonomia symptoms, the education materials may focus on the 4 pillars of active nonpharmacologic management: liberalizing salt intake, increasing hydration, low level of physical activity, and the use of compression garments. For patients with gastrointestinal symptoms of dysautonomia, eating small and frequent meals and eating slowly in a low-stress environment may help alleviate some of the symptoms. For patients with heat intolerance, cold showers and ice packs applied to the face and neck may be important.

Referral to post-COVID or other subspecialty clinics: In response to the growing numbers of individuals presenting with long-COVID, multidisciplinary outpatient clinics have been formed throughout the United States and other countries. Using their experiences in the formation of such academic health clinics centers at Johns Hopkins and the University of California, San Francisco, Santhoth and colleagues suggest a framework focused on addressing clinical needs through coordination across multiple subspecialties to address impairments in physical function, cognitive function and mental health, longitudinal follow-up, and integration of research efforts to foster greater understanding of evolving disease processes.[51] As the pandemic continues, addressing optimal resource allocation, the focus of care (primary vs specialty), and the ability to scale-up will also become increasingly challenging.[81] Earlier referral may be appropriate in younger patients, more complex patients in whom the diagnosis is unclear and the treatment challenging, in patients for whom the disability impact of illness is severe, and in patients in whom local clinical support is limited.

DISCUSSION OF NEXT STEPS, CHALLENGES, AND UNANSWERED QUESTIONS

In recognition of the significant public health impact of long COVID, the National Institutes of Health launched a major initiative in February 2021 to support research efforts to better understand the cause of long COVID, and to identify best methods of prevention and treatment for affected individuals.[82] Additional efforts toward systematic collection of large-scale clinical data to examine the medium- and long-term consequences of COVID-19 have also come from the WHO, through their creation of a post-COVID case report form.[83]

Collections of individuals afflicted with long COVID have made an important contribution to the research response. Key initial reports of the defining symptoms of long COVID have come from such groups of citizen scientists and the large-scale surveys to which they have contributed. The first detailed patient surveys of long COVID came from efforts from the international Patient-Led Research Collaborative born out of the Body Politic support group.[37] The study sample in this study consisted predominately of white females between the ages 30 and 49 years. . A higher proportion of females has since been documented in subsequent peer-reviewed survey studies of long COVID symptoms[11]More research is needed to better understand the biological and psychosocial factors that may explain any differences in risk of long COVID symptsom by sex and/or gender. Another important challenge in long COVID research is that across many of the studies, the proportion of the study sample with laboratory confirmed SARS-CoV-2 infection will vary depending on the phase of the pandemic, the local availability of COVID-19 testing, the sensitivity and specificity of the specific COVID-19 tests used. Challenges with attribution of reported symptoms to the sequelae of COVID-19 infection were further revealed in a recent cross-sectional analysis of 26,823 individuals participating in the French population-based CONSTANCES cohort.[84] After adjusting for key metrics, including age, sex, income, self-reported health, level of education, and depressive symptoms, linear regression models revealed that the presence of a persistent long COVID symptom lasting for greater than 8 weeks was more strongly associated with a belief in having had COVID-19 than with having serologically confirmed COVID-19 infection. The limited sensitivity of COVID-19 serology performed after a long delay from symptom onset should, however, be kept in mind in interpreting this study.[84]

As of this writing, little of the published research on long COVID has been conducted in low- and middle-income countries. In addition, despite the disproportionate impact of COVID-19 on historically disadvantaged populations in the United States, the impact of long COVID in Black, Indigenous, and People of color community settings have been underexplored.

SUMMARY

The long-term sequelae of COVID-19 are protean, impacting multiple organ systems to varying degrees. The multiorgan dysfunction induced by COVID-19 has the potential to result in significant morbidity in affected individuals. The growing proportion of patients recovering from COVID-19 makes an improved understanding of risk factors, mechanistic pathways, sequelae, and potential mitigating factors important research and clinical goals.

CLINICS CARE POINTS

- Provide patients with physical fatigue, cognitive symptoms, and/or postexertional malaise educational materials about the importance of energy conservation
  - 4 *P's*: pacing, prioritization, planning, positioning.[71]
- Consider referring patients with cognitive complaints to specialist with expertise in cognitive rehabilitation therapies (eg, speech therapist, occupational therapist, neuropsychologist).[72]
- Assess the impact of the symptoms on the patient's ability to return to normal daily activities and consider early disability accommodations to facilitate recovery.
- For individuals with autonomic dysfunction without evidence or history of congestive heart failure, pericarditis, myocarditis, coronary artery disease, or essential hypertension, nonpharmacologic management can include[75]:
  - Liberalizing salt and electrolyte intake
  - Increase fluid intake
  - Compression garments
  - Individualized return to physical activity including consideration of recumbent or supine exercises.

DISCLOSURE

T.H. Evering, author, is a consultant for Tonix Pharmaceuticals. Aluko A. Hope is funded by the NIH (K01 HL 140279). I am waiting to hear from Teresa regarding her NIH funding sources.

REFERENCES

1. Datta SD, Talwar A, Lee JT. A Proposed Framework and Timeline of the Spectrum of Disease Due to SARS-CoV-2 Infection: Illness Beyond Acute Infection and Public Health Implications. JAMA 2020;324(22):2251–2.

2. Nalbandian A, Sehgal K, Gupta A, et al. Post-acute COVID-19 syndrome. Nat Med 2021;27(4):601–15.
3. Morris SB, Schwartz NG, Patel P, et al. Case Series of Multisystem Inflammatory Syndrome in Adults Associated with SARS-CoV-2 Infection - United Kingdom and United States, March-August 2020. MMWR Morb Mortal Wkly Rep 2020;69(40):1450–6.
4. Feldstein LR, Rose EB, Horwitz SM, et al. Multisystem Inflammatory Syndrome in U.S. Children and Adolescents. N Engl J Med 2020;383(4):334–46.
5. Lerner AM, Robinson DA, Yang L, et al. Toward Understanding COVID-19 Recovery: National Institutes of Health Workshop on Postacute COVID-19. Ann Intern Med 2021;174(7):999–1003.
6. Centers for Disease Control. Centers for Disease Control & Prevention Post COVID Conditions. Available at: https://www.cdc.gov/coronavirus/2019-ncov/long-term-effects/index.html?CDC_AA_refVal=https%3A%2F%2Fwww.cdc.gov%2Fcoronavirus%2F2019-ncov%2Flong-term-effects.html.
7. Shah W, Hillman T, Playford ED, et al. Managing the long term effects of covid-19: summary of NICE, SIGN, and RCGP rapid guideline. BMJ 2021;372:n136.
8. World Health Organization. Post-COVID Case Definition. Available at: https://www.who.int/publications/i/item/WHO-2019-nCoV-Post_COVID-19_condition-Clinical_case_definition-2021.1.
9. Crook H, Raza S, Nowell J, et al. Long covid-mechanisms, risk factors, and management. BMJ 2021;374:n1648.
10. Townsend L, Dowds J, O'Brien K, et al. Persistent Poor Health after COVID-19 Is Not Associated with Respiratory Complications or Initial Disease Severity. Ann Am Thorac Soc 2021;18(6):997–1003.
11. Sudre CH, Murray B, Varsavsky T, et al. Attributes and predictors of long COVID. Nat Med 2021;27(4):626–31.
12. Drew DA, Nguyen LH, Steves CJ, et al. Rapid implementation of mobile technology for real-time epidemiology of COVID-19. Science 2020;368(6497):1362–7.
13. Greenhalgh T, Knight M, A'Court C, et al. Management of post-acute covid-19 in primary care. BMJ 2020;370:m3026.
14. Tenforde MW, Kim SS, Lindsell CJ, et al. Symptom Duration and Risk Factors for Delayed Return to Usual Health Among Outpatients with COVID-19 in a Multistate Health Care Systems Network - United States, March-June 2020. MMWR Morb Mortal Wkly Rep 2020;69(30):993–8.
15. Logue JK, Franko NM, McCulloch DJ, et al. Sequelae in Adults at 6 Months After COVID-19 Infection. JAMA Netw Open 2021;4(2):e210830.
16. Fernandez-de-Las-Penas C, Palacios-Cena D, Gomez-Mayordomo V, et al. Long-term post-COVID symptoms and associated risk factors in previously hospitalized patients: A multicenter study. J Infect 2021;83(2):237–79.
17. Fernandez-de-Las-Penas C. Long COVID: current definition. Infection 2021.
18. Carvalho-Schneider C, Laurent E, Lemaignen A, et al. Follow-up of adults with noncritical COVID-19 two months after symptom onset. Clin Microbiol Infect 2021;27(2):258–63.
19. Carfi A, Bernabei R, Landi F, et al. Persistent Symptoms in Patients After Acute COVID-19. JAMA 2020;324(6):603–5.
20. Huang C, Huang L, Wang Y, et al. 6-month consequences of COVID-19 in patients discharged from hospital: a cohort study. Lancet 2021;397(10270):220–32.
21. Goertz YMJ, Van Herck M, Delbressine JM, et al. Persistent symptoms 3 months after a SARS-CoV-2 infection: the post-COVID-19 syndrome? ERJ Open Res 2020;6(4).

22. Blomberg B, Mohn KG, Brokstad KA, et al, Bergen COVID-19 Research Group. Long COVID in a prospective cohort of home-isolated patients. Nat Med 2021; 27(9):1607–13.

23. Groff D, Sun A, Ssentongo AE, et al. Short-term and Long-term Rates of Postacute Sequelae of SARS-CoV-2 Infection: A Systematic Review. JAMA Netw Open 2021;4(10):e2128568.

24. Ceban F, Ling S, Lui LMW, et al. Fatigue and cognitive impairment in Post-COVID-19 Syndrome: A systematic review and meta-analysis. Brain Behav Immun 2021; 101:93–135.

25. Siripanthong B, Nazarian S, Muser D, et al. Recognizing COVID-19-related myocarditis: The possible pathophysiology and proposed guideline for diagnosis and management. Heart Rhythm 2020;17(9):1463–71.

26. Blitshteyn S, Whitelaw S. Postural orthostatic tachycardia syndrome (POTS) and other autonomic disorders after COVID-19 infection: a case series of 20 patients. Immunol Res 2021;69(2):205–11.

27. Bisaccia G, Ricci F, Recce V, et al. Post-Acute Sequelae of COVID-19 and Cardiovascular Autonomic Dysfunction: What Do We Know? J Cardiovasc Dev Dis 2021;8(11).

28. Jennings G, Monaghan A, Xue F, et al. A Systematic Review of Persistent Symptoms and Residual Abnormal Functioning following Acute COVID-19: Ongoing Symptomatic Phase vs. Post-COVID-19 Syndrome. J Clin Med 2021;10(24).

29. Iadecola C, Anrather J, Kamel H. Effects of COVID-19 on the Nervous System. Cell 2020;183(1):16–27 e1.

30. Rogers JP, Chesney E, Oliver D, et al. Psychiatric and neuropsychiatric presentations associated with severe coronavirus infections: a systematic review and meta-analysis with comparison to the COVID-19 pandemic. Lancet Psychiatry 2020;7(7):611–27.

31. Colatutto D, Sonaglia A, Zabotti A, et al. Post-COVID-19 Arthritis and Sacroiliitis: Natural History with Longitudinal Magnetic Resonance Imaging Study in Two Cases and Review of the Literature. Viruses 2021;13(8).

32. Sultan S, Altayar O, Siddique SM, et al. AGA Institute Rapid Review of the Gastrointestinal and Liver Manifestations of COVID-19, Meta-Analysis of International Data, and Recommendations for the Consultative Management of Patients with COVID-19. Gastroenterology 2020;159(1):320–334 e27.

33. Lopez-Leon S, Wegman-Ostrosky T, Perelman C, et al. More than 50 long-term effects of COVID-19: a systematic review and meta-analysis. Sci Rep 2021; 11(1):16144.

34. Serviente C, Decker ST, Layec G. From heart to muscle: Pathophysiological mechanisms underlying long-term physical sequelae from SARS-CoV-2 infection. J Appl Physiol 1985;2022.

35. Chopra V, Flanders SA, O'Malley M, et al. Sixty-Day Outcomes Among Patients Hospitalized With COVID-19. Ann Intern Med 2021;174(4):576–8.

36. Iwashyna TJ, Kamphuis LA, Gundel SJ, et al. Continuing Cardiopulmonary Symptoms, Disability, and Financial Toxicity 1 Month After Hospitalization for Third-Wave COVID-19: Early Results From a US Nationwide Cohort. J Hosp Med 2021.

37. Davis HE, Assaf GS, McCorkell L, et al. Characterizing long COVID in an international cohort: 7 months of symptoms and their impact. EClinicalMedicine 2021; 38:101019.

38. Singh I, Joseph P, Heerdt PM, et al. Persistent Exertional Intolerance After COVID-19: Insights From Invasive Cardiopulmonary Exercise Testing. Chest 2022;161(1):54–63.

39. George PM, Barratt SL, Condliffe R, et al. Respiratory follow-up of patients with COVID-19 pneumonia. Thorax 2020;75(11):1009–16.
40. Qin W, Chen S, Zhang Y, et al. Diffusion capacity abnormalities for carbon monoxide in patients with COVID-19 at 3-month follow-up. Eur Respir J 2021;58(1).
41. Younger DS. Post-acute sequelae of SARS-CoV-2 infection (PASC): peripheral, autonomic, and central nervous system features in a child. Neurol Sci 2021; 42(10):3959–63.
42. Gupta A, Madhavan MV, Sehgal K, et al. Extrapulmonary manifestations of COVID-19. Nat Med 2020;26(7):1017–32.
43. Fleming KC, Volcheck MM. Central sensitization syndrome and the initial evaluation of a patient with fibromyalgia: a review. Rambam Maimonides Med J 2015; 6(2):e0020.
44. Bierle DM, Aakre CA, Grach SL, et al. Central Sensitization Phenotypes in Post Acute Sequelae of SARS-CoV-2 Infection (PASC): Defining the Post COVID Syndrome. J Prim Care Community Health 2021;12. 21501327211030826.
45. Schou TM, Joca S, Wegener G. Bay-Richter C. Psychiatric and neuropsychiatric sequelae of COVID-19 - A systematic review. Brain Behav Immun 2021;97: 328–48.
46. Merikanto I, Dauvilliers Y, Chung F, et al. Disturbances in sleep, circadian rhythms and daytime functioning in relation to coronavirus infection and Long-COVID - A multinational ICOSS study. J Sleep Res 2021;e13542.
47. Dani M, Dirksen A, Taraborrelli P, et al. Autonomic dysfunction in 'long COVID': rationale, physiology and management strategies. Clin Med (Lond) 2021;21(1):e63–7.
48. Graham EL, Clark JR, Orban ZS, et al. Persistent neurologic symptoms and cognitive dysfunction in non-hospitalized Covid-19 "long haulers. Ann Clin Transl Neurol 2021;8(5):1073–85.
49. Patel MB, Morandi A, Pandharipande PP. What's new in post-ICU cognitive impairment? Intensive Care Med 2015;41(4):708–11.
50. Katz BZ, Collin SM, Murphy G, et al. The International Collaborative on Fatigue Following Infection (COFFI). Fatigue 2018;6(2):106–21.
51. Ho-Yen DO. Patient management of post-viral fatigue syndrome. Br J Gen Pract 1990;40(330):37–9.
52. Beyond Myalgic Encephalomyelitis/Chronic Fatigue Syndrome: Redefining an Illness. Washington (DC)2015.
53. Kumar A, Narayan RK, Prasoon P, et al. COVID-19 Mechanisms in the Human Body-What We Know So Far. Front Immunol 2021;12:693938.
54. Cristillo V, Pilotto A, Cotti Piccinelli S, et al. Premorbid vulnerability and disease severity impact on Long-COVID cognitive impairment. Aging Clin Exp Res 2022.
55. Asadi-Pooya AA, Akbari A, Emami A, et al. Risk Factors Associated with Long COVID Syndrome: A Retrospective Study. Iran J Med Sci 2021;46(6):428–36.
56. Bai F, Tomasoni D, Falcinella C, et al. Female gender is associated with long COVID syndrome: a prospective cohort study. Clin Microbiol Infect 2021.
57. Sigfrid L, Drake TM, Pauley E, et al. Long Covid in adults discharged from UK hospitals after Covid-19: A prospective, multicentre cohort study using the ISARIC WHO Clinical Characterisation Protocol. Lancet Reg Health Eur 2021;8:100186.
58. Boglione L, Meli G, Poletti F, et al. Risk factors and incidence of long-COVID syndrome in hospitalized patients: does remdesivir have a protective effect? QJM 2022;114(12):865–71.
59. Menni C, Valdes AM, Freidin MB, et al. Real-time tracking of self-reported symptoms to predict potential COVID-19. Nat Med 2020;26(7):1037–40.

60. Martin-Loeches I, Motos A, Menendez R, et al. ICU-Acquired Pneumonia Is Associated with Poor Health Post-COVID-19 Syndrome. J Clin Med 2021;11(1).
61. Hoffmann M, Kleine-Weber H, Schroeder S, et al. SARS-CoV-2 Cell Entry Depends on ACE2 and TMPRSS2 and Is Blocked by a Clinically Proven Protease Inhibitor. Cell 2020;181(2):271–280 e8.
62. Gaebler C, Wang Z, Lorenzi JCC, et al. Evolution of antibody immunity to SARS-CoV-2. Nature 2021;591(7851):639–44.
63. Cheung KS, Hung IFN, Chan PPY, et al. Gastrointestinal Manifestations of SARS-CoV-2 Infection and Virus Load in Fecal Samples From a Hong Kong Cohort: Systematic Review and Meta-analysis. Gastroenterology 2020;159(1):81–95.
64. Vonbank K, Lehmann A, Bernitzky D, et al. Predictors of Prolonged Cardiopulmonary Exercise Impairment After COVID-19 Infection: A Prospective Observational Study. Front Med (Lausanne) 2021;8:773788.
65. Peluso MJ, Lu S, Tang AF, et al. Markers of Immune Activation and Inflammation in Individuals With Postacute Sequelae of Severe Acute Respiratory Syndrome Coronavirus 2 Infection. J Infect Dis 2021;224(11):1839–48.
66. Plassmeyer M, Alpan O, Corley MJ, et al. Caspases and therapeutic potential of caspase inhibitors in moderate-severe SARS-CoV-2 infection and long COVID. Allergy 2022;77(1):118–29.
67. Ehrenfeld M, Tincani A, Andreoli L, et al. Covid-19 and autoimmunity. Autoimmun Rev 2020;19(8):102597.
68. Desai AD, Lavelle M, Boursiquot BC, et al. Long-term complications of COVID-19. Am J Physiol Cell Physiol 2022;322(1):C1–11.
69. Acosta-Ampudia Y, Monsalve DM, Rojas M, et al. Persistent Autoimmune Activation and Proinflammatory State in Post-COVID Syndrome. J Infect Dis 2022.
70. de Boer E, Petrache I, Goldstein NM, et al. Decreased Fatty Acid Oxidation and Altered Lactate Production during Exercise in Patients with Post-acute COVID-19 Syndrome. Am J Respir Crit Care Med 2022;205(1):126–9.
71. Herrera JE, Niehaus WN, Whiteson J, et al. Multidisciplinary collaborative consensus guidance statement on the assessment and treatment of fatigue in postacute sequelae of SARS-CoV-2 infection (PASC) patients. PM R 2021;13(9):1027–43.
72. Fine JS, Ambrose AF, Didehbani N, et al. Multi-disciplinary collaborative consensus guidance statement on the assessment and treatment of cognitive symptoms in patients with post-acute sequelae of SARS-CoV-2 infection (PASC). PM R 2022;14(1):96–111.
73. Maley JH, Alba GA, Barry JT, et al. Multi-disciplinary collaborative consensus guidance statement on the assessment and treatment of breathing discomfort and respiratory sequelae in patients with post-acute sequelae of SARS-CoV-2 infection (PASC). PM R 2022;14(1):77–95.
74. Freeman R, Wieling W, Axelrod FB, et al. Consensus statement on the definition of orthostatic hypotension, neurally mediated syncope and the postural tachycardia syndrome. Clin Auton Res 2011;21(2):69–72.
75. Lahrmann H, Cortelli P, Hilz M, et al. EFNS guidelines on the diagnosis and management of orthostatic hypotension. Eur J Neurol 2006;13(9):930–6.
76. Invernizzi A, Torre A, Parrulli S, et al. Retinal findings in patients with COVID-19: Results from the SERPICO-19 study. EClinicalMedicine 2020;27:100550.
77. Invernizzi A, Schiuma M, Parrulli S, et al. Retinal vessels modifications in acute and post-COVID-19. Sci Rep 2021;11(1):19373.
78. Murugan AK, Alzahrani AS. SARS-CoV-2: Emerging Role in the Pathogenesis of Various Thyroid Diseases. J Inflamm Res 2021;14:6191–221. https://doi.org/10.2147/jir.S332705.

79. Antonelli M, Penfold RS, Merino J, et al. Risk factors and disease profile of post-vaccination SARS-CoV-2 infection in UK users of the COVID Symptom Study app: a prospective, community-based, nested, case-control study. Lancet Infect Dis 2022;22(1):43–55.

80. Vance H, Maslach A, Stoneman E, et al. Addressing Post-COVID Symptoms: A Guide for Primary Care Physicians. J Am Board Fam Med 2021;34(6):1229–42.

81. Yu E, Kelly B. The Next Challenge for Post-COVID-19 Clinics: Scale. Chest 2022; 161(1):e63.

82. Natinal Institutes of Health. NIH launches new initiative to study "Long COVID". Available at: https://www.nih.gov/about-nih/who-we-are/nih-director/statements/nih-launches-new-initiative-study-long-covid.

83. World Health Organization. Global COVID-19 Clinical Platform Case REport Form for Post COVID condition (Post COVID-19 CRF). Available at: https://www.who.int/publications/i/item/global-covid-19-clinical-platform-case-report-form-(crf)-for-post-covid-conditions-(post-covid-19-crf-. Accessed December 29, 2021.

84. Matta J, Wiernik E, Robineau O, et al. Association of Self-reported COVID-19 Infection and SARS-CoV-2 Serology Test Results With Persistent Physical Symptoms Among French Adults During the COVID-19 Pandemic. JAMA Intern Med 2022;182(1):19–25.

COVID-19 in the Immunocompromised Host, Including People with Human Immunodeficiency Virus

Niyati Jakharia, MD[a,]*, Aruna K. Subramanian, MD[a],
Adrienne E. Shapiro, MD, PhD[b,c]

KEYWORDS

- HIV • Immunocompromise • CD4 • COVID-19 • SARS-CoV-2
- Solid organ transplant • Immunosuppression • Hematopoietic stem cell transplant

KEY POINTS

- Persons with immunocompromising conditions are at elevated risk of severe outcomes, hospitalization, and death from severe acute respiratory distress syndrome (SARS)-coronavirus 2 (CoV-2) infection.
- Immunocompromising conditions are associated with decreased protective immunity after an initial infection with SARS-CoV-2 and decreased efficacy of COVID-19 vaccines.
- Persons with certain immunocompromising conditions should receive an additional dose(s) of initial vaccine series and should be prioritized for receipt of therapeutics and consideration of other preventive interventions.

HUMAN IMMUNODEFICIENCY VIRUS

Epidemiology

Incidence of COVID-19 in people with human immunodeficiency virus
There is conflicting evidence regarding whether COVID-19 incidence is higher in people with human immunodeficiency virus (HIV) (PWH) compared with people without HIV, after controlling for medical and structural risks that increase exposure to severe acute respiratory distress syndrome (SARS)–coronavirus 2 (CoV-2) and affect likelihood of progression to detected disease. A large study using linked clinical data from adults attending public sector health facilities from March 2020 to June 2020 in South Africa found a similar crude prevalence of laboratory-diagnosed COVID-19

[a] Department of Medicine, Division of Infectious Disease, Stanford University School of Medicine, 300 Pasteur Drive, Lane L134, Stanford, CA 94305, USA; [b] Department of Global Health, University of Washington, 325 Ninth Avenue, Box 359927, Seattle, WA 98104, USA; [c] Department of Medicine, Division of Allergy and Infectious Diseases, University of Washington, Seattle, WA, USA
* Corresponding author.
E-mail address: nnarsana@stanford.edu

Infect Dis Clin N Am 36 (2022) 397–421
https://doi.org/10.1016/j.idc.2022.01.006   id.theclinics.com
0891-5520/22/© 2022 Elsevier Inc. All rights reserved.

in PWH compared with people without HIV but was unable to control for age and immune status.[1] By contrast, public health surveillance data in San Francisco found an increased proportion of positive tests among PWH tested for COVID-19 compared with people without HIV (4.5% vs 3.5%; $P < .001$).[2] This discrepancy in the risk of infection was attributed to structural factors increasing exposure among PWH; the investigators noted a greater proportion of tested PWH were living in congregate housing or were homeless. Routine COVID-19 testing services in a federally qualified health center population in Chicago found the test positivity between March 2020 and July 2020 in PWH (10.6%) and HIV-negative patients (7.1%) was not significantly different in adjusted models.[3] Data from an insured Kaiser Permanente cohort in the United States found that PWH were twice as likely to be diagnosed with COVID-19, despite being younger and having fewer comorbidities than others in their network.[4] In the Center for AIDS Research Network of Integrated Clinical Systems (CNICS) multisite cohort of PWH in the United States, the strongest predictors of having COVID-19 in 2020 were self-identifying as black or Hispanic, female sex, and having diabetes or hypertension. The only HIV-specific predictor of having COVID-19 in this cohort was having a history of having a CD4[+] cell count less than or equal to $350/mm^3$ or a low current CD4/CD8 ratio; current CD4[+] cell count, being on antiretroviral therapy (ART), and viral suppression were not associated with COVID-19 incidence in this cohort.[5] Wider serosurveillance studies are necessary to determine absolute risk of infection conferred by HIV, with adequate controlling for structural factors that affect exposure as well as clinical risks that may affect symptom manifestation.

Descriptive epidemiology of the natural history of COVID-19 disease in people with human immunodeficiency virus

Infection with SARS-CoV-2 has differential consequences in PWH compared with persons without HIV. Several global registry data and cohorts have demonstrated a higher risk of severe disease and mortality from COVID-19 in PWH, with World Health Organization (WHO) global registry data estimating an adjusted mortality hazard ratio (HR) of 1.29 (95% CI, 1.23–1.35) in PWH, although most estimates did not adjust directly for CD4[+] cell count.[1,6,7] Some cohorts with a relatively higher proportion of PWH without immunosuppression have not observed increased mortality with HIV.[8] After infection with SARS-CoV-2, PWH can develop robust antibody and T-cell responses comparable to those seen in people without HIV; however, low CD4[+] cell count and low CD4:CD8 ratio, indicators of T-cell immunocompromise, are associated with impaired IgG antibody response, neutralization, and T-cell responses following infection.[9,10]

Time to clearance of SARS-CoV-2 may be prolonged in immunocompromised PWH compared with typical clearance time in immunocompetent persons. Cases have been documented of prolonged infectious viral shedding in immunosuppressed PWH with unsuppressed HIV viral loads, resulting in persistent illness and allowing accumulation of immune escape mutations in the viral genome.[11,12]

Many PWH experience an acute decrease in CD4[+] cell count at the time of SARS-CoV-2 infection, as a component of generalized lymphopenia that is a consequence of COVID-19. There is conflicting evidence about the effect of acute SARS-CoV-2 on HIV viral suppression in PWH. A small case series (n = 35) from Wuhan, China, found evidence of HIV viral blips (transiently detectable low-level viremia) during acute COVID-19 despite continuous ART.[13] Similarly, another study comparing PWH serum samples pre-COVID and serum samples in PWH with polymerase chain reaction (PCR)-proved COVID-19, using highly sensitive single-copy HIV viral assays, detected a trend toward increased detectable, low-level viremia in PWH with COVID-19.[14] The clinical significance of these viral blips in each setting likely is minimal but suggests an immunomodulatory effect of SARS-CoV-2 on HIV immune control, which has unclear long-term implications.

No significant differences have emerged in non–HIV-specific inflammatory markers (eg, cytokines, C-reactive protein, D dimer, and other laboratory markers) or clinical presentation of COVID-19 in PWH compared with HIV-negative controls in larger cohorts.[15,16]

Predictors of severe disease and death in people with human immunodeficiency virus
Although studies conducted early in the COVID-19 pandemic did not detect a strong association between CD4 count and severity of COVID-19 outcomes,[17,18] subsequent well-characterized cohorts have established a strong and consistent association between HIV-associated immune suppression and increased risk of severe COVID-19 outcomes (hospitalization, intensive care, and mortality). In studies that better quantified the relationship of CD4$^+$ cell count to risk of COVID-19 hospitalization and death, however, CD4$^+$ cell count less than 200/mm^3 was consistently associated with increased risk of hospitalization[7,8,19] and death[7,19]; in the CNICS cohort of more than 15,000 PWH, CD4$^+$ cell count less than 350/mm^3 was significantly associated with an adjusted relative risk of 2.68 (95% CI, 1.93–3.71) for hospitalization.[20] The relationship between lack of ART or unsuppressed viral load and COVID-19 outcomes is less clearly defined, in part because the proportion of many PWH in US cohorts who are not on ART or virally unsuppressed is relatively small. In studies in which there is power to evaluate it, there seems to be a trend toward increased risk of hospitalization and mortality in PWH not on ART or virally unsuppressed.[7,21]

In PWH, non–HIV-specific comorbidities, including diabetes, obesity, liver disease, renal disease, and cardiovascular disease,[16,19,22,23] confer similar elevated risk of poor COVID-19 outcomes as in people without HIV.

Treatment Considerations for people with Human Immunodeficiency Virus

Treatment of PWH hospitalized with COVID-19 is not different from treatment of non-immunosuppressed persons or persons without HIV. Treatment guidelines for the use of the antiviral remdesivir and corticosteroids, including dexamethasone, and consideration of immunomodulatory therapies, such as tocilizumab all are independent of HIV status or degree of immune compromise.[24] In contrast, for ambulatory PWH with COVID-19 and no supplemental oxygen requirement, given the demonstrated elevated risk of COVID-19 disease progression seen in PWH overall and most strongly among PWH with untreated HIV or with CD4$^+$ cell count less than 350/mm^3, these immunocompromised PWH meet National Institutes of Health (NIH) COVID-19 treatment guidelines recommendations criteria for consideration of early therapies, including approved neutralizing monoclonal antibodies (mAbs) with efficacy against the presumed infecting SARS-CoV-2 variant.[25] Oral antivirals (molnupiravir and nirmatrelvir/ritonavir) also may be appropriate early therapies for PWH, although the use of a ritonavir booster in the nirmatrelvir combination may have limiting interactions with certain antiretrovirals; the US Food and Drug Administration (FDA) Emergency Use Authorization (EUA) for nirmatrelvir/ritonavir indicates that ritonavir- or cobicistat-containing ART regimens should be continued unmodified, with clinical monitoring for adverse effects.[26,27] PWH with immune compromise or uncontrolled viremia should be urgently prioritized for early therapeutics that have demonstrated efficacy in reducing the risk of severe outcomes, including hospitalization and death.

Prevention Considerations for People with Human Immunodeficiency Virus

PWH should be prioritized for receipt of preventive vaccines. PWH with CD4$^+$ cell counts less than 200/mm^3 were excluded from initial phase 3 vaccine efficacy trials, but many trials included PWH without advanced HIV. Vaccine efficacy in PWH in trials was similar to people without HIV receiving the ChAdOx1 nCov-19 vaccine (AstraZeneca, United Kingdom) and the BNT162b2 (Pfizer-BioNTech, United States) vaccine.[28–30] A study of 100 PWH and 100 matched HIV-uninfected controls found PWH had lower IgG antibody responses and viral neutralization assays responses after receipt of mRNA vaccines, with a stronger effect seen among PWH with lower $CD4^+$ cell counts or unsuppressed viral loads.[31] Given this observation of decreased vaccine-induced antibody responses in PWH with immunosuppression, PWH meeting these criteria are recommended to receive an additional vaccine dose as part of the initial series as well as a subsequent booster dose. A multicountry cohort of 6952 PWH showed COVID-19 vaccine uptake among PWH globally has broadly mirrored uptake in the general population for many countries, although this corresponds to wide variations in vaccination prevalence by country, with residence in a high-income country the most significant predictor of receipt of a vaccine.[32]

Health Care Access and Continuity of Care

Globally, the COVID-19 pandemic has had a devastating effect on continuity of care for PWH, including maintenance of ART and diagnosis and treatment of opportunistic infections.[33] Adapting care models during the pandemic to include telemedicine and telephone appointments has been successful in retaining some PWH in care[34] and limiting loss of viral suppression,[35] but these benefits were not experienced uniformly among PWH. Clinics patients with lower financial and technological resources were disproportionately less able to access care during shelter-in-place periods, with concomitant increased risk of loss of viral suppression seen in persons experiencing homelessness.[36] Increasing home postal delivery of ART enabled maintenance of viral load suppression in an Australian clinic cohort.[37]

Urgent Research Questions

Key research questions remain for addressing COVID-19 in PWH, in particular PWH with current or historic immunosuppression. Vaccines currently provide the best intervention for preventing severe disease in PWH, but vaccines might have lower efficacy in immunosuppressed PWH. Many questions remain regarding the relative immunogenicity of different vaccine types (mRNA, Ad5 vector, Ad26 vector, protein subunit, and whole-inactivated) for PWH, in particular PWH with $CD4^+$ cell count less than $350/mm^3$ or untreated HIV with persistent HIV viremia, the persistence of vaccine-induced immunity, and the optimal dosing and boosting interval for vaccines. Studies, such as the recently initiated COVID-19 Prevention Trials Network (CoVPN) 3008 protocol, evaluating the immunogenicity of the mRNA-1273 (Moderna, United States) vaccine in sub-Saharan Africa in countries with a high prevalence of HIV, are well poised to answer some of these questions, but additional global cohorts of vaccinated PWH should be engaged to assess immunologic markers while clinical and immunologic outcomes are awaited.[38]

Also critical to preventing COVID-19 and severe disease in PWH are additional research into use and indications for prophylactic therapies, including new oral antivirals and neutralizing mAbs, and identifying the PWH who would most benefit from these preventive therapeutics (eg, $CD4^+$ cell count thresholds, other historical immune indicators).

Finally, post-COVID sequelae (long COVID, or postacute sequelae of SARS-CoV-2 [PASC]), characterized by persistent neuropsychiatric, cardiovascular, pulmonary, and other symptoms after the acute phase of COVID-19 has resolved and replicating virus no longer can be demonstrated, is emerging as a significant source of morbidity among people who have had COVID-19.[39] PASC is beginning to be studied in the general population; however, the incidence, prevalence, and predictors of PASC in PWH currently are unknown. One small study characterized PASC in an Indian cohort of 94 PWH, finding a PASC prevalence of 43.6% and increased risk among persons who had had moderate to severe COVID-19 compared with those who had had mild disease.[40] There is an urgent need to characterize risk and manifestations of PASC more broadly, including the relationship between immunosuppression and incidence of PASC, in PWH in larger, more diverse global cohorts. This information is critical to guide post-COVID HIV care, to understand potential interactions between HIV and COVID, and to inform interventional strategies to prevent and treat PASC in PWH.

Clinics Care Points

- PWH with CD4$^+$ T-cell counts less than 350/mm^3 or low CD4$^+$ T-cell count nadirs are at elevated risk for severe disease outcomes with COVID-19 and should be prioritized for vaccination (including additional doses), preventive therapeutic options, and early therapies (antiviral antibodies and mAbs) in the event of infection with SARS-CoV-2.
- To reduce all-cause and COVID-19–specific morbidity and mortality for PWH, it is essential to maintain access to routine HIV care during pandemic COVID-19, especially initiating and continuing ART to achieve and maintain virologic suppression of HIV. Approaches, including telemedicine, extended monthly dispensing, and home delivery of medications, should be explored to prioritize ART continuity.

COVID-19 IN SOLID ORGAN TRANSPLANTION
Epidemiology

Incidence of infection
SARS-CoV-2 infection has led to high mortality and morbidity in solid organ transplant (SOT) patients.[41–43] The incidence of COVID-19 SOT patients is higher than in immunocompetent patients.[44,45] In a large US cohort of 18,121 SOT patients, the incidence of clinically detected COVID was 10.2% from January 2020 to November 2020.[45] A large UK cohort study showed a positivity rate of 3.8% (197/5184) in waitlisted patients and 1.3% (597/46,789) of SOT recipients between February 2020 and May 2020.[42] A study (TANGO) from 12 transplant centers from March 2020 to May 2020, across the United States Italy, and Spain, showed 1.5% positivity rate (144/9845) in hospitalized kidney transplant patients.[46]

Effects of immunosuppression
SARS-CoV-2 infection induces both memory B-cell production and long-lasting functionally replete memory T-cell responses.[47,48] Community-acquired respiratory viral infections in SOT recipients usually are more severe in the early post-transplant period or after receiving lymphocyte-depleting therapies.[49] The pathogenesis of COVID-19 infection involves an early phase of highly replicating virus followed by a late phase of hyperactive or dysregulated immune system that leads to severe systemic effects. The immunosuppression in this population may impair development of T-cell immunity to SARS-CoV-2 virus.[50] Prolonged viral shedding has been observed beyond day 30 in transplant patients. The SARS-CoV-2 plasma viral load also has been associated with mortality in the kidney transplant population.[51] Immunosuppressive therapies may help with curbing severe immune responses in the late phases of COVID-19.[50,52] The effect of immunosuppressive therapies varies with the type and intensity and with phase of

illness. Most centers practice reduction or holding immunosuppression. Most retrospective cohort studies did not reveal any significant impact of immunosuppression on mortality,[41,46,53] except within a liver transplant cohort, in which mycophenolate-containing regimens were an independent risk predictor of severe disease (relative risk = 3.94), especially at doses of greater than 1000 mg/d.[44] These were retrospective studies, however, and must be interpreted with caution. The impact of type and degree of immunosuppression on the course of COVID-19 remains unclear. Further randomized controlled trials (RCTs) are needed to address this question.[54]

Predictors of severe disease and death

The mortality in the SOT population has ranged in studies from 6% to 27% (**Table 1**). The various risk factors associated with mortality in this population are increasing age (>60 years), chronic heart failure, chronic lung disease, obesity, lymphopenia, mycophenolate-containing regimens for immunosuppression, and lung transplantation.[41,42,44,53] In the lung transplant population, chronic lung allograft dysfunction was an independent predictor of mortality.[55] The rate of hospitalization for COVID-19 in SOT recipients also is high, ranging from 30% to 89%. Acute kidney injury has been reported in 24% to 52% of patients. A meta-analysis showed that age, male sex, diabetes mellitus, hypertension, chronic kidney disease, and cardiovascular disease are associated with acute kidney injury in transplant patients and also lead to increased mortality.[56] The reported rate of rejection associated with SARS-CoV-2 infection is low: 1.5% to 6%.

Treatment considerations

Antiviral

Remdesivir. Remdesivir is an inhibitor of viral RNA–based RNA polymerase, which is essential for viral replication of SARS-CoV-2. The Adaptive COVID-19 Treatment Trial (ACTT)-1) showed reduced time to clinical recovery in patients with severe COVID, especially on supplemental oxygen.[62] The WHO solidarity trial did not show any decrease in the in-hospital mortality in hospitalized patients compared with standard of care.[63] There was no significant difference in the outcomes between a 5-day versus 10-day course of remdesivir.[64] Treatment of SOT populations with remdesivir does not differ from that of the general population, although some consider the extended 10-day course for patients without improving clinical status, due to risk for increased duration of viral replication in this population.

Nirmatrelvir/ritonavir and molnupiravir. The FDA granted EUA for both the nirmatrelvir/ritonavir and molnupiravir antivirals in December 2021.

Nirmatrelvir is a SARS-CoV-2 protease inhibitor that inhibits viral replication. It is administered with ritonavir, which inhibits cytochrome P450 3A4, and raises nirmatrelvir levels to a therapeutic range. In the EPIC-HR(Evaluation of Protease Inhibition for Covid-19 in High-Risk Patients) trial, ritonavir-boosted nirmatrelvir (Paxlovid) reduced the risk of hospitalization or death by 88% compared with placebo in nonhospitalized high-risk adults with laboratory-confirmed SARS-CoV-2 infection and within 5 day of symptom onset.[65] This drug must be used with caution, however, in the transplant population, due to the drug interactions between ritonavir and calcineurin inhibitors (CNIs). In the MOVe-OUT (Molnupiravir for Oral Treatment of Covid-19 in Nonhospitalized Patients)trial, molnupiravir reduced the rate of hospitalization or death by 30% compared with placebo in high-risk adults within 5 days of symptom onset, and the recommendations for its use in SOT recipients do not differ from those in the general population.[66]

Table 1
Studies of clinical outcomes of COVID-19 in solid organ transplantation

Study Name	Hospitalization Rates	Mortality (%)	Acute Kidney Injury (%)	Acute Rejection/ Graft Loss (%)	Predictors of Severe Disease or Death
Kates et al.[41] Total n = 482 Lung, liver, heart, kidney	78%	20.5	37.8	6	1. Age > 65 y 2. Chronic heart failure 3. Chronic lung disease 4. Obesity 5. Lymphopenia 6. Abnormal chest imaging
Vinson et al.[45] Total n = 1925 Lung, liver, kidney	42.9%		35.3	1.5	
Colmenero et al.[44] Total n = 111 Liver	86.5%	18			1. Mycophenolate-containing regimen (doses >1000 mg/d) 2. Male gender 3. Charlson comorbidity index 4. Dyspnea at diagnosis
Ravanan et al.[42] Total n = 597 All SOT		25.8%			Increased age
Coll et al.[53] Total n = 778 Kidney, liver, lungs, heart, pancreas	89%	27			1. Lung transplantation 2. Age >60 y 3. Hospital-acquired COVID-19
Cravedi et al.[46] Total n = 144 Kidney	All hospitalized patients	32	52		1. Older patients 2. High LDH, IL-6, and procalcitonin levels 3. High respiratory rate

(continued on next page)

Table 1
(continued)

Study Name	Hospitalization Rates	Mortality (%)	Acute Kidney Injury (%)	Acute Rejection/ Graft Loss (%)	Predictors of Severe Disease or Death
Favà et al.[57] Total n = 104 Kidney	All hospitalized patients	27	47		1. Age 2. ARDS 3. Increased baseline LDH
Webb et al.[58] Total n = 151 Liver	82%	19	38		Age
Hadi et al.[59] Total n = 2307 Kidney, liver, heart, and lung	30.97%	6.45	24.73		
Fisher et al.[60] Total n = 128 Kidney, liver, heart, pancreas	All hospitalized patients	21.9	33.6		1. Male sex 2. Age 3. Diabetes mellitus 4. ANC and D-dimer on presentation 5. Level of respiratory support (WHO index 3 and 4) on presentation
Pereira et al.[61] Total n = 117 Kidney, liver, heart, kidney-pancreas	All hospitalized patients	23			

Abbreviations: ANC, absolute neutrophil count; ARDS, acute respiratory distress syndrome; LDH, lactate dehydrogenase.

Monoclonal antibodies
Various mAbs to the spike protein of SARS-CoV-2 have received EUA by the FDA for treatment of nonhospitalized patients with COVID-19, who are at a high risk of progression to severe disease. Real-world experience in SOT patients showed a decrease in hospitalization and respiratory failure compared with patients who did not receive mAbs (**Table 2**).with
   Accumulating evidence indicates no role for neutralizing mAbs for treatment of COVID in nonimmunocompromised people with moderate to severe COVID-19 requiring hospital care and/or oxygen therapy; however, the role of mAbs for SARS-CoV-2 seronegative, highly immunosuppressed people with moderate to severe COVID-19 still is unclear and may have benefit.[67,68] MAbs generally are not authorized for use in hospitalized patients and, as such, require individual consideration for use in transplant populations.

Convalescent plasma
The FDA issued an EUA for treatment of hospitalized patients with COVID with convalescent plasma from donors who have recovered from COVID-19, which contains antibodies to SARS-CoV-2. In immunocompromised patients, there are only a few case series and retrospective studies that suggest some benefit, however, and RCTs are lacking.[73,74] In a double-blind, placebo-controlled RCT, administration of high-titer (>1:1000 anti–SARS-CoV-2 antibodies) convalescent plasma to older adults within 72 hours of onset of mild symptoms of COVID led to relative risk reduction of development of severe COVID by 48%.[75] In December 2021, the FDA extended the EUA for convalescent plasma to include immunocompromised nonhospitalized patients.

Table 2
Studies of monoclonal antibodies in solid organ transplant patients

Study	Population	Monoclonal Antibody	Outcomes
Yetmar et al.[69]	73 patients with lung, liver, kidney, and heart transplant	Bamlanivimab	1. 12.3% of patients required hospitalization for median of 4 d. 2. No deaths
Klein et al.[70]	20 of 95 kidney transplant patients	Balmanivimab	1. mAb administration led to 15% vs 76% emergency department/hospital visits ($P < .001$).
Del Bello et al.[71]	16/48 patients with kidney, kidney-liver, kidney-heart	5 bamlanivimab 9 bamlanivimab + etesevimab 2 casirivimab + imdevimab	1. 0 vs 46% patients developed severe respiratory failure in the non-mAb group ($P = .007$).
Jenks et al.[72]	175/617 high-risk patients	83% received bamlanivimab + etesevimab 16% bamlanivimab	1.7% vs 24% hospitalizations and 0 vs 2.7% deaths in mAb vs non-mAb groups, respectively

[a]Bamlanivimab or bamlanivimab + etesevimab research are presented for context, but these drugs no longer may be appropriate, depending on circulating variants of concern.

Immunomodulators

COVID-19–associated systemic inflammation results from cytokine release. Interleukin-6 (IL-6) is a proinflammatory cytokine that is released by various cells during systemic inflammation. It is hypothesized that modulating or inhibiting these levels may reduce the severity of COVID-19 infection.

A large, multicenter RCT (RECOVERY, Randomised Evaluation of COVID-19 Therapy) showed decreased 28-day mortality in hospitalized patients with COVID-19 on supplemental oxygen or invasive mechanical ventilation, who received 10 days of dexamethasone (an anti-inflammatory agent).[76]

Tocilizumab and sarilumab, mAbs to IL-6 receptor, are used in management of certain rheumatological disorders and cytokine release syndrome related to chimeric antigen receptor T-cell (CAR-T) therapy. In the RECOVERY and REMAP-CAP (A Randomised, Embedded, Multi-factorial, Adaptive Platform Trial for Community-Acquired Pneumonia) trials, tocilizumab was reported to have mortality benefit in COVID patients with respiratory decompensation, requiring oxygen or noninvasive ventilation.[76,77] These trials, however, did not include SOT patients. These drugs must be used with caution in the SOT population due to an increased risk of secondary infections.

Janus kinase (JAK) inhibitors prevent phosphorylation of proteins that lead to immune activation and inflammation. The COV-BARRIER (Efficacy and safety of baricitinib for the treatment of hospitalised adults with COVID-19) trial showed a decrease in the 28-day mortality, and the ACTT-2 trial showed improved time to recovery in patients who received baricitinib with remdesivir.[78,79] At this time, there is insufficient evidence to recommend for or against the use of these immunomodulators in immunocompromised patients.

Proposed treatment algorithm for solid organ transplant patients with COVID-19 as outlined below.

Prevention

Vaccine safety in solid organ transplant patients

A study of 741 SOT patients undergoing mRNA vaccination showed that the reactogenicity of this vaccine was similar to that seen in immunocompetent adults. There were no cases of anaphylaxis or new SARS-CoV-2 diagnosis. Only 1 patient developed acute rejection after the second dose.[80]

Immunogenicity of vaccines in solid organ transplantation

A significant proportion of organ transplant patients do not develop humoral response despite 2 doses of mRNA vaccine. In 658 transplant patients undergoing vaccination, 46% patients did not have an antispike protein antibody response after 2 doses of vaccine. Poor humoral response was associated with use of antimetabolite immunosuppression.[81] In another study of 127 SOT patients receiving mRNA-1273 (Moderna), anti–receptor binding domain of the antispike protein (RBD) antibody response was seen in 34%, neutralizing antibody in 29%. CD4+ T-cell responses were observed in 48% of patients,[82] and these responses were present in a significant proportion of patients who also were antibody negative.

Vaccine effectiveness

Various studies showed that vaccine effectiveness in immunocompromised patients was lower compared with immunocompetent patients (**Table 3**). The immunogenicity of vaccines is low in transplant patients, and although there lack sufficient vaccine efficacy data in this population, there is observation of reduced clinical effectiveness. The breakthrough infection rate ranged from 0.4% to 0.8%. A UK registry study of

Disease Severity	Recommendations
Nonhospitalized setting	1. Sotrovimab (for Omicron variant B.1.1.529) Other authorized mAbs, if activity against circulating variants of concern 2. Remdesivir 3. Paxlovid (nirmatrelvir/ritonavir)—monitor for drug-drug interactions 4. Molnupiravir (only if above options are not available)
Hospitalized, not requiring supplemental oxygen (not admitted for COVID-19)	1. Sotrovimab (for Omicron variant B.1.1.529) Other approved mAB with activity against circulating variants of concern 2. Remdesivir 3. Consider adjustment of immunosuppression based on severity of disease, risk of rejection, type of transplant, etc.
Hospitalized, requiring supplemental oxygen	1. Consider mAb use via expanded access protocol. 2. Start remdesivir and dexamethasone. 3. Consider adjustment of immunosuppression based on severity of disease, risk of rejection, type of transplant, etc.
Hospitalized, requiring oxygen via high-flow nasal cannula or noninvasive mechanical ventilation	1. Consider mAb use via expanded access protocol. 2. Start remdesivir and dexamethasone. 3. Consider adjustment of immunosuppression based on severity of disease, risk of rejection, type of transplant, etc. 4. There is insufficient evidence at this time about the risks and benefits of use of tocilizumab or baricitinib with dexamethasone in this population. Careful monitoring due to increased risk of secondary opportunistic infections
Hospitalized, requiring oxygen via invasive mechanical ventilation	1. Start dexamethasone 2. Consider adjustment of immunosuppression based on severity of disease, risk of rejection, type of transplant, etc.

SOT patients showed a lower mortality rate in vaccinated versus unvaccinated individuals.

Vaccine schedule and third vaccine dose
In transplant candidates, it is recommended that patients receive 3 dose series of mRNA vaccine at least 2 weeks prior to transplantation, or, if infeasible, 1 month post-transplant. In patients who receive B-cell– or T-cell–depleting therapies, post-poning to 3 months post-transplantation should be considered. The American Society of Transplantation and Centers for Disease Control and Prevention (CDC) both strongly recommend 3 dose series of the mRNA vaccine (Pfizer and Moderna) followed by a booster dose and an additional second dose of the Johnson and Johnson vaccine for all transplant recipients and the eligible household and close contacts of all transplant recipients.

A third dose of an mRNA vaccine is recommended 28 days after the most recent mRNA vaccine. An additional booster dose is recommended to be given 5 months after the last primary dose of the mRNA vaccine. Several small studies showed an improvement in humoral response after the third dose of the vaccine in transplant patients who did not develop adequate response after 2 doses (**Table 4**).

Table 3
Studies of vaccine effectiveness in solid organ transplant patients

Study	Results
Embi et al.[83] Multistate analysis across 7 health care systems	VE against COVID-19 associated hospitalization was lower (VE 77%) in immunocompromised patients compared with immunocompetent patients (VE 90%). VE was much lower (59%) in SOT and stem cell transplant patients.
Aslam et al.[84] 2151 SOT (912 vaccinated and 1239 controls)	Infections occurred in 61 of unvaccinated vs 4 of fully vaccinated patients. Vaccination led to 80% reduction in the incidence of symptomatic COVID-19.
Ravanan et al.[85] UK transplant registry Unvaccinated, n = 6748 Vaccinated, n = 39,727	The 28-d mortality rate was 12% in unvaccinated vs 7% in vaccinated individuals.
Malinis et al.[86] Fully vaccinated SOT individuals, n = 459	Breakthrough infection occurred in 3/459 (0.65%) fully vaccinated individuals.
Anjan et al.[87] Vaccinated SOT individuals (n = 2957)	Breakthrough infections occurred in 26 patients (0.87%). 5 (19.2%) had severe COVID-19 and 2 (7.6%) patients died.
Qin et al.[88] Fully vaccinated SOT individuals (n = 18,215)	Breakthrough infections occurred in 151 patients (0.83%). Of those, 87 (0.48%) were hospitalized. Of those, 14 (0.077%) died.
Mehta et al.[89] Fully vaccinated kidney transplant individuals (n = 1680)	Breakthrough infections in 8 patients and 3 were hospitalized

Abbreviation: VE, vaccine effectiveness.

Monoclonal antibodies for postexposure prophylaxis

Vaccines are effective in preventing severe COVID-19 infection in immunocompetent persons, but transplant patients do not always mount an adequate immune response and still may be at a risk of breakthrough infections, as discussed previously.

Two large RCTs showed that administration of mABs for postexposure prophylaxis was effective in prevention of COVID-19 in certain high-risk patients. Bamlanivimab monotherapy significantly reduced the incidence of COVID-19 (8%, vs 15% in placebo group) in 966 nursing and assisted living home residents with a confirmed index case.[94] In another RCT, administration of casirivimab and imdevimab to high-risk patients (household contacts) within 96 hours of exposure led to a reduction of acquiring symptomatic COVID-19 infection by 81% compared with placebo. This trial included immunosuppressed patients as well.[95] Based on these 2 trials, the FDA expanded the EUA indication to use certain mABs for postexposure prophylaxis in high-risk individuals, preferably within 7 days of exposure, assuming the mAb has activity against locally circulating variants.[96]

Pre-exposure prophylaxis

One important strategy for prevention of COVID-19 in persons with significant immunosuppression, who are not expected to mount a response to vaccines, is providing

Table 4
Studies showing immunogenicity of third vaccine dose in solid organ transplant patients

Study	Results
Hall et al.[90] An RCT of 120 patients, third dose of vaccine vs placebo	1. Increased anti-RBD antibody level in 55%, vs 18% in placebo group 2. After third dose, median percent virus neutralization was 71%, vs 13% in placebo group. 3. SARS-CoV-2–specific CD4$^+$ T-cell counts 432 vs 67 cells per 10^6
Kamar et al.[91] 101 SOT patients who received third dose of Pfizer vaccine	1. 26 of 59 (44%) patients who were seronegative prior to the third dose became seropositive. 2. Patients who were older, on higher immunosuppression, and had lower estimated glomerular filtration rate did not have an antibody response.
Benotmane et al.[92] Study of 159 kidney transplant patients who received a third dose of Moderna vaccine	1. Serologic response was observed after a third dose in patients who had a weak response after the second dose. 2. Patients who were on tacrolimus, mycophenolate, or steroids were less likely to develop an antibody response.
Stumpf et al.[93] 71 kidney transplant patients who received third dose of Pfizer vaccine	1. Increase in cumulative humoral response from 6% to 55% after first and third doses, respectively 2. Cellular response was present in 26% (9/35) patients.

mAb for pre-exposure prophylaxis. In November 2021, the FDA authorized (EUA) the AstraZeneca Evusheld (tixagevimab with cilgavimab) for pre-exposure prophylaxis for immunocompromised individuals. In a randomized placebo-controlled trial, administration of Evusield for pre-exposure prophylaxis led to 77% decrease in development of symptomatic COVID-19 compared with placebo.[97]

Impact of COVID-19 on Transplantation

There was a decline in transplantation all over the world during the first several months of pandemic, for various reasons.[50] Early in the pandemic, there was a national decline in the number of transplants by 35% from January 2020 to April 2020. There also was an increase in the waitlist deaths by 26%. These changes were more significant in regions with high COVID-19 burden. The largest reductions were seen in kidney (42%) and lung (40%) transplant patients.[98]

A survey was conducted to understand the impact of COVID-19 on transplant activity on organ transplants in 111 centers across the United States. Complete suspension of live kidney and liver transplantation was reported by 71% and 67% centers, respectively. Many centers were limiting their transplants to higher-acuity patients. Some transplants were limited by supplies, personnel, and capacity. In-person outpatient visits were limited by 98% of respondents, laboratory draws were stopped/limited by 20%, and 96% reported using telemedicine.[99] There also was a decline in the availability of ICU beds, because they were occupied by the critically ill COVID patients. Pretransplant COVID screening measures for donors and recipients were implemented by most centers. There was an 11% decline in donor organ authorization by families from March 2020 to May 2020. Donor cause of death due to substance abuse increased by 35% and trauma decreased by 5% in that time period.[100]

The transplantation societies have issued guidance for safe donation and transplantation practices, and there is an increased use of telemedicine for outpatient care to minimize hospital exposure.

Organ Transplantation from COVID-positive Donors

Little is known about the transmissibility of SARS-CoV-2 virus during organ transplantation. All deceased organ donors are tested for SARS-CoV-2 PCR by nasopharyngeal swab within 72 hours prior to transplantation, as per the Organ Procurement and Transplantation Network (OPTN) policy. Lower respiratory tract (LRT) testing of COVID by bronchoalveolar lavage is recommended in all potential lung donors, because there is a likelihood of missing an active infection with an upper respiratory tract (URT) sample alone. Between May 27, 2021, and July 31, 2021, OPTN identified 12 donors who had negative URT but positive LRT SARS-CoV-2 tests.[101] There were 3 reported cases of transmission of COVID via lung transplantation, where the URT sample was negative but the LRT sample returned positive from the donor after transplantation. One of the recipients died.[102,103] Hence, it is recommended that all lung donors must be tested for SARS-CoV-2 by LRT samples prior to transplantation. There was no transmission reported in the nonlung organ transplantation from these donors. A recent report of 10 patients who received kidneys from SARS-CoV-2–positive donors reported good outcomes in all patients, without the development of active COVID infection.[104] Long-term data in large samples, however, still are lacking. Based on these data, accepting lungs from SARS-CoV-2–positive donors must be deferred. Nonlung organs from COVID-positive donors may be considered in recipients, depending on the risk of mortality or complications from delaying transplantation.

COVID-19 IN HEMATOPOIETIC STEM CELL TRANSPLANT PATIENTS
Epidemiology

Risk of infection and natural history of disease

Much of the data regarding natural history of disease in hematopoietic cell transplant (HCT) patients were gathered early in the pandemic. Incidence of COVID-19 infection in HCT patients around the world varied by local rates of infection and infection prevention practices. A group of HCT patients in New York City were followed weekly for 2 months, in the spring of 2020, with access to testing and early treatment. Of the 254 patients tracked, 24 reported symptoms that prompted testing, and 6 of the 254 were diagnosed with COVID-19, all of whom received prompt care with good outcomes.[105]

A report from the Center for International Blood and Marrow Transplant Research (CIBMTR) of 318 HCT patients with COVID-19, from March 2020 to August 2020, found moderate to severe disease in greater than 50% of patients, with 14% requiring mechanical ventilation overall.[106] Those with allogeneic HCT had a 30-day survival rate of 68%, and those with autologous HCT had a 67% 30-day survival rate after COVID-19 diagnosis.[107] A similar survey from Europe, which included 382 HCT recipients diagnosed with COVID-19 prior to July 31, 2020, found 6-week survival rates of 78% in allogeneic HCT recipients and 72% in autologous recipients; in this group, 83% developed LRT disease, and 22.5% required ICU care.[107] The reported median time to viral resolution was 24 days, with the longest time to resolution 210 days, consistent with long-term viral replication in immunosuppressed hosts.[107]

In a smaller series, a group from Turkey found a mortality rate of 15.6% in patients who were hospitalized for COVID-19 with HCT and 11.8% in those with cancer without HCT, compared with 5.6% in those without cancer.[108] In Spain, mortality of 20% was reported in allogeneic HCT recipients and 24% in autologous HCT. Shah and colleagues[109] found an overall survival rate of 78% in a series of 77 allogeneic HCT, autologous HCT, and CAR-T recipients with a diagnosis of COVID-19. Overall, 48%, 26%, and 22% had mild, moderate, and severe disease, respectively.[109]

Predictors of severe disease and death
In the CIBMTR study, age greater than 50 years of age (HR 2.53, $P = .02$), male sex (HR 3.53, $P = .006$), and development of COVID-19 within 12 months of transplantation (HR 2.67, $P = .005$) were associated with a higher risk of mortality among allogeneic HCT recipients. In those with autologous transplantation, those with lymphoma had a higher risk of mortality that those with plasma cell disorder or myeloma (HR 2.41, $P = .033$).[106] In the European survey by Ljungman and colleagues,[107] age and level of immunodeficiency as calculated by a scoring index were found to be associated with an overall increased risk of death, and ongoing immunosuppression was the only risk factor in the allogeneic HCT recipients associated with need for ICU care. Not surprisingly, better performance status was associated with an overall decreased risk of death.[106]

In the series from Turkey, HCT recipients on immunosuppressive agents had a higher mortality rate than those who were not receiving exogenous immunosuppression (33% vs 11.5%,).[108] As was seen in the study by Shah and colleagues,[109] active malignancy was associated with worse outcomes in hospitalized HCT patients with COVID-19. In those without active malignancy, however, survival rates were similar to the general population hospitalized in the same area. Clinical variables associated with either need for ventilatory support or death included the number of comorbidities (HR for ≥2 vs 0 comorbidities 5.41, $P = .004$), presence of infiltrates on chest imaging (HR 3.08, $P = .032$), and neutropenia (HR 1.15, $P = .04$).[109]

Treatment Considerations

For HCT and cellular immunotherapy candidates, current guidelines recommend deferring transplantation or immunotherapy procedures, including peripheral blood stem cell mobilization, bone marrow harvest, T-cell collection, and conditioning or lymphodepletion in patients who test positive for SARS-CoV-2 or who have clinical symptoms that are consistent with infection. Final decisions should be made on a case-by-case basis while weighing the risks of delaying or altering therapy for the underlying disease, including the ability to give anti–SARS-Cov-2 mAb, which can be given as early treatment of infection or postexposure prophylaxis prior to lymphodepletion.

SARS-Cov-2 VACCINATION IN HEMATOPOIETIC CELL TRANSPLANT

A few studies of antibody response to 2 doses of mRNA vaccines after HCT helped inform the decision to offer third doses to immunocompromised people, including HCT patients. A study from France found that after a second dose of the Pfizer BNT162b2 vaccine, 83% of 117 HCT patients had detectable antispike IgG antibodies, but only 62% had antibodies at the level detected in immunocompetent control participants. Factors associated with nonresponse to vaccine were being a haploidentical transplant recipient, vaccination within 1 year after HCT, lymphopenia (<1000 cells/mL), and receipt of immunosuppression or chemotherapy at the time of vaccination.[110] Another study of 63 HCT recipients in Switzerland who received either of the SARS-CoV-2 mRNA vaccines found that 76% had some humoral response after 2 doses. Age greater than 60 years, vaccination within 6 months of HCT, or use of antithymocyte globulin during conditioning all were associated with lack of response to vaccination in this group.[111] As in other populations not expected to mount adequate vaccine responses, use of authorized anti–SARS-CoV-2 mAbs for pre-exposure prophylaxis may be warranted.

Timing of vaccination after hematopoietic cell transplant

Vaccination should be delayed for 3 months following HCT or CAR-T therapy to maximize vaccine efficacy, according to National Comprehensive Cancer Network (NCCN) guidelines. The European Society for Blood and Marrow Transplantation (EBMT) guidelines recommend waiting for at least 3 months in high transmission areas, preferably for 6 months if the transmission is low. It also is recommended to repeat the vaccine series if vaccinated prior to HCT.

Currently, the CDC and international societies, including the NCCN, CIBMTR, and EBMT, all recommend a third dose of mRNA vaccine for those who received 2 doses of an mRNA SARS-CoV-2 vaccine after transplant, after a minimum 4-week interval from the prior dose.[112,113] Boosters continue to be recommended following completion of the initial series, as in nonimmunocompromised persons.

QUALITY OF LIFE DURING THE PANDEMIC

A survey study of 101 patients post-HCT was done to assess their supportive care needs. Largely, there were unmet physical and psychological needs of the patients. Compliance with exercise programs was low. Women had more unmet psychological needs compared with men, and measures of their quality of life were low.[114] A cross-sectional analysis of 205 patients undergoing HCT enrolled in a supportive care trial found that enrollment during COVID-19 was not associated with pre-HCT symptoms of depression, anxiety, posttraumatic stress disorder, fatigue, or quality of life impairment. During the COVID-19 era, patients reported negative implications, such as increased isolation and increased family and caregiver distress, and positive implications, such as engagement in meaningful activities and increased support from caregivers.[115] Telehealth services can be helpful to provide increased support and interventions to meet patient needs and reduce distress.

COVID-19 IN OTHER IMMUNOCOMPROMISED POPULATIONS

In a large registry (COVID-19 and Cancer Consortium) of 928 cancer patients with confirmed SARS-CoV-2 infection, the factors that were associated with increased 30-day mortality were increased age, male sex, comorbidities, smoking, and having active cancer. Type of cancer or chemotherapy was not associated with mortality.[116] Another prospective observational study of COVID patients with active cancer and symptomatic COVID-19 reported mortality of 28%. Risk of death was associated with advancing age, male sex, and presence of comorbidities, such as hypertension and cardiovascular disease. There was no significant effect of chemotherapy, immunotherapy, or radiation therapy on mortality.[117]

In a recent report from COVID-19 Global Rheumatology Alliance physician registry, of 2869 people with COVID-19 on disease-modifying antirheumatic drugs, 21% required hospitalization and 5.5% died. Patients on rituximab or JAK inhibitors had higher rates of hospitalization and deaths compared with tumor necrosis factor (TNF)-α inhibitors.[118] An international registry (SECURE-IBD, Surveillance Epidemiology of Coronavirus Under Research Exclusion - Inflammatory Bowel Disease) to record outcomes of COVID-19 in patients with inflammatory bowel disease of 525 patients, 31% were hospitalized and 3% died. Risk factors for severe COVID-19 were increased age, greater than 2 comorbidities, and use of systemic steroids. Use of TNF-α inhibitors was not associated with severe disease.[119] Another study from the same registry, with 1400 patients, showed that thiopurine monotherapy and combination of TNF-α antagonists with thiopurine monotherapy had higher risk of severe COVID-19 compared with TNF-α monotherapy.[120]

A case series of 7 immunocompromised patients (5 with common variable immunodeficiency [CVID] and 2 with agammaglobulinemia) described mild symptoms in agammaglobulinemia compared with severe disease in CVID patients; 1 patient died and 3 required ICU admission.[121] In another report of 10 patients with CVID from New York City, only 1 patient was hospitalized and none died. All these patients were on regular immunoglobulin replacement.[122] Pre-exposure and postexposure prophylaxis should be prioritized for any of these groups at risk of poor vaccine response and higher risk of disease progression as well as prioritized for early treatment of infection with mAbs and/or antivirals.

SUMMARY

COVID-19 has had a major impact on the SOT population. Although developed policies and practices have been developed for better management during this pandemic, there still is a need for better preventive measures due to the depressed immune response in this vulnerable population. There also is a need for better therapeutic agents for management of this infection. There still are some uncertainties about some practices, such as management of immunosuppression, vaccine responses, and role of immunomodulators, which need to be studied.

CLINICS CARE POINTS

- Three-dose primary series of vaccination and a booster, along with masking, social distancing, and avoiding large indoor crowds, are recommended for all immunocompromised patients to prevent severe COVID-19 infection.

- Anti–SARS-CoV-2 mAbs use can be considered for pre-exposure and postexposure prophylaxis and for early treatment in high-risk patients who are not expected to have developed an antibody response despite having received appropriate vaccine series.

- The use of nonlung organs from SARS-CoV-2–positive donors may be considered; however, more robust data are needed to evaluate the safety and transmission.

DISCLOSURE

A.E. Shapiro received grant funding from Vir Biotechnology, Inc., and NIH K23AI140918. A. K. Subramanian received grant funding from Gilead Sciences, Regeneron Pharmaceuticals, and Janssen Pharmaceuticals.

REFERENCES

1. Boulle A, Davies M-A, Hussey H, et al. Risk factors for coronavirus disease 2019 (COVID-19) death in a population cohort study from the western cape province, South Africa. Clin Infect Dis 2021;73(7):e2005–15.
2. Sachdev D, Mara E, Hsu L, et al. COVID-19 susceptibility and outcomes among people living with HIV in San Francisco. J Acquir Immune Defic Syndr 2021; 86(1):19–21.

3. Pyra M, Rusie L, Houlberg M, et al. COVID-19 testing results by HIV status, March–July 2020, Chicago, USA. Open Forum Infect Dis 2021;8(7):ofab053.

4. Chang JJ, Bruxvoort K, Chen LH, et al. Brief Report: COVID-19 testing, characteristics, and outcomes among people living with HIV in an integrated health system. J Acquir Immune Defic Syndr 2021;88(1):1–5.

5. Bender Ignacio R, Shapiro A, Nance R, et al. Racial and ethnic disparities in COVID-19 disease incidence independent of comorbidities, among people with HIV in the US. medRxiv 2021. https://doi.org/10.1101/2021.12.07.21267296.

6. Bertagnolio S, Thwin SS, Silva R, et al. WHO Global Clinical Platform forx COVID-19.Clinical features and prognostic factors of COVID-19 in people living with HIV hospitalized with suspected or confirmed SARS-CoV-2 infection. 2021;

7. Yang X, Sun J, Patel RC, et al. Associations between HIV infection and clinical spectrum of COVID-19: a population level analysis based on US National COVID Cohort Collaborative (N3C) data. Lancet HIV 2021;8(11):e690–700.

8. Yendewa GA, Perez JA, Schlick K, et al. Clinical Features and outcomes of coronavirus disease 2019 among people with human immunodeficiency virus in the United States: a multicenter study from a large global health research network (TriNetX). Open Forum Infect Dis 2021;8(7):ofab272.

9. Alrubayyi A, Gea-Mallorquí E, Touizer E, et al. Characterization of humoral and SARS-CoV-2 specific T cell responses in people living with HIV. Nat Commun 2021;12(1). https://doi.org/10.1038/s41467-021-26137-7.

10. Spinelli MA, Lynch KL, Yun C, et al. SARS-CoV-2 seroprevalence, and IgG concentration and pseudovirus neutralising antibody titres after infection, compared by HIV status: a matched case-control observational study. Lancet HIV 2021;8(6):e334–41.

11. Karim F, Moosa MY, Gosnell B, et al. Persistent SARS-CoV-2 infection and intrahost evolution in association with advanced HIV infection. medRxiv 2021. https://doi.org/10.1101/2021.06.03.21258228.

12. Yousaf M, Hameed M, Alsoub H, et al. COVID-19: prolonged viral shedding in an HIV patient with literature review of risk factors for prolonged viral shedding and its implications for isolation strategies. Clin Case Rep 2021;9(3):1397–401.

13. Hu R, Yan H, Liu M, et al. Brief report: virologic and immunologic outcomes for HIV patients with coronavirus disease 2019. J Acquir Immune Defic Syndr 2021;86(2):213–8.

14. Peluso MJ, Bakkour S, Busch MP, et al. A high percentage of people with human immunodeficiency virus (HIV) on antiretroviral therapy experience detectable low-level plasma HIV-1 RNA following coronavirus disease 2019 (COVID-19). Clin Infect Dis 2021;73(9):e2845–6.

15. Laracy J, Zucker J, Castor D, et al. HIV-1 Infection does not change disease course or inflammatory pattern of SARS-CoV-2-infected patients presenting at a large urban medical center in New York City. Open Forum Infect Dis 2021;8(2):ofab029.

16. Vizcarra P, Perez-Elias MJ, Quereda C, et al. Description of COVID-19 in HIV-infected individuals: a single-centre, prospective cohort. Lancet HIV 2020;7(8):e554–64.

17. Inciarte A, Gonzalez-Cordon A, Rojas J, et al. Clinical characteristics, risk factors, and incidence of symptomatic coronavirus disease 2019 in a large cohort of adults living with HIV: a single-center, prospective observational study. AIDS 2020;34(12):1775–80.

18. Ceballos ME, Ross P, Lasso M, et al. Clinical characteristics and outcomes of people living with HIV hospitalized with COVID-19: a nationwide experience. Int J STD AIDS 2021;32(5):435–43.

19. Dandachi D, Geiger G, Montgomery MW, et al. Characteristics, comorbidities, and outcomes in a multicenter registry of patients with human immunodeficiency virus and coronavirus disease 2019. Clin Infect Dis 2021;73(7):e1964–72.

20. Shapiro AE, Bender Ignacio RA, Whitney BM, et al. Factors associated with severity of COVID-19 disease in a multicenter cohort of people with HIV in the United States, March-December 2020. medRxiv 2021. https://doi.org/10.1101/2021.10.15.21265063.

21. Nomah DK, Reyes-Urueña J, Díaz Y, et al. Sociodemographic, clinical, and immunological factors associated with SARS-CoV-2 diagnosis and severe COVID-19 outcomes in people living with HIV: a retrospective cohort study. Lancet HIV 2021;8(11):e701–10.

22. Ko JY, Danielson ML, Town M, et al. Risk factors for coronavirus disease 2019 (COVID-19)–associated hospitalization: COVID-19–associated hospitalization surveillance network and behavioral risk factor surveillance system. Clin Infect Dis 2021;72(11):e695–703.

23. Ambrosioni J, Blanco JL, Reyes-Urueña JM, et al. Overview of SARS-CoV-2 infection in adults living with HIV. Lancet HIV 2021;8(5):e294–305.

24. NIH.. COVID-19 treatment guidelines: clinical management summary. 2021. Available at: https://www.covid19treatmentguidelines.nih.gov/management/clinical-management/clinical-management-summary/. Accessed 16-DEC-2021.

25. Accelerating COVID-19 therapeutic interventions and vaccines (ACTIV). Available at: https://www.nih.gov/research-training/medical-research-initiatives/activ. Accessed 23 November, 2021.

26. Jayk Bernal A, Gomes Da Silva MM, Musungaie DB, et al. Molnupiravir for oral treatment of Covid-19 in nonhospitalized patients. N Engl J Med 2021. https://doi.org/10.1056/nejmoa2116044.

27. Fact sheet for healthcare providers: emergency use authorization for Paxlovid (2021).

28. Frater J, Ewer KJ, Ogbe A, et al. Safety and immunogenicity of the ChAdOx1 nCoV-19 (AZD1222) vaccine against SARS-CoV-2 in HIV infection: a single-arm substudy of a phase 2/3 clinical trial. Lancet HIV 2021;8(8):e474–85.

29. Woldemeskel BA, Karaba AH, Garliss CC, et al. The BNT162b2 mRNA vaccine elicits robust humoral and cellular immune responses in people living with human immunodeficiency virus (HIV). Clin Infect Dis 2021. https://doi.org/10.1093/cid/ciab648.

30. Levy I, Wieder-Finesod A, Litchevsky V, et al. Immunogenicity and safety of the BNT162b2 mRNA COVID-19 vaccine in people living with HIV-1. Clin Microbiol Infect 2021. https://doi.org/10.1016/j.cmi.2021.07.031.

31. Spinelli MA, Peluso MJ, Lynch KL, et al. Differences in Post-mRNA vaccination SARS-CoV-2 IgG concentrations and surrogate virus neutralization test response by HIV status and type of vaccine: a matched case-control observational study. Clin Infect Dis 2021. https://doi.org/10.1093/cid/ciab1009.

32. Fulda ES, Fitch KV, Overton ET, et al. COVID-19 vaccination rates in a global HIV cohort. J Infect Dis 2021. https://doi.org/10.1093/infdis/jiab575.

33. The Global Fund. Results Report. 2021. https://www.theglobalfund.org/media/11304/corporate_2021resultsreport_report_en.pdf

34. Wood BR, Lan KF, Tao Y, et al. Visit trends and factors associated with telemedicine uptake among persons with HIV during the COVID-19 pandemic. Open Forum Infect Dis 2021;8(11):ofab480.

35. Sorbera M, Fischetti B, Khaimova R, et al. Evaluation of virologic suppression rates during the COVID-19 pandemic with outpatient interdisciplinary HIV care. J Am Coll Clin Pharm 2021;4(8):964–8.

36. Spinelli MA, Brown LB, Glidden DV, et al. SARS-CoV-2 incidence, testing rates, and severe COVID-19 outcomes among people with and without HIV. AIDS 2021;35(15):2545–7.

37. Lee D, Chow EPF, Aguirre I, et al. Access to HIV Antiretroviral therapy among people living with HIV in melbourne during the COVID-19 pandemic. Int J Environ Res Public Health 2021;18(23):12765.

38. December 13, 2021, 2021. Accessed 15 December 2021. https://www.hvtn.org/en/media-room/news-releases/covid-19-vaccine-trial-sub-saharan-africa-first-study-efficacy-mrna-covid-19-vaccines-people-living-with-hiv.html

39. Xie Y, Bowe B, Al-Aly Z. Burdens of post-acute sequelae of COVID-19 by severity of acute infection, demographics and health status. Nat Commun 2021;12(1):6571.

40. Pujari S, Gaikwad S, Chitalikar A, et al. Long-coronavirus disease among people living with HIV in western India: an observational study. Immun Inflamm Dis 2021;9(3):1037–43.

41. Kates OS, Haydel BM, Florman SS, et al. Coronavirus Disease 2019 in Solid Organ Transplant: A Multicenter Cohort Study. Clin Infect Dis 2021;73(11):e4090–409943.

42. Ravanan R, Callaghan CJ, Mumford L, et al. SARS-CoV-2 infection and early mortality of waitlisted and solid organ transplant recipients in England: a national cohort study. Am J Transplant 2020;20(11):3008–18.

43. Heldman MR, Kates OS. COVID-19 in Solid Organ Transplant Recipients: a Review of the Current Literature. Curr Treat Options Infect Dis 2021;13:67–82. 72.

44. Colmenero J, Rodríguez-Perálvarez M, Salcedo M, et al. Epidemiological pattern, incidence, and outcomes of COVID-19 in liver transplant patients. J Hepatol 2021;74(1):148–55.

45. Vinson AJ, Agarwal G, Dai R, et al. COVID-19 in solid organ transplantation: results of the national COVID cohort collaborative. Transplant Direct 2021;7(11):e775.

46. Cravedi P, Mothi SS, Azzi Y, et al. COVID-19 and kidney transplantation: results from the TANGO international transplant consortium. Am J Transplant 2020;20(11):3140–8.

47. Rodda LB, Netland J, Shehata L, et al. Functional SARS-CoV-2-specific immune memory persists after mild COVID-19. Cell 2021;184(1):169–83.e17.

48. Sekine T, Perez-Potti A, Rivera-Ballesteros O, et al. Robust T Cell immunity in convalescent individuals with asymptomatic or Mild COVID-19. Cell 2020;183(1):158–68.e14.

49. Nam HH, Ison MG. Community-acquired respiratory viruses in solid organ transplant. Curr Opin Organ Transplant 2019;24(4):483–9.

50. Danziger-Isakov L, Blumberg EA, Manuel O, et al. Impact of COVID-19 in solid organ transplant recipients. Am J Transplant 2021;21(3):925–37.

51. Benotmane I, Gautier-Vargas G, Wendling MJ, et al. In-depth virological assessment of kidney transplant recipients with COVID-19. Am J Transplant 2020;20(11):3162–72.

52. Kates OS, Fisher CE, Stankiewicz-Karita HC, et al. Earliest cases of coronavirus disease 2019 (COVID-19) identified in solid organ transplant recipients in the United States. Am J Transplant 2020;20(7):1885–90.

53. Coll E, Fernández-Ruiz M, Sánchez-Álvarez JE, et al. COVID-19 in transplant recipients: the spanish experience. Am J Transplant 2021;21(5):1825–37.

54. Heldman MR, Kates OS, Fisher CE, et al. Immunosuppression in solid organ transplant recipients with Covid-19: More data, but still complicated. Transpl Infect Dis 2021;23(4):e13650.

55. Heldman MR, Kates OS, Safa K, et al. COVID-19 in hospitalized lung and non-lung solid organ transplant recipients: A comparative analysis from a multicenter study. Am J Transplant 2021;21(8):2774–84.

56. Fu EL, Janse RJ, de Jong Y, et al. Acute kidney injury and kidney replacement therapy in COVID-19: a systematic review and meta-analysis. Clin Kidney J 2020;13(4):550–63.

57. Favà A, Cucchiari D, Montero N, et al. Clinical characteristics and risk factors for severe COVID-19 in hospitalized kidney transplant recipients: A multicentric cohort study. Am J Transplant 2020;20(11):3030–41.

58. Webb GJ, Marjot T, Cook JA, et al. Outcomes following SARS-CoV-2 infection in liver transplant recipients: an international registry study. Lancet Gastroenterol Hepatol 2020;5(11):1008–16.

59. Hadi YB, Naqvi SFZ, Kupec JT, et al. Outcomes of COVID-19 in Solid organ transplant recipients: a propensity-matched analysis of a large research network. Transplantation 2021;105(6):1365–71.

60. Fisher AM, Schlauch D, Mulloy M, et al. Outcomes of COVID-19 in hospitalized solid organ transplant recipients compared to a matched cohort of non-transplant patients at a national healthcare system in the United States. Clin Transplant 2021;35(4):e14216.

61. Pereira MR, Arcasoy S, Farr MA, et al. Outcomes of COVID-19 in solid organ transplant recipients: a matched cohort study. Transpl Infect Dis 2021;23(4): e13637.

62. Beigel JH, Tomashek KM, Dodd LE, et al. Remdesivir for the Treatment of Covid-19 - Final Report. N Engl J Med 2020;383(19):1813–26.

63. Pan H, Peto R, Henao-Restrepo AMF, et al, WHO Solidarity Trial Consortium. Repurposed antiviral drugs for Covid-19 - interim WHO solidarity trial results. N Engl J Med 2021;384(6):497–511.

64. Goldman JD, Lye DCB, Hui DS, et al. Remdesivir for 5 or 10 days in patients with severe Covid-19. N Engl J Med 2020;383(19):1827–37.

65. Food and Drug Administration. Fact sheet for healthcare providers: emergency use authorization for Paxlovid. 2021. Available at: https://www.fda.gov/media/155050/download.

66. Food and Drug Administration. Fact sheet for healthcare providers: emergency use authorization for molnupiravir. 2021. Available at: https://www.fda.gov/media/155054/download.

67. Horby PW, Mafham M, Peto LF, et al, RECOVERY Collaborative Group. Casirivimab and imdevimab in patients admitted to hospital with COVID-19 (RECOVERY): a randomised, controlled, open-label, platform trial. medRxiv 2021.

68. Self WH, Sandkovsky U, Reilly CS, et al. Efficacy and safety of two neutralising monoclonal antibody therapies, sotrovimab and BRII-196 plus BRII-198, for adults hospitalised with COVID-19 (TICO): a randomised controlled trial. Lancet Infect Dis 2021.

69. Yetmar ZA, Beam E, O'Horo JC, et al. Monoclonal antibody therapy for COVID-19 in solid organ transplant recipients. Open Forum Infect Dis 2021;8(6): ofab255.

70. Klein EJ, Hardesty A, Vieira K, et al. Use of anti-spike monoclonal antibodies in kidney transplant recipients with COVID-19: Efficacy, ethnic and racial disparities [published online ahead of print, 2021 Sep 30]. Am J Transplant 2021. https://doi.org/10.1111/ajt.16843.

71. Del Bello A, Marion O, Vellas C, et al. Anti-SARS-CoV-2 Monoclonal Antibodies in Solid-organ Transplant Patients. Transplantation 2021;105(10):e146–7.

72. Jenks JD, Aslam S, Horton L, et al. . Early monoclonal antibody administration can reduce both hospitalizations and mortality in high-risk outpatients with COVID-19. Clin Infect Dis. In press.

73. Fung M, Nambiar A, Pandey S, et al. Treatment of immunocompromised COVID-19 patients with convalescent plasma. Transpl Infect Dis 2021;23(2):e13477.

74. Thompson MA, Henderson JP, Shah PK, et al. Association of convalescent plasma therapy with survival in patients with hematologic cancers and COVID-19 [published correction appears in JAMA Oncol. 2021 Aug 1;7(8):1249]. JAMA Oncol 2021;7(8):1167–75.

75. Libster R, Pérez Marc G, Wappner D, et al. Early high-titer plasma therapy to prevent severe Covid-19 in older adults. N Engl J Med 2021;384(7):610–8.

76. Horby P, Lim WS, Emberson JR, et al, RECOVERY Collaborative Group. Dexamethasone in hospitalized patients with Covid-19. N Engl J Med 2021;384(8): 693–704.

77. Gordon AC, Mouncey PR, Al-Beidh F, et al. Interleukin-6 receptor antagonists in critically ill patients with Covid-19. N Engl J Med 2021;384(16):1491–502.

78. Kalil AC, Patterson TF, Mehta AK, et al. Baricitinib plus remdesivir for hospitalized adults with Covid-19. N Engl J Med 2021;384(9):795–807.

79. Marconi VC, Ramanan AV, de Bono S, et al. Efficacy and safety of baricitinib for the treatment of hospitalised adults with COVID-19 (COV-BARRIER): a randomised, double-blind, parallel-group, placebo-controlled phase 3 trial [published correction appears in Lancet Respir Med. Lancet Respir Med 2021;9(10):e102.

80. Ou MT, Boyarsky BJ, Motter JD, et al. Safety and reactogenicity of 2 doses of SARS-CoV-2 vaccination in solid organ transplant recipients. Transplantation 2021;105(10):2170–4.

81. Boyarsky BJ, Werbel WA, Avery RK, et al. Antibody response to 2-dose SARS-CoV-2 mRNA vaccine series in solid organ transplant recipients. JAMA 2021; 325(21):2204–6.

82. Hall VG, Ferreira VH, Ierullo M, et al. Humoral and cellular immune response and safety of two-dose SARS-CoV-2 mRNA-1273 vaccine in solid organ transplant recipients [published online ahead of print, 2021 Aug 4]. Am J Transplant 2021. https://doi.org/10.1111/ajt.16766.

83. Embi PJ, Levy ME, Naleway AL, et al. Effectiveness of 2-dose vaccination with mRNA COVID-19 vaccines against COVID-19-associated hospitalizations among immunocompromised adults - nine states, January-September 2021. MMWR Morb Mortal Wkly Rep 2021;70(44):1553–9.

84. Aslam S, Adler E, Mekeel K, et al. Clinical effectiveness of COVID-19 vaccination in solid organ transplant recipients. Transpl Infect Dis 2021;23(5):e13705.

85. Ravanan R, Mumford L, Ushiro-Lumb I, et al. Two doses of SARS-CoV-2 vaccines reduce risk of death due to COVID-19 in solid organ transplant recipients: preliminary outcomes from a UK registry linkage analysis. Transplantation 2021; 105(11):e263–4.

86. Malinis M, Cohen E, Azar MM. Effectiveness of SARS-CoV-2 vaccination in fully vaccinated solid organ transplant recipients. Am J Transplant 2021;21(8): 2916–8.

87. Anjan S, Natori Y, Fernandez Betances AA, et al. Breakthrough COVID-19 infections after mRNA vaccination in solid organ transplant recipients in miami, Florida. Transplantation 2021;105(10):e139–41.

88. Qin CX, Moore LW, Anjan S, et al. Risk of breakthrough SARS-CoV-2 infections in adult transplant recipients. Transplantation 2021;105(11):e265–6.

89. Mehta RB, Silveira FP. COVID-19 after two doses of mRNA vaccines in kidney transplant recipients [published online ahead of print, 2021 Jul 31]. Am J Transplant 2021. https://doi.org/10.1111/ajt.16778.

90. Hall VG, Ferreira VH, Ku T, et al. Randomized trial of a third dose of mRNA-1273 vaccine in transplant recipients. N Engl J Med 2021;385(13):1244–6.

91. Kamar N, Abravanel F, Marion O, et al. Three doses of an mRNA Covid-19 vaccine in solid-organ transplant recipients. N Engl J Med 2021;385(7):661–2.

92. Benotmane I, Gautier G, Perrin P, et al. Antibody response after a third dose of the mRNA-1273 SARS-CoV-2 vaccine in kidney transplant recipients with minimal serologic response to 2 doses. JAMA 2021;326(11):1063–5.

93. Stumpf J, Tonnus W, Paliege A, et al. Cellular and humoral immune responses after 3 doses of BNT162b2 mRNA SARS-CoV-2 vaccine in kidney transplant. Transplantation 2021;105(11):e267–9.

94. Cohen MS, Nirula A, Mulligan MJ, et al. Effect of bamlanivimab vs placebo on incidence of COVID-19 among residents and staff of skilled nursing and assisted living facilities: a randomized clinical trial. JAMA 2021;326(1):46–55.

95. O'Brien MP, Forleo-Neto E, Musser BJ, et al. Subcutaneous REGEN-COV antibody combination to prevent Covid-19. N Engl J Med 2021;385(13):1184–95.

96. Fact sheet for healthcare providers: emergency use authorization (EUA) of REGEN-COV (casirivimab and imdevimab). 2021. Available at: https://www.fda.gov/media/145611/download.

97. Available at: https://www.fda.gov/media/154701/download. Accessed January 2022.

98. Cholankeril G, Podboy A, Alshuwaykh OS, et al. Early impact of COVID-19 on solid organ transplantation in the United States. Transplantation 2020;104(11): 2221–4.

99. Boyarsky BJ, Po-Yu Chiang T, Werbel WA, et al. Early impact of COVID-19 on transplant center practices and policies in the United States. Am J Transplant 2020;20(7):1809–18.

100. Ahmed O, Brockmeier D, Lee K, et al. Organ donation during the COVID-19 pandemic. Am J Transplant 2020;20(11):3081–8.

101. https://optn.transplant.hrsa.gov/media/kkhnlwah/sars-cov-2-summary-of-evidence.pdf

102. Kaul DR, Valesano AL, Petrie JG, et al. Donor to recipient transmission of SARS-CoV-2 by lung transplantation despite negative donor upper respiratory tract testing. Am J Transplant 2021;21(8):2885–9.

103. Kumar D, Humar A, Keshavjee S, et al. A call to routinely test lower respiratory tract samples for SARS-CoV-2 in lung donors. Am J Transplant 2021;21(7): 2623–4.

104. Koval CE, Poggio ED, Lin YC, et al. Early success transplanting kidneys from donors with new SARS-CoV-2 RNA positivity: A report of 10 cases. Am J Transplant 2021;21(11):3743–9.

105. Lupo-Stanghellini MT, Xue E, Mastaglio S, et al. COVID-19 in recipients of allo-geneic stem cell transplantation: favorable outcome. Bone Marrow Transplant 2021;56(9):2312–5.

106. Sharma A, Bhatt NS, St Martin A, et al. Clinical characteristics and outcomes of COVID-19 in haematopoietic stem-cell transplantation recipients: an observa-tional cohort study [published correction appears in Lancet Haematol. 2021 Jun;8(6):e393]. Lancet Haematol 2021;8(3):e185–93.

107. Ljungman P, de la Camara R, Mikulska M, et al. COVID-19 and stem cell trans-plantation; results from an EBMT and GETH multicenter prospective survey. Leu-kemia 2021;35(10):2885–94.

108. Altuntas F, Ata N, Yigenoglu TN, et al. COVID-19 in hematopoietic cell transplant recipients. Bone Marrow Transplant 2021;56(4):952–5.

109. Shah GL, DeWolf S, Lee YJ, et al. Favorable outcomes of COVID-19 in recipients of hematopoietic cell transplantation. J Clin Invest 2020;130(12):6656–67.

110. Le Bourgeois A, Coste-Burel M, Guillaume T, et al. Safety and antibody response after 1 and 2 doses of BNT162b2 mRNA vaccine in recipients of allo-geneic hematopoietic stem cell transplant. JAMA Netw Open 2021;4(9): e2126344.

111. Mamez AC, Pradier A, Giannotti F, et al. Antibody responses to SARS-CoV2 vaccination in allogeneic hematopoietic stem cell transplant recipients. Bone Marrow Transplant 2021;56(12):3094–6.

112. https://www.nccn.org/docs/default-source/covid-19/2021_covid-19_vaccina-tion_guidance_v5-0.pdf?sfvrsn=b483da2b_74. Accessed Jan 2022.

113. https://www.ebmt.org/sites/default/files/2022-01/COVID%20vaccines% 20version%208.3%20-%202022-01-03.pdf. Accessed Jan 2022.

114. Yildiz Kabak V, Atasavun Uysal S, Duger T. Screening supportive care needs, compliance with exercise program, quality of life, and anxiety level during the COVID-19 pandemic in individuals treated with hematopoietic stem cell trans-plantation. Support Care Cancer 2021;29(7):4065–73.

115. Amonoo HL, Topping CEW, Clay MA, et al. Distress in a pandemic: association of the coronavirus disease-2019 Pandemic with distress and quality of life in he-matopoietic stem cell transplantation. Transplant Cell Ther 2021;27(12): 1015.e1–7.

116. Kuderer NM, Choueiri TK, Shah DP, et al. Clinical impact of COVID-19 on pa-tients with cancer (CCC19): a cohort study [published correction appears in Lancet. Lancet 2020;395(10241):1907–18.

117. Lee LY, Cazier JB, Angelis V, et al. COVID-19 mortality in patients with cancer on chemotherapy or other anticancer treatments: a prospective cohort study [pub-lished correction appears in Lancet. Lancet 2020;395(10241):1919–26.

118. Sparks JA, Wallace ZS, Seet AM, et al, COVID-19 Global Rheumatology Alli-ance. Associations of baseline use of biologic or targeted synthetic DMARDs with COVID-19 severity in rheumatoid arthritis: results from the COVID-19 global rheumatology alliance physician registry. Ann Rheum Dis 2021;80:1137–46.

119. Brenner EJ, Ungaro RC, Gearry RB, et al. Corticosteroids, but Not TNF antago-nists, are associated with adverse COVID-19 outcomes in patients with inflam-matory bowel diseases: results from an international registry. Gastroenterology 2020;159(2):481–91.e3.

120. Ungaro RC, Brenner EJ, Gearry RB, et al. Effect of IBD medications on COVID-19 outcomes: results from an international registry. Gut 2021;70(4):725–32.

121. Quinti I, Lougaris V, Milito C, et al. A possible role for B cells in COVID-19? Lesson from patients with agammaglobulinemia. J Allergy Clin Immunol 2020; 146(1):211–3.e4.
122. Cohen B, Rubinstein R, Gans MD, et al. COVID-19 infection in 10 common variable immunodeficiency patients in New York City. J Allergy Clin Immunol Pract 2021;9(1):504–7.e1.

COVID-19 and Pregnancy

Sonja A. Rasmussen, MD, MS[a,b,c,]*, Denise J. Jamieson, MD, MPH[d]

KEYWORDS

- Pregnancy • COVID-19 • SARS-CoV-2 vaccine • Intrauterine transmission
- SARS-CoV-2 • Pregnancy complications • mRNA vaccine

KEY POINTS

- Pregnant persons are at increased risk for severe disease from COVID-19.
- SARS-CoV-2 crosses the placenta rarely, but adverse effects of maternal disease on the fetus and newborn have been observed.
- Studies show that SARS-CoV-2 vaccines during pregnancy are effective at preventing disease in the mother and the fetus. Antibodies to SARS-CoV-2 have been found in umbilical cord blood and breast milk following vaccination during pregnancy, suggesting protection of the infant after maternal vaccination.

INTRODUCTION

Since the emergence of SARS-CoV-2 in late 2019, the virus and the response to it have had catastrophic effects on the world's health, societies, and economies. Early on, data on the effects of SARS-CoV-2 on the pregnant person and fetus were limited. Data on the effects during pregnancy of previous coronaviruses (severe acute respiratory syndrome [SARS] and Middle East respiratory syndrome [MERS]) are sparse, but those data along with information on other respiratory infections such as influenza raised concerns about the potential effects of COVID-19 during pregnancy.[1] Here we review available information on the effects of SARS-CoV-2 infection during pregnancy and the effectiveness and safety of the SARS-CoV-2 vaccines in protecting pregnant persons and their newborns from COVID-19.

[a] Department of Pediatrics, University of Florida College of Medicine, 1600 Archer Road, Box 100296, Gainesville, Florida, 32610; [b] Department of Obstetrics and Gynecology, University of Florida College of Medicine, Gainesville, FL, USA; [c] Department of Epidemiology, University of Florida College of Public Health and Health Professions and College of Medicine, Gainesville, FL, USA; [d] Emory University School of Medicine, Department of Gynecology and Obstetrics, Woodruff Memorial Research Building, 101 Woodruff Circle, Suite 4208, Atlanta, GA 30322, USA
* Corresponding author:
E-mail address: sonja.rasmussen@peds.ufl.edu

Infect Dis Clin N Am 36 (2022) 423–433
https://doi.org/10.1016/j.idc.2022.01.002
0891-5520/22/© 2022 Elsevier Inc. All rights reserved.

id.theclinics.com

EFFECTS OF SARS-CoV-2 INFECTION DURING PREGNANCY

An initial question after emergence of a novel pathogen is whether pregnancy is a risk factor for infection or severe disease. Successful pregnancy requires changes in the pregnant person's immune system to tolerate a genetically foreign fetus. These changes in the immune system as well as alterations in the cardiac, pulmonary, and other systems can result in increased susceptibility to or increased morbidity and mortality with infection during pregnancy.[2] Understanding the susceptibility to infection during pregnancy is challenging, given that the number of infections observed depends not only on susceptibility but also on the level of exposure to the pathogen. Pregnant persons might be more cautious about risk, resulting in a lower level of exposure, which could seem as decreased susceptibility. To adequately address this question, a comparison of incident rates between pregnant persons and women of the same age with similar levels of SARS-CoV-2 exposure would be needed. A prospective cohort analysis of incident disease among pregnant persons identified through weekly self-collected testing showed an incidence during pregnancy that was similar to the modeled estimates for US adults of reproductive age during the same time period.[3] Thus, currently available data do not support increased susceptibility to SARS-CoV-2 infection during pregnancy,[4] but conclusions are difficult, given issues with potential differences in exposure levels between pregnant and nonpregnant persons.

Studies to determine whether pregnancy increases the risk for severe disease are also challenging, given the increased surveillance and enhanced clinical response to illness that occur during pregnancy, as well as potential confounding factors (eg, pregnancy being a marker of better health).[5] Several early studies did not include appropriate comparison groups; however, later studies that have compared pregnant persons with nonpregnant women of reproductive age have suggested that pregnancy is a risk factor for severe disease.[4] A systematic review and meta-analysis showed increased odds of admission to an intensive care unit (ICU) (odds ratio [OR] 2.13, 95% confidence interval [CI] 1.53–2.95, 7 studies, n = 601,108), of invasive ventilation (OR 2.59, 95% CI 2.28–2.94, 6 studies, n = 601,044), and of the need for extracorporeal membrane oxygenation (ECMO) (OR 2.02, 95% CI 1.22–3.34, 2 studies, n = 461,936) for pregnant and recently pregnant persons compared with nonpregnant women of reproductive age.[6] These findings are similar to those in a study from the Centers for Disease Control and Prevention (CDC) of more than 400,000 women of reproductive age with symptomatic COVID-19, which also showed a significantly elevated adjusted risk ratio (aRR) for death among pregnant persons (aRR = 1.7, 95% CI 1.2–2.4), compared with nonpregnant women of reproductive age; however, pregnancy status was missing in more than half of reported cases.[7] A study from Colombia also showed a significantly increased risk of death among pregnant persons, compared with nonpregnant women of reproductive age (aRR = 1.82, 95% CI 1.60–2.07, n = 371,363).[8] Several risk factors for severe disease during pregnancy have been identified, including higher maternal age, high body mass index, nonwhite ethnicity, and prepregnancy comorbid conditions, such as diabetes and hypertension.[4]

Studies of COVID-19 suggest that the postpartum period is also one of increased risk, similar to what was seen with 2009 H1N1 influenza.[9] For example, analysis of a prospective cohort from New York City showed a high risk of severe disease during the postpartum period; among patients with an asymptomatic presentation during pregnancy, clinical worsening or new symptoms occurred during the first 7 days after birth in 13% of women.[10] The risk for postpartum complications (eg, fever, hypoxia, or need for readmission) was higher among patients with COVID-19 (12.9%) compared with those without COVID-19 (4.5%, P < .001).[10] In a multivariate analysis in Brazil that compared nonpregnant SARS-CoV-2-infected women with those who were pregnant or postpartum (defined as up to 42 days after childbirth), the postpartum period was associated with the highest odds for death (OR = 1.90, 95% CI 1.53–2.35). Among those who were postpartum, age greater than 35 years and diabetes were independently associated with increased risk of death. Postpartum status was also associated with an increased rate of ICU admission and invasive ventilation.[11]

Because SARS-CoV-2 testing is often performed as part of screening for hospital admission at delivery, pregnant and recently pregnant persons who test positive for SARS-CoV-2 infection are less likely to report symptoms (OR 0.28, 95% CI 0.13–0.62).[6] In a prospective cohort of individuals tested weekly for SARS-CoV-2, 99 participants tested positive, with 20 (20%) reporting no symptoms throughout their infections. Among those with detailed symptom data, nasal congestion (72%), cough (64%), headache (59%), and changes in taste or smell (54%) were most commonly reported; a measured or subjective fever was reported in 28%.[3]

TREATMENT OF COVID-19 DURING PREGNANCY

The National Institutes of Health has developed treatment guidelines for care of patients with COVID-19, which are updated regularly (https://www. covid19treatmentguidelines.nih.gov/). Many clinical trials evaluating novel treatments for COVID-19 have excluded pregnant persons; however, treatment recommended for the nonpregnant population should not be withheld from pregnant persons; this includes treatment with remdesivir, dexamethasone, and monoclonal antibodies. Given that pregnancy is a risk factor for progression to serious disease, pregnant persons are eligible to receive outpatient treatment or postexposure prophylaxis with anti-SARS-CoV-2 monoclonal antibodies under the Emergency Use Authorization.[4,12]

Clinical algorithms for care of pregnant and nonpregnant patients with COVID-19 are generally similar; however, use of algorithms specific to pregnancy can account for some important differences. For example, peripheral oxygen saturation during pregnancy should be maintained at 95% or greater to ensure a favorable oxygen diffusion gradient across the placenta.[13] Timing of delivery for pregnant patients needs to be individualized, weighing the benefits and the risks to the patient and fetus.[13] In the setting of a patient with refractory hypoxemia at or after 32 weeks gestation or in the setting of worsening or persistent critical illness, it is reasonable to consider delivery. In a recent study of pregnant patients with COVID-19–related acute respiratory distress syndrome (ARDS), delivery resulted in a small improvement of Po_2/Fio_2 ratio, an indicator of ARDS severity.[14] However, the investigators emphasized that this study was not generalizable to patients without ARDS who are at significantly lower morbidity and mortality risk.

EFFECTS OF SARS-CoV-2 ON PREGNANCY OUTCOMES

Several studies have shown that SARS-CoV-2 infection during pregnancy increases the risk of pregnancy complications. In a systematic review and meta-analysis that included 42 studies of 438,548 pregnant persons, COVID-19 was associated with an increased risk for preeclampsia, preterm birth, and stillbirth, compared with no SARS-CoV-2 infection during pregnancy. Severe COVID-19 disease (defined as presence of dyspnea, respiratory rate of ≥30 breaths per minute and an oxygen saturation of 93% or less on room air, or findings consistent with pneumonia) was strongly associated with preeclampsia, gestational diabetes, cesarean delivery, preterm birth, low birth weight, and admission to the neonatal intensive care unit, compared with mild disease (defined as a positive test for SARS-CoV-2 without severe symptoms).[15] In a large study using data from 499 US academic health centers or community affiliates published after the systematic review, COVID-19 diagnosis was not associated with an increased risk of cesarean delivery ($P = .57$); however, the association between diagnosis of COVID-19 and preterm birth remained ($P < .001$).[16] A systematic review and meta-analysis focusing on the effects of SARS-CoV-2 infection during pregnancy and preeclampsia showed increased odds for preeclampsia; preeclampsia with severe features; eclampsia; and hemolysis, elevated liver enzymes, and low platelet count (HELLP) syndrome among pregnant persons with SARS-CoV-2 infection compared with those without SARS-CoV-2 infection. Increased odds of preeclampsia were seen in patients with both asymptomatic and symptomatic SARS-CoV-2 infection; however, the odds were higher among symptomatic patients.[17] In a recent study of nearly 500,000 hospitalizations in 703 US hospitals, pregnant persons with a documented COVID-19 diagnosis were only slightly more likely to have a cesarean delivery (33.5 vs 32.0%, $P = .0093$) and preterm labor with a preterm delivery (aRR 1.2, 95% CI 1.1–1.3) than those without a COVID-19 diagnosis. The investigators noted that differences in the risks of cesarean delivery and preterm birth might be related to different obstetric intervention practices across populations and geographic areas.[18]

INTRAUTERINE TRANSMISSION OF SARS-CoV-2

When a newborn infant tests positive for SARS-CoV-2, it can be difficult to determine whether transmission was intrauterine (during pregnancy and before labor onset), intrapartum (during labor and delivery), or postnatal, either through contact with the mother or others or through breastfeeding. Criteria to evaluate whether intrauterine transmission has occurred have been developed and include documentation of maternal infection, identification of SARS-CoV-2 in the first 24 hours of life, and evidence of persistence of infection in the neonate.[19–21] Although intrauterine transmission of SARS-CoV-2 has been documented,[22] it seems to be rare. In a systematic review that included 1141 neonates born to infected pregnant persons, 58 newborns had documented SARS-CoV-2 infection; 4 of these were believed to be congenital (2 confirmed, 1 probable, and 1 "not sure"), 41 were acquired postpartum, and 13 were unclassified because of missing information.[23] The reasons for the low frequency of intrauterine transmission of SARS-CoV-2 are not fully understood but might be related to low levels of viremia with SARS-CoV-2 infection[24] and the lack of placental coexpression of factors that facilitate SARS-CoV-2 entry into cells (ie, angiotensin-converting enzyme 2 and transmembrane serine protease 2),[25,26] although not all studies have been consistent on this issue.[27]

A recent study has suggested that the placental immune response to SARS-CoV-2 infection differs depending on the sex of the fetus. When the fetus was male, maternal SARS-CoV-2 antibody titers were lower, and antibody transfer across the placenta was impaired.[28] Whether these differences result in increased vulnerability of male infants to early life SARS-CoV-2 infection is unknown.

SARS-CoV-2 VACCINES AND PREGNANCY

Three vaccines have received emergency use authorization or full approval in the United States by the Food and Drug Administration (FDA): 2 messenger RNA (mRNA) vaccines (made by Pfizer/BioNTech and Moderna) and one viral vector vaccine made by Janssen (Johnson and Johnson). The clinical trials for these vaccines excluded pregnant persons. However, given the data on safety of other vaccines during pregnancy and the known increased risk to pregnant persons of serious disease from COVID-19, CDC, American College of Obstetricians and Gynecologists (ACOG), and the Society for Maternal-Fetal Medicine (SMFM) all made initial recommendations to ensure that pregnant persons could choose to be vaccinated.[29] Since that time, information has become available on the effectiveness and safety of the SARS-CoV-2 vaccines during pregnancy, leading ACOG and SMFM to change to a strong recommendation for vaccination during pregnancy on July 30, 2021, followed by CDC on August 11, 2021. After a record number of 22 deaths among pregnant persons in the United States in the month of August 2021 alone, CDC issued an urgent public health advisory on September 29, 2021, urging people who are pregnant, recently pregnant, or who might become pregnant in the future to get vaccinated.[30]

In 2021, the FDA also authorized booster doses of all 3 available vaccines for certain populations (boosters for Pfizer/BioNTech were authorized on September 22 and boosters for Moderna and Johnson and Johnson vaccines were authorized on October 20, 2021). Booster doses are recommended for all persons 12 years and older, including pregnant persons, at least 5 months after the second dose of the Pfizer/BioNTech and Moderna vaccines, and at least 2 months after the first dose of the Janssen vaccine.

SARS-CoV-2 Vaccine Effectiveness During Pregnancy

With regard to effectiveness, antibody responses during pregnancy were found to have similar immunogenicity and reactogenicity to those in nonpregnant women.[31,32] The second dose of the vaccine was essential for pregnant persons to achieve adequate immune responses similar to those of nonpregnant women.[33] An analysis of responses against the B.1.1.7 (Alpha) and B.1.351 (Beta) variants of concern showed reduced antibody titers, but preserved T-cell responses.[34] In addition, vaccine-generated antibodies during pregnancy were found to be significantly higher than those induced by SARS-CoV-2 infection during pregnancy.[31] In a large retrospective cohort study from Israel, the likelihood of infection in vaccinated versus unvaccinated pregnant persons suggested significant protection from the vaccine (adjusted hazard ratio of 0.22 [95% CI 0.11–0.43]).[35] Vaccine effectiveness after the second dose of vaccine during pregnancy was found to be similar to that seen in the general population: 96% (95% CI 89%–100%) for any documented infection, 97% (95% CI 91%–100%) for symptomatic infection, and 89% (95% CI 43%–100%) for COVID-19-associated hospitalization against alpha and ancestral variants.[36]

SARS-CoV-2 Vaccine Safety During Pregnancy

Safety data on mRNA vaccine–exposed pregnancies from 3 vaccine safety systems in the United States have been reassuring. Pregnant persons were less likely to report headache, myalgia, chills, and fever and more likely to report pain at the injection site. The frequencies of adverse pregnancy and neonatal outcomes were similar to those seen in studies before the COVID-19 pandemic, suggesting no increase in adverse outcomes related to vaccination.[37] Similar findings were seen in studies from Israel. A study of more than 500 pregnant persons who were vaccinated throughout pregnancy showed no increase in the rate of obstetric complications.[38] In a study of more than 700 pregnant persons vaccinated in the third trimester of pregnancy, adverse maternal outcomes were not increased; however, those who were vaccinated had a higher rate of elective cesarean delivery and a lower rate of vacuum-assisted vaginal delivery. A composite score for adverse neonatal outcomes showed a lower risk among those vaccinated compared with unvaccinated.[39] Three studies have specifically addressed the risk of pregnancy loss after receiving the SARS-CoV-2 vaccine and have found no increased risk. These included data from a CDC COVID-19 vaccine pregnancy registry,[40] a case-control analysis from 8 health systems in the United States,[41] and a case-control study using several Norwegian national health registries.[42] These studies primarily focused on the use of mRNA vaccines, although a small proportion of pregnancies in the study from Norway were exposed to the ChAdOx1-S/nCoV-19 (recombinant) vaccine.

SARS-CoV-2 Vaccines During Pregnancy and Protection of the Infant

Other vaccines (ie, inactivated influenza and the tetanus toxoid, reduced diphtheria toxoid, and acellular pertussis) are recommended during pregnancy because of their ability to protect infants from influenza and pertussis, respectively, during the first few months of life. Therefore, another important question is whether SARS-CoV-2 vaccine during pregnancy provides immune protection to the infant. SARS-CoV-2 antibodies were seen in umbilical cord blood and breast milk after vaccination with mRNA vaccines during pregnancy in several studies, suggesting that maternal vaccination might provide some protection to the infant.[31,34,43–45] In one study, infants whose mothers had a longer time period between vaccination and delivery and who had received both doses of the vaccine had higher levels of immunoglobulin G (IgG) antibodies. In 3 infants (one set of twins) who did not have IgG in umbilical cord blood, mothers were vaccinated less than 3 weeks before delivery.[43] In another study, IgG antibodies were detected in maternal and umbilical cord blood samples of all pregnancies by 4 weeks after the vaccine dose, except for one. IgG was detectable in 44% and 99% of cord blood samples in which the pregnant person had received only 1 vaccine dose and 2 doses of vaccine, respectively,[46] again emphasizing the importance of pregnant persons receiving the full vaccine series.

SARS-CoV-2 Vaccine Hesitancy During Pregnancy

Despite the availability of reassuring data on effectiveness and safety of the SARS-CoV-2 vaccines, the uptake of SARS-CoV-2 vaccines has been lower than that of the general population. As of October 23, 2021, less than 35% of pregnant people in the United States reported being fully vaccinated for COVID-19 before or during pregnancy. Rates varied by race and ethnicity, ranging from the highest rate in non-Hispanic Asians (49.8%) to the lowest rate in non-Hispanic Black persons (19.2%).[47] In a study of vaccine uptake among health care workers in a medical center in Israel during the first months after vaccine roll-out, the most common reason for declining the vaccine was concerns about risks during pregnancy.[48]

Other studies have identified factors associated with the likelihood of receiving COVID-19 vaccination during pregnancy. In an analysis of pregnant patients in Israel, those who received both doses of the vaccine were likely to be older and to have had previous miscarriages, previous cesarean deliveries, or fertility treatments.[39] In a study of persons giving birth at a hospital in the United Kingdom, lower vaccine uptake was seen among younger persons, persons of lower socioeconomic background, and people not identified as White. Higher vaccine uptake was seen in pregnant persons with prepregnancy diabetes.[49]

In a survey of pregnant persons in Italy, 28.2% agreed to be vaccinated. Most noted that pregnancy influenced their decision, even though the majority (90.1%) reported being generally in favor of vaccines. The main reason for declining the vaccine was fear of the effects on their baby's health.[50] In a study from Germany conducted between March 30 and April 19, 2021, most (57.4%) of the pregnant respondents were not in favor of receiving the vaccine, 28.8% were unsure, and only 13.8% would get vaccinated. Nearly half (47.2%) of the pregnant respondents were in favor of receiving the vaccine if more scientific evidence on vaccine safety were available. The main reasons for vaccine hesitancy were concerns about limited information about the vaccine, limited information on vaccine safety, and fear of harm to the fetus or infant. When asked who the best contact person would be for questions regarding COVID-19 vaccination, pregnant persons named their gynecologist.[51]

A study conducted at a single academic health center in Missouri from April 27 to May 20, 2021 addressed whether improving vaccine access would result in increased SARS-CoV-2 vaccine uptake by comparing time periods when SARS-CoV-2 vaccines were available onsite versus before onsite vaccine availability. No difference in vaccine uptake was noted during these time periods, suggesting that vaccine hesitancy, not convenience, was the critical issue causing low vaccination rates in their population.[52]

Shook and colleagues[53] recently proposed a framework to address vaccine hesitancy during pregnancy. Their framework included addressing the "four Cs": confidence, complacency, convenience, and compassion. Increasing vaccine confidence by addressing concerns about safety, combatting complacency due to the perception that a pregnant person is at low-risk, increasing vaccine convenience by offering the vaccine at the time of a prenatal appointment, and the need for compassionate conversations between obstetric care providers and vaccine-hesitant pregnant persons are all believed to be important to increase vaccination rates among this population.

One reason frequently cited for declining COVID-19 vaccination has been concerns about fertility. The issue regarding female fertility initially arose from a blog post that noted a similarity between the spike protein of SARS-CoV-2 and a protein on the placenta, syncytin-1, with a hypothesis that vaccine-induced antibodies could target the placental protein and result in infertility. Although the similarity between the 2 proteins is minimal and no evidence for infertility had been seen among women following COVID-19 infection, who also would have exposure to antibodies to the spike protein, this false information spread quickly. Several pieces of information can be used to address this rumor. First, convalescent serum from patients with COVID-19 does not react with syncytin-1 protein. Second, no evidence of fertility issues was seen in the developmental and reproductive toxicology studies done on animals before vaccine authorization. Third, despite pregnant people being excluded from the clinical trials and participants being were asked to avoid pregnancy, 57 pregnancies occurred, with similar numbers of inadvertent pregnancies in the vaccinated and placebo groups. Finally, no increases in rates of miscarriage have been seen following vaccination in pregnancy, a finding that might be expected if antibodies were causing damage to the placenta.[54] More recently, concerns, again unfounded, have been raised about male infertility. Studies have shown no decreases in any sperm parameters after receipt of a COVID-19 mRNA vaccine.[55] Thus, based on available data, there is no evidence to support any negative effects on female or male fertility related to SARS-CoV-2 vaccines.

SUMMARY

Pregnant persons are at increased risk for severe disease during pregnancy, with increased risk of admission to an ICU, increased need for mechanical ventilation, need for ECMO, and likely increased risk of death. In general, treatment of COVID-19 during pregnancy is similar to nonpregnant persons, with a few modifications. Treatment should not be withheld based on pregnancy status, but rather pregnant persons should be prioritized for early treatments such as antivirals and monoclonal antibodies to prevent severe outcomes. Intrauterine transmission of SARS-CoV-2 occurs but is rare, possibly related to the low rate of SARS-CoV-2 viremia and an absence of coexpression of receptors on the placenta that facilitate SARS-CoV-2's entry into cells. However, even in the absence of intrauterine transmission, SARS-CoV-2 infection during pregnancy increases the risk of adverse pregnancy outcomes, especially among those severely affected. Available data on SARS-CoV-2 vaccines during pregnancy suggest that they are safe and effective. In addition, SARS-CoV-2 antibodies have been identified in umbilical cord blood and in breast milk following vaccination during pregnancy, suggesting that maternal vaccination provides some degree of protection to the infant. However, coverage rates among pregnant persons remain low as of late 2021; available data suggest that concerns regarding the safety of the vaccine on the fetus are key to vaccine hesitancy during pregnancy. Additional studies are needed to better understand ways to address vaccine hesitancy among pregnant persons.

CLINICS CARE POINTS

- Effective COVID-19 treatments such as remdesivir, dexamethasone, and monoclonal antibodies should not be withheld from pregnant persons. Pregnancy is a high-risk condition, which is considered a priority indication for early treatment or prophylaxis with SARS-CoV-2 monoclonal antibodies and antivirals.

- Because COVID-19 is associated with an increased risk of poor pregnancy outcomes such as preeclampsia, preterm birth, and stillbirth, pregnant persons with COVID-19 infection should be closely monitored, particularly those with severe disease.

- Health care providers should emphasize to their pregnant patients the importance of being fully vaccinated for COVID-19 and of receiving booster doses of vaccine.

DISCLOSURES

None.

REFERENCES

1. Rasmussen SA, Smulian JC, Lednicky JA, et al. Coronavirus disease 2019 (COVID-19) and pregnancy: what obstetricians need to know. Am J Obstet Gynecol 2020;222(5):415–26.
2. Jamieson DJ, Theiler RN, Rasmussen SA. Emerging infections and pregnancy. Emerg Infect Dis 2006;12(11):1638–43.
3. Dawood FS, Varner M, Tita A, et al. Incidence, clinical characteristics, and risk factors of SARS-CoV-2 infection among pregnant individuals in the United States. Clin Infect Dis 2021;ciab713.
4. Jamieson DJ, Rasmussen SA. An update on COVID-19 and pregnancy. Am J Obstet Gynecol 2022;226(2):177–86.
5. Savitz DA, Bengtson AM, Hardy E, et al. Pregnancy and the risk of severe coronavirus disease 2019 infection: methodological challenges and research recommendations. BJOG 2022;129(2):192–5.
6. Allotey J, Stallings E, Bonet M, et al. Clinical manifestations, risk factors, and maternal and perinatal outcomes of coronavirus disease 2019 in pregnancy: living systematic review and meta-analysis. BMJ 2020;370:m3320.

7. Zambrano LD, Ellington S, Strid P, et al. Update: characteristics of symptomatic women of reproductive age with laboratory-confirmed SARS-CoV-2 infection by pregnancy status - United States, January 22-October 3, 2020. MMWR Morb Mortal Wkly Rep 2020;69(44):1641–7.

8. Rozo N, Valencia D, Newton SM, et al. Severity of illness by pregnancy status among laboratory-confirmed SARS-CoV-2 infections occurring in reproductive-aged women in Colombia. Paediatr Perinat Epidemiol 2021. online ahead of print.

9. Louie JK, Jamieson DJ, Rasmussen SA. 2009 pandemic influenza A (H1N1) virus infection in postpartum women in California. Am J Obstet Gynecol 2011;204(2): 144 e1-6.

10. Prabhu M, Cagino K, Matthews KC, et al. Pregnancy and postpartum outcomes in a universally tested population for SARS-CoV-2 in New York City: a prospective cohort study. BJOG 2020;127(12):1548–56.

11. Knobel R, Takemoto MLS, Nakamura-Pereira M, et al. COVID-19-related deaths among women of reproductive age in Brazil: the burden of postpartum. Int J Gynaecol Obstet 2021;155(1):101–9.

12. Food and Drug Administration. Fact sheet for health care providers: emergency use authorization (EUA) of REGEN-COV™ (casirivimab and imdevimab). 2021. Available at: https://www.fda.gov/media/145611/download. [Accessed 11 November 2021]. Accessed.

13. Society for Maternal-Fetal Medicine. Management considerations for pregnant patients with COVID-19. 2021. Available at. https://www.smfm.org/covidclinical. [Accessed 11 November 2021]. Accessed.

14. Pineles BL, Stephens A, Narendran LM, et al. The relationship between delivery and the PaO2/FiO2 ratio in COVID-19: a cohort study. BJOG 2021;129(3):493–9.

15. Wei SQ, Bilodeau-Bertrand M, Liu S, et al. The impact of COVID-19 on pregnancy outcomes: a systematic review and meta-analysis. CMAJ 2021;193(16):E540–8.

16. Chinn J, Sedighim S, Kirby KA, et al. Characteristics and outcomes of women with COVID-19 giving birth at US academic centers during the COVID-19 pandemic. JAMA Netw Open 2021;4(8):e2120456.

17. Conde-Agudelo A, Romero R. SARS-CoV-2 infection during pregnancy and risk of preeclampsia: a systematic review and meta-analysis. Am J Obstet Gynecol 2022;226(1):68-89.e3.

18. Ko JY, DeSisto CL, Simeone RM, et al. Adverse pregnancy outcomes, maternal complications, and severe illness among US delivery hospitalizations with and without a coronavirus disease 2019 (COVID-19) Diagnosis. Clin Infect Dis 2021;73(Suppl 1):S24–31.

19. Blumberg DA, Underwood MA, Hedriana HL, et al. Vertical transmission of SARS-CoV-2: what is the optimal definition? Am J Perinatol 2020;37(8):769–72.

20. Shah PS, Diambomba Y, Acharya G, et al. Classification system and case definition for SARS-CoV-2 infection in pregnant women, fetuses, and neonates. Acta Obstet Gynecol Scand 2020;99(5):565–8.

21. World Health Organization. Definition andcategorization of the timing of mother-to-childtransmission of SARS-CoV-2 scientific brief, 8 February 2021. 2021. Available at: https://apps.who.int/iris/handle/10665/339422. [Accessed 11 November 2021]. Accessed on.

22. Vivanti AJ, Vauloup-Fellous C, Prevot S, et al. Transplacental transmission of SARS-CoV-2 infection. Nat Commun 2020;11(1):3572.

23. Dhir SK, Kumar J, Meena J, et al. Clinical features and outcome of SARS-CoV-2 infection in neonates: a systematic review. J Trop Pediatr 2021;67(3):fmaa059.

24. Wang W, Xu Y, Gao R, et al. Detection of SARS-CoV-2 in different types of clinical specimens. JAMA 2020;323(18):1843–4.
25. Pique-Regi R, Romero R, Tarca AL, et al. Does the human placenta express the canonical cell entry mediators for SARS-CoV-2? Elife 2020;9:e58716.
26. Edlow AG, Li JZ, Collier AY, et al. Assessment of maternal and neonatal SARS-CoV-2 viral load, transplacental antibody transfer, and placental pathology in pregnancies during the COVID-19 pandemic. JAMA Netw Open 2020;3(12): e2030455.
27. Weatherbee BAT, Glover DM, Zernicka-Goetz M. Expression of SARS-CoV-2 receptor ACE2 and the protease TMPRSS2 suggests susceptibility of the human embryo in the first trimester. Open Biol 2020;10(8):200162.
28. Bordt EA, Shook LL, Atyeo C, et al. Maternal SARS-CoV-2 infection elicits sexually dimorphic placental immune responses. Sci Transl Med 2021;13(617):eabi7428.
29. Rasmussen SA, Jamieson DJ. Pregnancy, postpartum care, and COVID-19 vaccination in 2021. JAMA 2021;325(11):1099–100.
30. CDC. Healthy Advisory Network: COVID-19 vaccination for pregnant people to prevent serious illness, deaths, and adverse pregnancy outcomes from COVID-19. released september 29, 2021. Accessed October 31, 2021. 2021.
31. Gray KJ, Bordt EA, Atyeo C, et al. Coronavirus disease 2019 vaccine response in pregnant and lactating women: a cohort study. Am J Obstet Gynecol 2021; 225(3):303 e1–03 e17.
32. Falsaperla R, Leone G, Familiari M, et al. COVID-19 vaccination in pregnant and lactating women: a systematic review. Expert Rev Vaccines 2021;1–10.
33. Atyeo C, DeRiso EA, Davis C, et al. COVID-19 mRNA vaccines drive differential Fc-functional profiles in pregnant, lactating, and non-pregnant women. Sci Transl Med 2021;13(617):eabi8631.
34. Collier AY, McMahan K, Yu J, et al. Immunogenicity of COVID-19 mRNA vaccines in pregnant and lactating women. JAMA 2021;325(23):2370–80.
35. Goldshtein I, Nevo D, Steinberg DM, et al. Association between BNT162b2 vaccination and incidence of SARS-CoV-2 infection in pregnant women. JAMA 2021; 326(8):728–35.
36. Dagan N, Barda N, Biron-Shental T, et al. Effectiveness of the BNT162b2 mRNA COVID-19 vaccine in pregnancy. Nat Med 2021;27(10):1693–5.
37. Shimabukuro TT, Kim SY, Myers TR, et al. Preliminary findings of mRNA Covid-19 vaccine safety in pregnant persons. N Engl J Med 2021;384(24):2273–82.
38. Bookstein Peretz S, Regev N, Novick L, et al. Short-term outcome of pregnant women vaccinated with BNT162b2 mRNA COVID-19 vaccine. Ultrasound Obstet Gynecol 2021;58(3):450–6.
39. Rottenstreich M, Sela HY, Rotem R, et al. Covid-19 vaccination during the third trimester of pregnancy: rate of vaccination and maternal and neonatal outcomes, a multicentre retrospective cohort study. BJOG 2022;129(2):248–55.
40. Zauche LH, Wallace B, Smoots AN, et al. Receipt of mRNA Covid-19 vaccines and risk of spontaneous abortion. N Engl J Med 2021;385(16):1533–5.
41. Kharbanda EO, Haapala J, DeSilva M, et al. Spontaneous abortion following COVID-19 vaccination during pregnancy. JAMA 2021;326(16):1629–31.
42. Magnus MC, Gjessing HK, Eide HN, et al. Covid-19 vaccination during pregnancy and first-trimester miscarriage. N Engl J Med 2021;385(21):2008–10.
43. Mithal LB, Otero S, Shanes ED, et al. Cord blood antibodies following maternal coronavirus disease 2019 vaccination during pregnancy. Am J Obstet Gynecol 2021;225(2):192–4.

44. Beharier O, Plitman Mayo R, Raz T, et al. Efficient maternal to neonatal transfer of antibodies against SARS-CoV-2 and BNT162b2 mRNA COVID-19 vaccine. J Clin Invest 2021;131(13):e150319.
45. Trostle ME, Aguero-Rosenfeld ME, Roman AS, et al. High antibody levels in cord blood from pregnant women vaccinated against COVID-19. Am J Obstet Gynecol MFM 2021;100481.
46. Prabhu M, Murphy EA, Sukhu AC, et al. Antibody Response to Coronavirus Disease 2019 (COVID-19) Messenger RNA Vaccination in Pregnant Women and Transplacental Passage Into Cord Blood. Obstet Gynecol 2021;138(2):278–80.
47. CDC. COVID-19 vaccination among pregnant people aged 18-49 years overall, by race/ethnicity, and date reported to CDC - Vaccine Safety Datalink, United States December 14, 2020–October 23, 2021. 2021. Available at: https://covid.cdc.gov/covid-data-tracker/#vaccinations-pregnant-womenCOVID-19.   [Accessed 31 October 2021]. Accessed.
48. Gilboa M, Tal I, Levin EG, et al. Coronavirus disease 2019 (COVID-19) vaccination uptake among healthcare workers. Infect Control Hosp Epidemiol 2021;1–6.
49. Blakeway H, Prasad S, Kalafat E, et al. COVID-19 vaccination during pregnancy: coverage and safety. Am J Obstet Gynecol 2021;226(2):236.e1–14.
50. Carbone L, Mappa I, Sirico A, et al. Pregnant women's perspectives on severe acute respiratory syndrome coronavirus 2 vaccine. Am J Obstet Gynecol MFM 2021;3(4):100352.
51. Schaal NK, Zollkau J, Hepp P, et al. Pregnant and breastfeeding women's attitudes and fears regarding the COVID-19 vaccination. Arch Gynecol Obstet 2021. online ahead of print.
52. Hirshberg JS, Huysman BC, Oakes MC, et al. Offering onsite COVID-19 vaccination to high-risk obstetrical patients: initial findings. Am J Obstet Gynecol MFM 2021;3(6):100478.
53. Shook L, Kishkovich T, Edlow A. Countering COVID-19 vaccine hesitancy in pregnancy: the "4 Cs. Am J Perinatol 2021. online ahead of print.
54. Male V. Are COVID-19 vaccines safe in pregnancy? Nat Rev Immunol 2021;21(4):200–1.
55. Lo SP, Hsieh TC, Pastuszak AW, et al. Effects of SARS CoV-2, COVID-19, and its vaccines on male sexual health and reproduction: where do we stand? Int J Impot Res 2021. online ahead of print.

Severe Acute Respiratory Syndrome Coronavirus 2 Infections in Children

Eric J. Chow, MD, MS, MPH[a],*, Janet A. Englund, MD[b]

KEYWORDS

- SARS-Cov-2 • COVID-19 • Pediatrics • Adolescents • MIS-C • Vaccinations
- Children

KEY POINTS

- Children are at risk for Coronavirus disease 2019 (COVID-19) although the proportion of severe disease is lower than in adults; optimal treatment for pediatric COVID-19 has not been fully vetted through clinical trials.
- Pediatric COVID-19 vaccines that are authorized by the Food and Drug Administration and approved by the Advisory Committee on Immunization Practices or World Health Organization are available in the United States and in other countries, with varying indications for booster doses. Severe acute respiratory syndrome coronavirus 2 (SARS-CoV-2) vaccinations are safe and effective in preventing severe COVID-19, and as of early 2022, vaccinations have been authorized for use in children aged ≥5 years.
- The identification of SARS-CoV-2 variants may impact the severity of pediatric COVID-19 and community transmissibility, as well as modify the effectiveness of approved vaccine and COVID-19 therapeutics; studies of new biologics to address COVID-19 caused by viral mutations are ongoing.
- The multisystem inflammatory syndrome in children (MIS-C) is a hyperinflammatory condition resulting in significant morbidity but low mortality.
- The pandemic has affected child health, contributing to delays in health care, decreases in routine childhood vaccination rates, disruption to education, and impact on mental health.

INTRODUCTION

Since the start of the severe acute respiratory syndrome coronavirus 2 (SARS-CoV-2) pandemic in 2020, acute coronavirus disease 2019 (COVID-19) has affected children of all ages.[1,2] Overall, the number and incidence of reported infections and cases of

[a] Division of Allergy and Infectious Diseases, Department of Medicine, University of Washington, 1959 NE Pacific Street, Box 356423, Seattle, WA 98195, USA; [b] Division of Pediatric Infectious Diseases, Department of Pediatrics, University of Washington, Seattle Children's Research Institute, 4800 Sand Point Way NE - MA7.234, Seattle, WA 98105, USA
* Corresponding author.
E-mail address: ejchow@uw.edu

Infect Dis Clin N Am 36 (2022) 435–479
https://doi.org/10.1016/j.idc.2022.01.005   id.theclinics.com
0891-5520/22/© 2022 Elsevier Inc. All rights reserved.

severe disease in children are fewer than those reported in adults.[3] Treatment of pediatric COVID-19 has largely been extrapolated from adult trials, but management has been focused on prevention and mitigation of transmission. Among the many complications associated with COVID-19, the multisystem inflammatory syndrome in children (MIS-C) has drawn much attention due to the hyperinflammatory findings and acuity at hospital presentation. SARS-CoV-2 vaccinations will likely play an important role in infection prevention in children as more are vaccinated. By the beginning of 2022, the safety and efficacy of vaccinations in the <5-year-old age group remain under evaluation. New studies will expand our knowledge of SARS-CoV-2 epidemiology, change our understanding of disease processes, and improve clinical management recommendations. Here, we summarize the current epidemiology, clinical features, and management of SARS-CoV-2 infection in children.

EPIDEMIOLOGY

Children of all ages are at risk for SARS-CoV-2 infection and severe COVID-19[4,5]; however, the number of infections and disease severity vary by age, with a higher number of infections and cases of severe disease in older age groups. There have been fewer reported cases of COVID-19 in children than in adults, and assessments of the true SARS-CoV-2 incidence in the pediatric population have been challenging, as early data relied on observational studies and convenience sampling. Children more frequently experience asymptomatic and mild disease, and early SARS-CoV-2 testing was prioritized to cases of severe disease,[6–8] leading to underreporting of pediatric cases at the start of the pandemic.[9] Lock-down procedures may have disproportionately mitigated transmission in children. As schools and childcare centers closed, children remained at home, reducing their exposure to SARS-CoV-2, thus likely reducing the role children played in community transmission early in the pandemic. By the fall of 2021, children returned to in-person school attendance in many locales, although the effect on community SARS-CoV-2 burden remains unclear. Stark differences in pediatric cases between communities of high and low vaccination rates illustrate the importance of vaccination campaigns in pediatric disease mitigation. The spread of SARS-CoV-2 variants is also likely to alter the epidemiology of COVID-19, including its impact on pediatric infections. As further steps are taken to reopen communities by governments around the world, additional impact of SARS-CoV-2 in pediatric populations is anticipated.

There are limited data on the global pediatric COVID-19 burden due to highly variable SARS-CoV-2 testing and changes in community mitigation efforts throughout the course of the pandemic. As of December 2021, UNICEF estimated that 0.4% of global deaths due to COVID-19 occurred in individuals younger than 20 years with 58% of those deaths occurring in adolescents aged 10 to 19 years and 42% in children aged 0 to 9 years.[10] These data likely underestimate the total COVID-19 mortality, given the disparities of resources, testing capability, differential reporting between regions, and the lack of inclusion of new variant viruses. Among Sub-Saharan African countries, pediatric COVID-19 is estimated to be 9% of confirmed cases and 2.4% of reported deaths, with variations in testing protocols by country.[11] Seroprevalence studies involving the detection of antibodies in response to infection have been undertaken to expand our understanding of the true burden of COVID-19. These studies show that SARS-CoV-2 infections in children have been frequently underdiagnosed.[12–14] Many of these studies conducted in different countries before[15–18] and after vaccine availability[19] showed a lower number of infection-derived SARS-CoV-2 antibody detection in children compared with adults. However, country and regional study differences conducted at varying timepoints during the pandemic have reported mixed results.[20] In the United States, individuals younger than 18 years comprise 22% of the population,[21] yet only 13% of COVID-19 cases have been reported in children.[3] Although the true incidence of pediatric SARS-CoV-2 infections is unknown, the US Centers for Disease Control and Prevention (CDC) estimates the cumulative incidence in the United States to be 25,844,005 total infections among those aged 0 to 17 years, with an infection rate of 35,490 per 100,000 individuals between February 2020 and September 2021 (**Table 1**).[22] In a summary of reported SARS-CoV-2 infections from March 1 to December 12, 2020, 17.4% of infections occurred in individuals aged 0 to 4 years, 25.7% among those aged 5 to 10 years, 18.6% in those aged 11 to 13 years, and 39.3% among those aged 14 to 17 years.[2]

Early in the pandemic from March 1 to July 25, 2020, age groups comprising the greatest proportion of hospitalized children in the United States were 12 to 17 years (42%), 0 to 2 months (19%) and 5 to 11 years (17%) with a hospitalization rate of 8 per 100,000 individuals.[5] The appearance and spread of SARS-CoV-2 variants had led to subsequent waves of infection across all age groups. By mid-June 2021, US pediatric hospitalizations were at their lowest with a rate of 0.3 per 100,000 children before the spread of the Delta (B.1.617.2 lineage)[23] SARS-CoV-2 variant.[24] Thereafter, the predominance of the Delta variant led to higher numbers of US pediatric emergency room visits and hospital admissions, particularly in regions where community-wide vaccinations were low.[25] In August 2021, the cumulative hospitalization rate for pediatric COVID-19 rose to 49.7 per 100,000 individuals.[24] Similarly, SARS-CoV-2 seropositivity had increased in children in England, coinciding with the spread of the Delta variant, reduction of lock-down procedures, and the start of the academic school year.[26] On November 26, 2021, the Omicron (B.1.1.529) SARS-CoV-2 variant was designated by the World Health Organization (WHO) as a variant of concern due to early evidence of increased transmissibility[27] and viral mutations allowing the evasion of prior immunity leading to rapid global spread and a spike in infection numbers.[28] In the United States, the spread of the Omicron variant[29] was associated with a rapid increase in COVID-19–associated pediatric hospitalizations.[30] With communities pursuing varying stages of re-opening, the identification of new variants and the increased availability of vaccinations for younger age groups, fluctuations in SARS-CoV-2 cases are likely to continue.

Table 1
SARS-CoV-2 point estimates of cumulative incidence and rates of COVID-19 outcomes by age group: United States, February 2020 to September 2021

Age-Group	Infections		Hospitalizations		Deaths	
	Estimated Cumulative Incidence	Estimated Rates per 100,000	Estimated Cumulative Incidence	Estimated Rates per 100,000	Estimated Cumulative Incidence	Estimated Rates per 100,000
0–17 y	25,844,005	35,490	266,597	366	645	0.9
18–49 y	75,179,070	54,860	1,996,830	1457	60,355	43.7
50–64 y	27,407,088	43,656	2,009,141	3200	159,489	253.5
≥65 y	18,012,882	32,363	3,232,213	5807	700,882	1296.5
Overall	146,585,169	44,650	7,506,029	2286	921,371	280.7

From Centers for Disease Control and Prevention. Estimated COVID-19 Burden. Accessed January 12, 2022. https://www.cdc.gov/coronavirus/2019-ncov/cases-updates/burden.html

The pandemic has accentuated racial and ethnic disparities among people in the United States.[31–36] A disproportionate number of children with COVID-19 who experience severe outcomes including hospitalizations and death come from communities of underrepresented racial and ethnic groups.[5,36,37] Among American Indian and Alaskan Natives, incidence of COVID-19 among those younger than 18 years was 3 times that of white, non-Hispanic individuals.[38] Hispanic and Latinx adults and children have experienced some of the highest rates of SARS-CoV-2 test positivity,[39,40] particularly during community-wide shelter-in-place directives.[35] Among individuals younger than 18 years with SARS-CoV-2 infection, rates of hospitalization were highest among Hispanic and Latinx children.[5,39] The cause of these disparities is likely multifactorial, including disproportionate burden of chronic conditions,[33] decreased access to health care and testing,[41] difficulty with social distancing in multigenerational households,[35] and greater representation in essential and in-person occupations with exposure risk to COVID-19[42] within the Hispanic and Latinx communities.[39] Survey studies also suggest that Black and Hispanic parents had a lower willingness to immediately vaccinate their children against COVID-19, highlighting the need for outreach, education, and messaging of the benefits of vaccination to these specific communities.[43] See Hernandez Acosta and colleagues' article, "Awakening: The unveiling of historically unaddressed social inequities during the COVID-19 pandemic in the United States", in this issue.

PEDIATRIC SEVERE ACUTE RESPIRATORY SYNDROME CORONAVIRUS 2 TRANSMISSION

Lock-down procedures, including closure of schools,[44] were first implemented in 2020 to reduce community transmission.[45,46] As communities have reopened and schools resumed in-person learning, questions remain about how best to limit the ongoing spread of SARS-CoV-2 and establish the role children play in community transmission.[47–49] Past experiences with other viruses demonstrate that children carry the community burden of influenza and respiratory syncytial viral infections,[48] and public health interventions,[50] such as vaccination of children, can reduce community-wide infections.[51–53] Thus far, data show fewer and milder pediatric SARS-CoV-2 infections compared with adult cases.

The primary mode of person-to-person transmission of SARS-CoV-2 is by respiratory spread,[54] and the use of face coverings, social distancing, and school closures contributed to community mitigation of infection early in the pandemic.[44,55–57] Children are both at risk for acquiring infection and spreading SARS-CoV-2.[49,58,59] Factors influencing individual transmissibility include symptomology, viral load, and behavioral patterns.[60] Both biological and social-behavioral factors vary by age, as a child younger than 5 years has different risks than adolescents. Vaccination status likely modifies an individual's risk of transmission, and vaccine availability to younger age groups will further influence SARS-CoV-2 epidemiology. The impact vaccines play in transmission by children will become evident as uptake and availability in younger age groups continues.

The first reports of pediatric COVID-19 were identified within household transmission investigations,[61–64] in which pediatric index cases of household SARS-CoV-2 infections were less common.[58,59,64–66] One study of household transmissions in which the index case was a child, showed fewer index cases in those aged 0 to 3 years, but a higher risk of household transmission in that age group than in index cases aged 14 to 17 years.[58] These findings suggest an individual's risk of transmission may have nuanced age-related associations. Younger age groups may be less likely to socially distance, cover their mouths when sneezing or coughing, or consistently wear masks, behaviors expected of older children and adults.[49] Furthermore, families are likely to physically interact more with younger ill children, leading to an increased risk for viral transmission.[49,67] Secondary attack rates (SAR) are calculated as the rate of infection among susceptible individuals from an index case and can be a helpful measure of person-to-person transmission. A systematic review of factors associated with SAR demonstrated higher rates for adult contacts than for children; pooled SAR was not associated with the index case's age.[68] These studies were limited to smaller sample sizes[69] and more finely defined age data were not available.

The risk of SARS-CoV-2 transmission has also been shown to be higher in exposed contacts of cases with higher viral loads.[70–72] In one community-based surveillance study, SARS-CoV-2 viral loads were similar regardless of symptoms and age.[73] Children experienced fewer symptoms for shorter duration when ill with COVID-19 and the presence of symptoms was correlated with a higher viral load than asymptomatic cases. Given that more children experience asymptomatic SARS-CoV-2, and viral load is lower in asymptomatic cases, children may play a smaller role in transmission than adults. The possibility of fecal-oral transmission has been raised, as infectious SARS-CoV-2 virus has been cultured from fecal samples of infected individuals[74] with prolonged shedding and higher levels of viral particles in pediatric fecal samples.[75,76] Thus far, significant fecal-oral transmission in close contacts of children with persistent fecal detection of SARS-CoV-2 has not been reported.[75] SARS-CoV-2 reinfection has been documented in children, although the degree at which it occurs is unknown.[77] With the appearance of novel variants, immune evasion may become more common.

The understanding of school and daycare-based transmission dynamics of SARS-CoV-2 is evolving. One systematic review of SAR found lower pediatric rates in school than household settings.[78] One early investigation in Ireland, where reported SARS-CoV-2 cases were screened for recent school attendance, reported no confirmed cases among school contacts.[79] An analysis of childcare centers in Washington, DC, found a limited number of outbreaks associated with each facility, with most cases acquired outside the facility.[80] A Delta variant outbreak investigation at a California elementary school involving an unvaccinated teacher as the index case found higher risks of infection with seating proximity to the teacher.[81] All students were unvaccinated at the time and had a reported high adherence to social distancing and mask wearing. A study in Los Angeles schools found that school-associated SARS-CoV-2 case rates among those aged 5 to 17 years were lower than community case rates but fluctuated with changes in the general community incidence.[82] In a series of school-based studies, the risk of a SARS-CoV-2 outbreak was 3.7 times higher in schools without mask requirements,[83] and larger increases of county case rates were seen when school mask mandates were optional.[84] These findings suggest that school-based transmission and community-wide case counts can be mitigated by implementing public health interventions as children return to school.

To minimize disruptions to attendance of in-person learning, some grade schools implemented the "Test to Stay" (TTS) strategy in which unvaccinated individuals who experienced a school-related SARS-CoV-2 exposure were allowed to stay in school if certain criteria were met. TTS required that both the index case and the close contact had to have been masked when exposed, and during the quarantine period, the close contact may remain in school provided they remained asymptomatic while wearing a mask and practiced social distancing and submitted to regular testing after the exposure. Schools adopting TTS between August and October 2021 in Illinois and California found a low SAR and low tertiary transmission after TTS implementation while minimizing loss of in-person school days.[85,86]

SEVERE ACUTE RESPIRATORY SYNDROME CORONAVIRUS 2 VACCINATIONS IN CHILDREN

The most significant public health breakthrough during the pandemic has been the development of SARS-CoV-2 vaccines (**Table 2**). As of December 17, 2021, the WHO has approved 9 vaccines against COVID-19 under their Emergency Use Listing process[87] including the Pfizer-BioNTech (BNT162b2) vaccine for those aged ≥12 years[88] (see William O. Hahn and Zanthia Wiley's article, "COVID-19 Vaccines," in this issue). More recently, individual countries have granted emergency use authorization (EUA) to vaccinations for younger children (vaccines produced by Pfizer-BioNTech, Cadila, Bharat, Sinopharm, and Sinovac). Given limited vaccine availability in many countries, WHO has prioritized vaccine use for those most at risk for severe disease, including adults and children aged 12 to 17 years who have high-risk underlying conditions. The CDC Advisory Committee on Immunization Practices (ACIP) recommends the SARS-CoV-2 vaccine for all individuals aged ≥5 years.[89–91] Since December 11, 2020, the mRNA-based SARS-CoV-2 vaccine produced by Pfizer-BioNTech at a 30-μg dose has been approved for individuals ≥16 years,[92] receiving full FDA approval on August 23, 2021.[93] On May 10, 2021, this vaccine was granted EUA in those aged 12 to 15 years,[94] with a 10 micro gram dose receiving EUA on October 29, 2021, for those ages 5 to 11 years.[95] Booster doses of vaccine were first authorized by the FDA on November 19, 2021, to adults, followed by approval for those aged 16 and 17 years on December 9, 2021,[96] and for those aged 12 to 15 years on January 3, 2022.[97] Booster doses administered ≥5 months after completion of the primary series are increasingly important with the spread of the Omicron variant.[98] A third primary dose of Pfizer-BioNTech has been authorized by the FDA for moderately or severely immunocompromised children aged ≥5 years.[97] On December 8, 2021, the FDA granted EUA to tixagevimab/cilgavimab (Evusheld), a combination monoclonal antibody, for those aged ≥12 years and weighing ≥40 kg who are not currently infected with SARS-CoV-2, have moderately to severely compromised immune systems, or a history of severe adverse reactions to the approved SARS-CoV-2 vaccines, as preexposure prophylaxis.[99] As of January 2022, pediatric data with this new long-acting monoclonal antibody have not been published, but approval offers an alternative to vaccinations in those who are unable to mount sufficient immunity to approved vaccines or those for whom current vaccines are not clinically recommended.

Vaccine trials and real-world effectiveness studies have shown that SARS-CoV-2 mRNA vaccines are highly effective against COVID-19. Before the predominance of SARS-CoV-2 variants, the Pfizer-BioNTech vaccine reported vaccine efficacy of 95% against confirmed COVID-19 in those aged ≥16 years.[100] In a subsequent analysis on the safety and efficacy of the same vaccine in participants aged 12 to 15 years, vaccine efficacy was 100% against confirmed COVID-19 after completion of the 2-dose series.[101] The Phase 2 to 3 vaccine trial (conducted between June 7, 2021 and October 8, 2021) evaluating the Pfizer-BioNTech mRNA vaccine in the 5-year-old to 11-year-old age group found a vaccine efficacy of 91% with no observation of myocarditis or pericarditis up to 2 months after the second dose of the vaccine.[102] Similarly, clinical trials with the Moderna (mRNA-1273) vaccine conducted between December 9, 2020, and February 28, 2021, showed no cases of acute COVID-19 in adolescents aged 12 to 17 years 2 weeks after the second injection, whereas 4 cases were reported in the placebo group.[103] Although early booster studies only included children aged 16 to 17 years, a reduction in confirmed SARS-CoV-2 infections and severe illness was seen in those who received a booster dose of the Pfizer-BioNTech vaccine than those who did not.[104]

Table 2
SARS-CoV-2 vaccines available in the United States

Vaccine Name	Manufacturer	Vaccine Type	Reported Vaccine Efficacy in Children	Schedule	Approval for Children	Approval Dates
BNT162b2 (Comirnaty)	Pfizer-BioNTech	mRNA (Intramuscular)	1. 100% vaccine efficacy against confirmed COVID-19 in individuals aged 12–15 y[101] 2. 90.7% vaccine efficacy against confirmed COVID-19 in individuals aged 5–11 y[102]	1. 2-dose primary series separated by 21 d 2. 1 additional primary dose in immunocompromised persons[a] (≥28 d since 2nd dose) 3. Booster dose ≥5 mo after last dose in primary series	1. FDA approved for individuals ≥16 y 2. FDA EUA for individuals 5–15 y 3. Booster dose approval for individuals aged ≥12 y 4. Third primary series dose for certain immunocompromised children ≥5 y	1. December 11, 2020: FDA EUA for individuals ≥16 y[92] 2. May 10, 2021: FDA EUA for individuals 12–15 y[94] 3. August 12, 2021: FDA EUA for third primary dose for certain immunocompromised individuals[a],[257] 4. August 23, 2021: FDA approved for individuals ≥16 y[93] 5. September 22, 2021: FDA updated EUA to allow for single booster dose for high-risk populations[b] aged ≥18 y administered at least 6 mo after completion of primary series[258] 6. October 20, 2021: FDA updated EUA to allow for heterologous booster dose in eligible individuals

(continued on next page)

Table 2
(continued)

Vaccine Name	Manufacturer	Vaccine Type	Reported Vaccine Efficacy in Children	Schedule	Approval for Children	Approval Dates
						7. October 29, 2021: FDA EUA for individuals 5–11 y[95]
						8. November 19, 2021: FDA updated EUA to allow for single booster dose for all individuals aged ≥18 y[259]
						9. December 9, 2021: FDA updated EUA to allow for single booster dose in individuals aged 16–17 y[96]
						10. January 3, 2022: FDA updated EUA to expand use of booster dose in individuals aged 12–15 y; shorten time interval for booster dose to ≥5 mo and allow for third primary series dose for certain immunocompromised children aged 5–11 y[97]
mRNA-1273	Moderna	mRNA (Intramuscular)	Vaccine efficacy against COVID-19 in adolescents aged 12–17 y showed 100%	1. 2-dose primary series separated by 28 d 2. 1 additional	Not approved by FDA for children	1. December 18, 2020: FDA EUA for individuals ≥18 y[260]

efficacy 14 d after second primary dose, although not statistically significant given low incidence of infection (4 cases in placebo group and none in vaccine arm)[103]

primary dose in immunocompromised persons[a] (≥28 d since 2nd dose)
3. Booster dose ≥5 mo after last dose in primary series

2. August 12, 2021: FDA EUA for third primary dose for certain immunocompromised individuals[a,260]
3. October 20, 2021: FDA updated EUA to allow for booster dose for high-risk populations[b] aged ≥18 y administered at least 6 mo after completion of primary series, including the use of a heterologous booster dose in eligible individuals[260]
4. November 19, 2021: FDA updated EUA to allow for single booster dose for all individuals aged ≥18 y[260]
5. January 7, 2022: FDA updated EUA to shorten interval between completion of primary vaccine series to booster to ≥5 mo for all individuals ≥18 y[261]

| Ad26.COV2.S | Janssen/ Johnson & Johnson | Viral vector (Intramuscular) | Data not available | 1. Single primary dose 2. Booster dose ≥2 mo after primary dose | Not approved by FDA for children | 1. February 27, 2021: FDA EUA for individuals ≥18 y[262] 2. October 20, 2021: FDA updated EUA to allow for a single booster dose |

(continued on next page)

Table 2
(continued)

Vaccine Name	Manufacturer	Vaccine Type	Reported Vaccine Efficacy in Children	Schedule	Approval for Children	Approval Dates
						at least 2 mo after completion of the single-dose primary series for all individuals aged ≥18 y and allows for the use of a heterologous booster dose in eligible individuals[262]
						3. December 16, 2021: CDC ACIP recommendations updated, preferring approved mRNA vaccines over Janssen vaccine for primary and booster vaccinations[263]

Abbreviations: ACIP, Advisory Committee on Immunization Practices; CDC, Centers for Disease Control and Prevention; COVID-19, coronavirus disease 2019; EUA, emergency use authorization; FDA, Food and Drug Administration; mRNA, messenger RNA.

a Moderately to severely immunocompromised persons may include (not limited to) individuals undergoing active treatment for solid tumor and hematologic malignancies, receiving a solid organ transplant and taking immunosuppressive therapy, receiving chimeric antigen receptor T-cell or hematopoietic cell transplant; individuals who have moderate or severe primary immunodeficiency, advanced or untreated human immunodeficiency virus infection, receiving active treatment with high-dose corticosteroids, alkylating agents, antimetabolites, transplant-related immunosuppressive drugs, cancer chemotherapeutics agents classified as severely immunosuppressive, tumor necrosis factor blockers, and other immunosuppressive or immunomodulatory biologic agents.

b High-risk populations include individuals 65 y and older; individuals 18 to 64 y with an underlying medical condition putting them at high risk for severe COVID-19, and individuals 18 to 64 y with frequent institutional or occupational exposure to SARS-CoV-2 putting them at risk for serious complications of COVID-19, including severe COVID-19. Interim updated CDC list of high-risk underlying conditions include but are not limited to asthma, cancer, cerebrovascular disease, chronic kidney disease, certain types of chronic lung diseases, certain types of chronic liver disease, cystic fibrosis, diabetes mellitus (type 1 and type 2), Down syndrome, heart conditions, human immunodeficiency virus, hypertension, immune deficiencies, certain mental health disorders (ie, mood disorders, schizophrenia spectrum disorders), obesity (body mass index [BMI] ≥30 kg/m²) and overweight (BMI ≥25 kg/m² but < 30 kg/m²), pregnancy and recent pregnancy, sickle cell disease, smoking (current and former), solid organ or blood stem cell transplantation, substance use disorders, thalassemia, tuberculosis, and use of corticosteroids or other immunosuppressive medications (an ongoing updated list of high-risk underlying conditions can be found on the CDC Web site)[141].

Vaccine effectiveness (VE) studies have been integral in understanding the effectiveness of vaccines in real-world settings at various stages of the pandemic. In one VE study in adolescents aged 12 to 18 years from June to September 2021 when the Delta variant was the predominant virus, the Pfizer-BioNTech vaccine was found to have a VE of 93% against COVID-19 hospitalizations.[105] Another VE study of the Pfizer-BioNTech vaccine in adolescents aged 12 to 17 years from July to December 2021 (when the Delta variant was widespread but before the predominance of the Omicron variant), VE against SARS-CoV-2 infection was 92%.[106] In a population-based study of SARS-CoV-2 infection, incidence rates also occurring during the Delta variant wave, the incidence rate ratio of laboratory-confirmed SARS-CoV-2 infections was 8.9 comparing unvaccinated with vaccinated adolescents aged 12 to 17 years.[107] Furthermore, early data show the protective effects of SARS-CoV-2 vaccination against MIS-C with a lower incidence with vaccination[108] and an estimated VE of 91% in adolescents 12 to 18 years who had completed a primary vaccine series with the Pfizer-BioNTech vaccine.[109] Despite vaccine availability and effectiveness, the percentage of vaccinated eligible children was less than 65% as of December 30, 2021, with fewer than 15% of children aged 5 to 11 years full vaccinated.[110] In some situations, there may be discordance in vaccine hesitancy between parents and guardians and their children. There remains regional variability of minor consent laws in which minors are allowed to consent to medical interventions that include vaccines.[111]

Overall, SARS-CoV-2 vaccines have had a favorable safety profile among children aged 5 to 17 years.[100,101,112] Most vaccine reactions to the Pfizer-BioNTech vaccine reported were local or mild systemic reactions,[112,113] with the exception of a small group of individuals, overwhelmingly male adolescents and younger adults, who reported self-limited cases of myocarditis and pericarditis.[114] In a nationwide study, the Pfizer-BioNTech vaccine was associated with an excess risk of 1 to 5 events per 100,000 vaccinated persons of all ages compared with the excess risk of 11.0 events per 100,000 persons after SARS-CoV-2 infection.[115] Myocarditis after SARS-CoV-2 vaccination was more common in younger age groups, whereas pericarditis was more common in older individuals, with onset generally within 3 days of vaccination.[116,117] Among individuals younger than 30 years with data reported to the Vaccine Adverse Event Reporting System, cases of myocarditis, pericarditis, and myopericarditis after SARS-CoV-2 vaccines occurred in individuals with a median age of 19 years (range: 12–29 years) with 96% hospitalized and no deaths.[118] Given the severe outcomes of SARS-CoV-2 infection including myocarditis,[119] the ACIP concluded that the benefits of vaccination outweighed the risk posed by these rare adverse events.

CLINICAL COURSE AND MANIFESTATIONS OF ACUTE CORONAVIRUS DISEASE 2019 IN CHILDREN

The clinical picture and severity of SARS-CoV-2 infection in children of all ages can vary from no symptoms to critical illness. When symptoms develop, most children will experience respiratory tract symptoms or an exacerbation of underlying conditions. Children with COVID-19 not requiring hospitalization have more subclinical, asymptomatic infection, and upper respiratory tract symptoms than adults.[8,120] One systematic review of early studies on pediatric COVID-19 found that 2% of SARS-CoV-2 infections in children were categorized as severe, whereas 0.6% had critical COVID-19,[121] although the spread of variants and increased exposure to SARS-CoV-2 may lead to increased numbers of infection and severe presentations of disease.

As in adults, the incubation period likely ranges from 2 to 14 days (mean, 6 days).[122,123] Illness duration is estimated to be a median of 6 days, but prolonged illness greater than 28 days can occur.[124] Overall, symptom duration is shorter in younger children.[124] Symptoms vary by age group (**Table 3**) and study type. In an early surveillance report of pediatric COVID-19, fever and cough were the most commonly reported symptoms, with headache a common symptom in older children.[9] In a longitudinal cohort study of infected school-aged children, headache and fatigue were the most common symptoms identified, with sore throat, altered taste or smell, and fever also frequently reported.[124] Neonates and infants may experience nonspecific symptoms, such as feeding difficulty with fever, so COVID-19 should be considered in the workup for infectious etiologies.[125] The presence of gastrointestinal (GI) symptoms, such as abdominal pain, nausea, vomiting, and diarrhea, are also common in pediatric acute COVID-19. Altered taste or smell is more commonly reported in older age groups.[9,124]

The National Institutes of Health (NIH) developed COVID-19 severity categories to unify treatment recommendations: asymptomatic or presymptomatic, mild, moderate, severe, and critical acute COVID-19 (**Table 4**).[126] Given these definitions are

Table 3
Symptom frequency in pediatric patients with acute COVID-19

Symptoms	CDC Surveillance Report - United States[9]			Longitudinal Cohort of School-Aged Children - UK[124]		
		Age Group			Age Group	
	Overall	0–9 y	10–19 y	Overall	5–11 y	12–17 y
	%	%	%	%	%	%
Cough	40	37	41	26	25	26
Fever	38	46	35	38	44	35
Headache	34	15	42	62	55	66
Sore throat	24	13	29	46	36	51
Myalgias	24	10	30	16	9	20
Diarrhea	14	14	14	7	8	7
Shortness of breath	13	7	16	10	4	12
Nausea	10	10	10	17	16	17
Runny nose	8	7	8	—	—	—
Change in sense of taste or smell	7	1	10	40	22	48
Abdominal pain	7	7	8	21	28	17
Fatigue	—	—	—	55	44	61
Dizziness	—	—	—	22	14	26
Anorexia	—	—	—	22	20	22
Eye soreness	—	—	—	19	15	22
Voice change	—	—	—	13	11	14
Chest pain	—	—	—	10	6	12
Confusion	—	—	—	6	3	7
Red welts	—	—	—	3	3	3
Blisters	—	—	—	2	1	2

Abbreviations: CDC, Centers for Disease Control and Prevention; COVID-19, coronavirus disease 2019.

Table 4
Definitions of acute COVID-19 severity and available treatment

Severity of COVID-19	General Definition	Pediatric Considerations	Treatment Recommendations	
Asymptomatic infection	An individual who tests positive for SARS-CoV-2 but does not exhibit any symptoms over the course of the infection.	Diagnosis of asymptomatic or presymptomatic SARS-CoV-2 infections in infants and toddlers are reliant on clinical history gathering and specific questions to the child's caregiver. Symptoms may be subtle and difficult to ascertain in the nonverbal child.	Supportive care and ensuring caregivers and close contacts take appropriate precautions including encouraging SARS-CoV-2 vaccine uptake, if eligible. SARS-CoV-2–directed therapies should be used only in the context of a clinical trial.	Monoclonal antibodies are available by EUA to individuals ≥12 y and ≥40 kg who are at risk for severe disease,[a] but preferably be used in the context of a clinical trial. The EUA for bamlanivimab-etesevimab has been extended to children of all ages including hospitalized children from birth to 2 y of age; with the Omicron variant, sotrovimab is the only approved monoclonal antibody with maintained efficacy against the new virus and should be administered within 10 d of symptom onset.
Presymptomatic infection	An individual who tests positive for SARS-CoV-2 and does not exhibit symptoms at the time, but then develops symptoms later in the illness course.		Supportive care and ensuring caregivers and close contacts take appropriate precautions including encouraging SARS-CoV-2 vaccine uptake, if eligible. SARS-CoV-2–directed therapies should be used only in the context of a clinical trial; when symptoms develop, treatment provided based on level of severity.	
Mild	An individual who tests positive for SARS-CoV-2 and has signs or symptoms consistent with COVID-19, which may include fever, cough, sore throat, malaise, headache, muscle pain, nausea, vomiting, diarrhea, or change in sense of taste or smell. These individuals have no evidence of lower respiratory tract disease, including no shortness of breath, dyspnea, or abnormal chest imaging.	Children, particularly younger age groups, may also have nonspecific symptoms of feeding refusal, fussiness, runny nose, or nasal congestion.	Supportive care and ensuring caregivers and close contacts take appropriate precautions, including encouraging SARS-CoV-2 vaccine uptake, if eligible. Remdesivir and other therapies, including nirmatrelvir/ritonavir, should be used only in the context of a clinical trial; if remdesivir is used in an outpatient setting, this would be an off-label indication; molnupiravir is not approved for use in children, given concerns for interference with normal bone and cartilage development.	
Moderate	An individual who tests positive for SARS-CoV-2 and has signs or symptoms consistent with	In young children, a weak cry, grunting, tracheal tugging, nasal flaring, head bobbing,	Supportive care and ensuring caregivers and close contacts take appropriate precautions,	

(continued on next page)

Table 4
(continued)

Severity of COVID-19	General Definition	Pediatric Considerations	Treatment Recommendations
	lower respiratory tract disease, including shortness of breath or dyspnea or abnormal chest imaging. These individuals have normal baseline oxygen saturation typically ≥94% on room air.	and sternal or intercostal retractions are additional indicators of respiratory distress, and may also suggest a lower respiratory tract infection.	including encouraging SARS-CoV-2 vaccine uptake, if eligible. Remdesivir and other therapies including nirmatrelvir/ritonavir should be used only in the context of a clinical trial; if remdesivir is used in an outpatient setting, this would be an off-label indication; molnupiravir is not approved for use in children given concerns for interference with normal bone and cartilage development.
Severe	An individual who tests positive for SARS-CoV-2 and has oxygen saturation <94% or below baseline, ratio of arterial partial pressure of oxygen to fraction of inspired oxygen (Pao_2/Fio_2) <300 mm Hg, respiratory rate > 30 breaths/min, or lung infiltrates >50%.	Radiographic abnormalities may be common in children and findings should be considered in the context of other symptoms, including hypoxemia. Normal respiratory rate by age group[264]. Newborn 40–60 breaths/min <1 y 24–38 breaths/min 1–3 y 22–30 breaths/min 4–6 y 20–24 breaths/min 7–9 y 18–24 breaths/min 10–14 y 16–22 breaths/min 14–18 y 14–20 breaths/min	1. Caregivers and close contacts take appropriate precautions including encouraging SARS-CoV-2 vaccine uptake, if eligible. 2. Remdesivir can be used as an antiviral in those with severe or critical acute COVID-19 weighing at least 3.5 kg. A multicenter pediatric COVID-19 guideline committee suggests using respiratory support requirement as the indicator for its use.[177] 3. Dexamethasone[b] can be considered in critical disease, particularly in older age groups. 4. Interleukin-6 (eg, tocilizumab) or interleukin-1 (eg, anakinra) inhibitors can be considered in critical disease, preferably in the setting of a clinical trial.
Critical	An individual who tests positive for SARS-CoV-2 and develops respiratory failure, septic shock or organ dysfunction.	Careful consideration should be made to distinguish cases of critical COVID-19 and multisystem inflammatory syndrome in children (MIS-C). See **Table 5**.	

Abbreviations: COVID-19, coronavirus disease 2019; EUA, emergency use authorization; SARS-CoV-2, severe acute respiratory syndrome coronavirus 2.

a Risk factors based on the consensus by a multicenter panel of pediatric providers include children with medical complexity, young age less than 1 y, older age greater than 12 y, immunocompromised state, underlying severe cardiac or pulmonary disease, obesity, and diabetes.[177]

extrapolated to pediatric infections, normal vital signs and symptoms will differ by age. The diagnosis of asymptomatic or presymptomatic infection in younger children will rely on clinical history provided by the caregiver and findings on physical examination. Minimally symptomatic children will require careful assessment of vital signs and physical examination to ensure appropriate counseling is given. Weak cry, grunting, retractions, nasal flaring, and head bobbing may also be indicators of respiratory distress, and acute COVID-19 should be suspected in younger children, especially in the absence of alternative explanation. Rapid clinical deterioration with abrupt changes in respiratory status may occur a week into the illness course.[127] In children with critical illness, careful consideration should be given in distinguishing cases of acute COVID-19, MIS-C, and other diseases as evaluation and management may differ.

There remains a paucity of data on risk factors associated with severe outcomes of pediatric acute COVID-19. Data extrapolated from adult reports and observational studies highlight several chronic diseases in children that increase risk for infection, hospitalization, admission to the intensive care unit (ICU) and death.[128–132] In a study of hospitalized children younger than 18 years with COVID-19 when the Delta variant was widespread, 67.5% had one or more underlying medical conditions.[133] In another study of individuals younger than 21 years, at least one underlying medical condition was associated with 75% of SARS-CoV-2.[129] There does not appear to be a significant risk of severe disease associated with male gender, as there is in adults.[134] Some studies suggest that younger children (infants aged <1 year) did not have increased risk for severe disease[131] although early reports showed higher proportions of severe and critical illness in the younger age groups.[1,132] In a cross-sectional study of children with acute COVID-19, risk of hospitalization or severe COVID-19 was highest in those with obesity, sleeping disorders, diabetes (type 1 or type 2), congenital heart disease, neurodevelopmental disorders, psychiatric illness, hypertension and seizure disorders.[135] Among children aged 12 to 18 years, those with asthma were at increased risk for severe illness.[135] Other possible conditions at risk for severe outcomes in children include complex medical conditions,[135] genetic disorders such as trisomy 21,[136] sickle cell disease,[137] congenital heart disease[138] and immunosuppression.[139,140] However, few published reports of pediatric patients with these conditions are available, making statistical inferences challenging. Experience with other viral infections suggest that individuals with these chronic conditions should be treated as having a higher risk of severe disease. The CDC maintains a list of underlying medical conditions with higher risk of severe COVID-19 reported in the literature, although this list is not specific to pediatric patients.[141] Although uncommon, newborns are also at risk for SARS-CoV-2 infection with the highest risk when the mother or other caregiver has COVID-19 onset around delivery. With proper precautions, mothers and newborns may room safely together.[142,143] In addition, there has been little evidence to suggest transmission via breast milk, and breastfeeding is encouraged for those who are interested.[143]

SARS-CoV-2 infection commonly results in respiratory tract illness with extrapulmonary manifestations documented in case reports or case series in children. A variety of neurologic complications associated with pediatric acute COVID-19 has been described, including encephalopathy, seizures, encephalitis, Guillain-Barre Syndrome, acute demyelinating syndromes, movement disorders, and psychiatric disorders.[144] Acute COVID-19 in children can also be complicated by cardiovascular events, including myocarditis,[145,146] pericarditis,[147,148] pulmonary embolic events,[149] arrhythmias,[150] and acute myocardial infarction.[151] So-called "COVID toes," or pseudo-chilblains, caused by inflammation of small blood vessels leading to painful sores can also be seen in pediatric acute COVID-19.[152,153] GI[154–156] and renal[157] complications have also been described. Invasive mold infections (eg, pulmonary aspergillosis and mucormycosis) are increasingly recognized complications of severe COVID-19 in adults,[158] although rarely reported in children.[159] There remains little information on COVID-19–associated fungal infections in children, possibly owing to fewer cases of severe COVID-19.

LABORATORY AND IMAGING FINDINGS

Diagnosis of SARS-CoV-2 infection requires laboratory confirmation. Suspected cases may be identified based on characteristic symptoms and exposure to an individual with laboratory-confirmed SARS-CoV-2 infection. Adult acute COVID-19 has been associated with characteristic laboratory abnormalities, including lymphopenia in early disease, elevated inflammatory markers, and findings of a hypercoagulable state[160] that have been used to predict severe disease. In pediatric acute COVID-19, laboratory findings have been more variable, differ by age, and are less predictive of severe disease.[140,161] In addition to lymphopenia and hypercoagulability, markers of inflammation in children may be abnormal, including D-dimer, lactate dehydrogenase, fibrinogen, ferritin, procalcitonin, interleukin (IL)-6, C-reactive protein (CRP), aspartate aminotransferase, alanine aminotransferase, and erythrocyte sedimentation rate.[160,162,163] Elevations of creatine kinase, pro B-type natriuretic peptide, and troponin can be seen in those with end-organ disease.[162] Significantly elevated inflammatory markers with cardiovascular involvement should also prompt clinical consideration of an MIS-C diagnosis. Chest radiographic findings including characteristic multifocal ground glass opacities and pulmonary consolidations may be the most common imaging abnormalities in pediatric acute COVID-19.[164,165] Children may have abnormalities of chest imaging even with asymptomatic and presymptomatic infection.[165] Except in cases of severe disease or workup of alternative conditions, computed tomography is unlikely to provide additional clinical information when a diagnosis of acute COVID-19 is already known.

CLINICAL MANAGEMENT CONSIDERATIONS AND CORONAVIRUS DISEASE 2019 THERAPEUTICS

Management of symptomatic acute COVID-19 depends on the severity of the illness (see **Table 4**), and special consideration should be given to the evolution of SARS-CoV-2 variants, including the appearance of the Omicron variant, as they alter the landscape of effective monoclonal antibodies and available therapeutics.[166] Most children will not require specific therapy, especially with milder disease. Children with underlying medical conditions may be at greater risk for severe outcomes, thus close follow-up and baseline control of chronic illnesses may help mitigate the effects of infections. The mainstay of management in children with mild to moderate acute COVID-19 is supportive care, although cases of poor feeding or dehydration may prompt admission to the hospital for nutritional resuscitation. Children whose symptoms worsen may require higher levels of care because of progression of disease, end-organ complications, and coinfections. If new or worsening symptoms evolve, workup should be pursued to identify the etiology of the clinical change. During the pandemic, the use of antibiotics has exceeded the estimated prevalence of bacterial coinfections, leading to overuse in cases of COVID-19.[167] Continuation of antibiotics should be guided by culture results and risk factors, and generally reserved for severe or critical COVID-19 with presumed or confirmed bacterial coinfection. Acute COVID-

19 can lead to a hypercoagulable state; the use of thromboprophylaxis should be considered based on individual risk factors for coagulopathy.

Monoclonal antibodies have been used for risk reduction of severe disease in adults, in those with predisposing factors, but some approved therapies have diminished effectiveness against novel variants, including the Omicron variant. Currently, bamlanivimab-etesevimab, casirivimab-imdevimab, and sotrovimab are the only therapies available through EUA for individuals aged ≥12 years and ≥40 kg who have mild to moderate acute COVID-19 at risk of severe COVID-19 and are not hospitalized for COVID-19 (see Jakharia and colleagues' article, "COVID-19 in the Immunocompromised Host, including People with HIV," in this issue). Bamlanivimab-etesevimab and casirivimab-imdevimab were authorized as postexposure prophylaxis for those exposed and at high risk of severe COVID-19. The EUA for bamlanivimab-etesevimab has also been extended to younger children (from birth and older), including those who are hospitalized between birth and 2 years of age for treatment of mild to moderate acute COVID-19, but circulating variants have limited their use.[168] Hospital admission thresholds may be lower for neonates and young children who develop mild to moderate COVID-19, hence the EUA extension of its use during hospitalization for this younger age group. There remain limited data regarding the use of monoclonal antibodies in children,[169] with pediatric experts recommending against its routine use in children, including those with risk factors for severe disease.[170]

Antiviral therapy has formed the basis for COVID-19 therapy early in the illness course. Remdesivir, a nucleoside analog and viral RNA polymerase inhibitor, has been available through EUA since May 1, 2020. On October 22, 2020, remdesivir became the first FDA-approved antiviral treatment for use in hospitalized individuals aged ≥12 years and weighing ≥40 kg with COVID-19.[171] It remains available under EUA to children weighing 3.5 kg to less than 40 kg or those younger than 12 years and weighing ≥3.5 kg.[171] The data to support the use of remdesivir in COVID-19 has been derived from clinical trials of adult COVID-19. A 5-day course of remdesivir was associated with a reduction in median time to recovery, but not mortality in severe COVID-19.[172–174] The NIH recommends remdesivir for children ≥12 years and weighing ≥40 kg with new or increasing oxygen requirement with risk factors for severe disease,[169] and allows for the off-label treatment of nonhospitalized children with mild to moderate COVID-19 at risk for severe disease within 7 days of symptom onset.[175] They also recommend remdesivir for children aged ≥16 years with acute COVID-19 and new or increasing oxygen requirement regardless of the presence of severe disease risk factors.[169] Although there are data to support early remdesivir to mitigate severe acute COVID-19 in outpatients with symptomatic SARS-CoV-2 infection,[176] a panel of pediatric experts recommends the use of remdesivir for mild to moderate acute COVID-19 only in the context of a clinical trial, and 5 days of remdesivir therapy in children with severe and critical acute COVID-19. Up to 10 days of remdesivir could be considered in critical acute COVID-19.[177] WHO has recommended against the use of remdesivir for children, citing a lack of important clinical differences in mortality and severe outcomes.[178] In general, remdesivir is well tolerated. Reports of sinus bradycardia associated with its use have been documented in pediatric cases of COVID-19,[179] which appears to self-resolve after drug discontinuation.

In December 2021, the FDA granted EUA to 2 additional antiviral agents for the treatment of mild to moderate acute COVID-19, which include molnupiravir,[180] a ribonucleoside analog, and nirmatrelvir/ritonavir (Paxlovid),[181] a novel combination protease inhibitor. Molnupiravir may be associated with abnormalities in bone and cartilage development in children and as such, only nirmatrelvir/ritonavir has been granted approval for use in pediatric patients aged ≥12 years of age and weight of ≥40 kg with SARS-CoV-2 infection and high risk for progression to severe disease within 5 days of symptom onset. Careful consideration should be given to its use, given the potential for drug-drug interactions.

Immune dysregulation likely contributes to the progression of severe disease, and various immunomodulators have been proposed as treatment to mitigate inflammatory effects. Trials show that glucocorticoids in adults, specifically dexamethasone, can reduce days of mechanical ventilation and mortality in those with severe or critical disease[182–184]; however, data in children are lacking.[185] The NIH recommends dexamethasone in patients requiring high-flow oxygenation, mechanical ventilation, or extracorporeal membrane oxygenation.[169] A panel of pediatric experts maintains that glucocorticoids be considered for critical disease preferentially in the context of a clinical trial, and should still be used in other non–COVID-19 conditions in which steroids are indicated (eg, asthma exacerbation).[186] Dexamethasone use, typically up to 10 days or until discharge,[185] may be of more importance in older children and adolescents who have immune system physiology similar to adults. Among other immunomodulators, including IL-6 inhibitors (eg, tocilizumab), IL-1 (eg, anakinra), and Janus kinase (JAK) inhibitors (eg, baracitinib) have shown some clinical benefit in adult COVID-19, but in children, these study data are also lacking. Guidance from a panel of pediatric experts encourage the use of IL-1 or IL-6 inhibitors in the setting of a clinical trial for the treatment of critical acute COVID-19, whereas they recommend against the use of JAK inhibitors except for in cases of a clinical trial,[186] despite their authorization for use in these younger age groups. Consultation with pediatric rheumatologists and infectious disease specialists may be helpful in stratifying patients benefiting most from these therapies when clinical trials are not available. Convalescent plasma has been used as an adjunctive therapy for many different viral infections, and the data supporting its use in COVID-19 is sparse. As such, NIH has recommended against its use generally in pediatric acute COVID-19 except in the setting of a clinical trial.[169]

Other antivirals and anti-inflammatory agents had been considered for COVID-19 treatment early in the pandemic, including hydroxychloroquine, lopinavir-ritonavir, and ivermectin. No data support the use of these medications for pediatric (or adult) acute COVID-19 of any severity. Treatment guidelines have routinely recommended against their use given the lack of efficacy in reducing severe outcomes.[169,177,178]

MULTISYSTEM INFLAMMATORY SYNDROME IN CHILDREN ASSOCIATED WITH SEVERE ACUTE RESPIRATORY SYNDROME CORONAVIRUS 2 INFECTION

MIS-C is a systemic hyperinflammatory condition seen after SARS-CoV-2 infection. It is one of the most dramatic manifestations associated with COVID-19 in which multiple organ systems are affected; shock can sometimes occur, prompting ICU admission.[187] In April 2020, European clinicians reported unusual clusters of pediatric patients admitted to the hospital with hyperinflammation[188] and clinical features resembling Kawasaki disease (KD),[189] toxic shock syndrome,[190] and myocarditis.[191] Many patients were previously healthy, with symptoms appearing 2 to 6 weeks after the first wave of COVID-19 in Europe. Although few patients tested positive by SARS-CoV-2 polymerase chain reaction (PCR), most cases had antibody evidence of prior infection.[187,192,193] US cases were soon reported in New York after the first surge of SARS-CoV-2 infections.[192] Initially called the pediatric inflammatory multisystem syndrome temporally associated with SARS-CoV-2 (PIMS-TS),[194,195] a new case definition and new name, MIS-C, was published by the CDC.[196] The name change was made to allow for cases in adults that have now been described.[197–200]

Several epidemiologic case definitions are published for MIS-C (**Table 5**) each requiring clinical, virologic, and inflammatory marker data.[194,196,201] Of note, the CDC case definition specifically requires severe illness and hospitalization highlighting an important distinction between the definitions. Although a clinically significant condition, MIS-C is thought to be rare. Early estimates in New York State showed that although laboratory-confirmed SARS-CoV-2 infection in people younger than 21 years old was 322 per 100,000 individuals, the number of MIS-C cases over the same time-frame was 2 per 100,000 individuals.[192] Using surveillance data from US jurisdictions reporting MIS-C cases, the incidence between April and June 2020 was estimated to be 5.1 persons per 1,000,000 person-months, with 316 MIS-C cases per 1,000,000 SARS-CoV-2 infections.[202] Few MIS-C cases were reported in China and other countries in eastern Asia early in the pandemic with possible explanations including differences in SARS-CoV-2 burden, changes in the virus, or the implementation of different public health interventions.[203] Cases of MIS-C have now been reported in these regions.

Despite efforts to uncover the underlying mechanism of disease, the pathophysiologic cause of the syndrome is not fully understood.[203] Hypotheses based on associations with KD, a form of childhood vasculitis that shares clinical features with MIS-C, and the clinical course after acute COVID-19, suggests an immune-mediated process possibly driven by auto-antibody activity.[204] Immune profiling in those with KD, acute COVID-19, and MIS-C show differences in cellular subtypes and inflammatory protein composition that distinguish the 3 different diagnoses.[204] Antibody profiling also showed evidence of possible cardiac-specific auto-recognition, suggesting a mechanism for the cardiovascular and coronary damage characteristic of both MIS-C and KD.[204] Additional research will be needed to further stratify the immune differences between these 2 conditions and to identify the mechanisms that may provide clues to future therapies.

Children with MIS-C tend to be older and more racially and ethnically diverse than those with KD.[205,206] One US population-based study of MIS-C found the median age of children with MIS-C to be 9 years,[207] with children as young as less than 1 month old reported in the literature.[192,205] Whether race is an important risk factor in developing MIS-C after acute COVID-19 is still being investigated. Early studies showed a disproportionate risk of MIS-C in communities of color,[190,207] initially considered a reflection of disparities seen in acute SARS-CoV-2 infection.[208,209] However, more recent studies comparing MIS-C and COVID-19 showed an unexplained independent risk of MIS-C that continues to exist for those of Hispanic ethnicity or Black race.[210,211] Children affected by MIS-C tend to have fewer underlying medical conditions, with obesity a common diagnosis if chronic conditions were present.[192,207] Although MIS-C case definitions allow for the use of SARS-CoV-2 PCR, antibodies, antigen, or exposure as virologic confirmation, most children will have evidence of prior infection via SARS-CoV-2 antibodies.[207] As more children are vaccinated, use of anti-SARS-CoV-2 antibody tests other than spike protein antibodies will be required to differentiate between immunity from prior infection and vaccination. In the absence of SARS-CoV-2 testing, exposure to an individual with diagnosed COVID-19 or COVID-19–compatible symptoms also satisfy case definition requirements.

Clinical features of MIS-C vary by case and by age group.[192] All current MIS-C case definitions require fever during the illness as part of the diagnosis. Fever may be subjective or measured ($\geq$38°C), and is commonly persistent, lasting approximately 6 days in most children.[193] Many children will present to the hospital still febrile.[192] Other common symptoms at hospital presentation include GI symptoms (eg, abdominal pain, diarrhea, nausea, and vomiting), headache and neck pain, lymphadenopathy, myalgias, fatigue, sore throat, and mucocutaneous findings (eg, rash, red tongue, cracked lips and conjunctivitis).[192,212–214] Severe GI complications (eg, adenomesenteritis, appendicitis, abdominal fluid collections, pancreatitis, and intussusception) were frequently diagnosed in children with acute COVID-19 and MIS-C.[213] Chest pain and symptoms of myocarditis are more common in older children and adolescents.[192] Patients with MIS-C may have respiratory symptoms such as cough and shortness of breath, but these are more common in patients with acute COVID-19.[207] At hospital admission, vital signs seen in patients with MIS-C include fever, tachycardia, and tachypnea, typically without hypoxemia.[192] Symptoms of shock, including hypotension, were seen in approximately one-third of the cases described in New York State.[192] Subsets of patients may fulfill criteria for the diagnosis of KD, particularly those in the younger age groups.[192]

Laboratory findings show evidence of severe systemic inflammation. Complete blood count results can include neutrophilia, lymphopenia, anemia, and thrombocytopenia.[192,193,212] Inflammatory markers are broadly elevated, which generally include CRP, erythrocyte sedimentation rate, fibrinogen, ferritin, D-dimer, lactate dehydrogenase, procalcitonin, alanine aminotransferase, and IL-6 levels.[192,193] Other laboratory abnormalities, such as hypoalbuminemia, hyponatremia, and prolonged international normalized ratio, may be present.[192,193] Evidence of cardiovascular injury with elevated troponin, brain natriuretic peptide (BNP), or N-terminal proBNP is also common.[192] Specific level cutoffs and the predictive ability of individual tests for MIS-C diagnosis have not been established, although one observational study found that patients with MIS-C may have lower absolute counts of lymphocytes and platelets as well as greater CRP concentrations than children without MIS-C who are evaluated for outpatient febrile illness.[215] MIS-C is frequently associated with echocardiographic findings, including evidence of ventricular dysfunction with depressed ejection fraction, pericardial effusion, valvular dysfunction, and coronary artery dilatation or aneurysms.[192,216] Given the prominent GI symptoms at presentation, children with MIS-C may also undergo abdominal imaging to rule out other etiologies, including appendicitis. Common abnormal findings seen on abdominal ultrasonography or CT include liver and spleen enlargement, mesenteric adenopathy, trace ascitic or pelvic fluid, and inflammation of the intestines and appendix with bowel-wall thickening and fluid-filled bowel loops.[192] In children who receive chest radiography, evidence of pulmonary opacities or infiltrates may be present.[217] The hospital course for children with MIS-C may include admission to the ICU for close clinical monitoring, vasopressor support, and less frequently mechanical ventilation.[192,193] Extracorporeal membrane oxygenation may be required in a small number of patients.[192,193] Despite the morbidity associated at hospital presentation, children with MIS-C are often discharged within a week of admission,[192] mortality remains low,[207] and long-term outcomes, including functional outcomes, have been minimal[218] with resolution of most cardiac findings at subsequent follow-up visits.[219] Among those with persistent cardiovascular abnormalities, aneurysmal changes were seen in one group of children followed longitudinally.[219] Whether MIS-C can reoccur in children who experience reinfection is unknown; however, one published case study showed no reoccurrence of MIS-C with subsequent SARS-CoV-2 infection.[77]

The American College of Rheumatology, American Academy of Pediatrics, and the PIMS-TS National Consensus Management Study Group have provided a tiered guidance approach for the workup and management of MIS-C (**Table 6**).[220–222] Cases of MIS-C likely constitute a spectrum of disease with mild cases less frequently represented in the literature. Children with evidence of critical illness require workup for alternative diagnoses including, but not limited to, acute COVID-19, acute non-

Table 5
Case definitions of MIS-C

Institution	US Centers for Disease Control and Prevention[196]	World Health Organization[201]	Royal College of Pediatrics and Child Health[194]
Age group	An individual aged <21 y presenting with the following:	Children and adolescents 0–19 y of age with the following:	A child presenting with the following:
Fever	fever ≥38.0°C for ≥24 h, or report of subjective fever lasting ≥24 h AND	fever ≥3 d AND	persistent fever >38.5°C AND
Inflammation	Laboratory evidence of inflammation including, but not limited to, 1 or more of the following: elevated C-reactive protein (CRP), erythrocyte sedimentation rate (ESR), fibrinogen, procalcitonin, D-dimer, ferritin, lactic acid dehydrogenase (LDH), or interleukin 6 (IL-6), elevated neutrophils, reduced lymphocytes and low albumin AND	Elevated markers of inflammation such as ESR, CRP, or procalcitonin AND	Inflammation (neutrophilia, elevated CRP, and lymphopenia) AND
Severity of illness	Evidence of clinically severe illness requiring hospitalization AND		
Organ system involvement	With multisystem (≥2) organ involvement (cardiac, renal, respiratory, hematologic, gastrointestinal, dermatologic, or neurologic)	2 of the following: (1) Rash or bilateral nonpurulent conjunctivitis or muco-cutaneous inflammation signs (oral, hands or feet). (2) Hypotension or shock. (3) Features of myocardial dysfunction, pericarditis, valvulitis, or coronary abnormalities (including echocardiogram findings or elevated troponin/NT-proBNP. (4) Evidence of	Evidence of single or multi-organ dysfunction (shock, cardiac, respiratory, renal gastrointestinal or neurologic disorder)

(continued on next page)

Table 5
(continued)

Institution	US Centers for Disease Control and Prevention[196]	World Health Organization[201]	Royal College of Pediatrics and Child Health[194]
	AND	coagulopathy (by PT, PTT, elevated d-Dimers). (5) Acute gastrointestinal problems (diarrhea, vomiting, or abdominal pain). AND	AND with additional features[a] AND
Alternative explanations	No alternative for plausible diagnoses AND	No other obvious microbial cause of inflammation, including the following: Bacterial sepsis Staphylococcal or streptococcal shock syndromes AND	Exclusion of any other microbial cause including the following: Bacterial sepsis Staphylococcal or streptococcal shock syndromes Infections associated with myocarditis (such as enterovirus) AND
Virologic testing	Positive for current or recent SARS-CoV-2 infection by RT-PCR, serology, or antigen test; or exposure to a suspected or confirmed COVID-19 case within the 4 wk before the onset of symptoms	Evidence of COVID-19 (RT-PCR, antigen test or serology positive), or likely contact with patients with COVID-19	SARS-CoV-2 PCR testing may be positive or negative
Additional comments	Some individuals may fulfill full or partial criteria for Kawasaki disease but should be reported if they meet the case definition for MIS-C Consider MIS-C in any pediatric death with evidence of SARS-CoV-2 infection		This may include children fulfilling full or partial criteria for Kawasaki disease

Abbreviations: COVID-19, coronavirus disease 2019; MIS-C, multisystem inflammatory syndrome in children; NT-proBNP, N-terminal pro brain natriuretic peptide; PT, prothrombin time; PTT, partial thromboplastin time; RT-PCR, reverse-transcriptase polymerase chain reaction; SARS-CoV-2, severe acute respiratory distress syndrome coronavirus 2.

a Additional features: abnormal fibrinogen, high D-dimer, high ferritin, hypoalbuminemia, acute kidney injury, anemia, coagulopathy, high interleukin (IL) 10,

SARS-CoV-2 infection, and KD. For children in whom MIS-C is considered, basic laboratory workup should be pursued. If there is evidence of inflammation, a broader scope of inflammatory markers should be obtained to help differentiate between MIS-C and other etiologies of inflammation. Chest and abdominal radiography can be considered, especially in the workup of other disease processes, but a diagnosis of MIS-C cannot be made based on these results alone. Given the prominence of cardiovascular findings, guidance extrapolated from the workup of KD has been recommended, which includes obtaining laboratory markers of cardiac injury (BNP and troponin), echocardiography, and electrocardiography. Treatment is also extrapolated from the management of KD; expert panelists note that not all patients will require immunomodulatory therapy. When therapy is considered, immunomodulators include intravenous immunoglobulin (IVIG) with or without glucocorticoids, as well as biologics are options. Biologics such as anakinra or infliximab are used if the patient's disease is refractory to the first-line therapies of IVIG and glucocorticoids. To date, there have been no clinical trial data available to guide the treatment of MIS-C. Observational data comparing IVIG with glucocorticoid and IVIG alone suggested that combined therapy was associated with fewer days of fever and may be associated with lower risk of new or persistent MIS-C–associated cardiovascular dysfunction.[223,224]

POST-ACUTE SEQUELAE OF CORONAVIRUS DISEASE 2019 IN CHILDREN

A picture of long-term symptoms experienced by children after SARS-CoV-2 infection is emerging. First recognized in adults, post-acute sequelae of COVID-19 (PASC) or "long COVID-19," is a constellation of persistent symptoms affecting different organ systems reported by patients recovering from all spectrums of acute COVID-19, including those with asymptomatic infection.[225,226] Currently, no formal definition or diagnostic criteria describes PASC, and individuals experiencing longer term symptoms likely represent a heterogeneous cohort. The prevalence of PASC is unknown, although a review of published reports show variability by study from 4% to 66%.[227] Among the few studies describing persistent symptoms in children, fatigue, persistent cough, difficulties with concentration, chest pain, heart palpitations, dyspnea, headache, dizziness, sore throat, and sleep disturbances were experienced up to 8 months after acute infection.[228–232] Short-term cognitive and psychiatric complications have also been observed in the aftermath of acute COVID-19, and whether these will persist in the long-term is not known.[233] Similar to adults, these symptoms may relapse and remit over the illness course. Information on the cause and optimal management of these patients is unknown and may require interdisciplinary rehabilitation[234] directed toward specific symptoms experienced by the individual. Long-term follow-up studies of children recovering from SARS-CoV-2 infection, including the UK CLoCK[235] and NIH RECOVER[236] studies, will be helpful to further characterize PASC in children.

OTHER HEALTH IMPACTS ON CHILDREN DURING THE CORONAVIRUS DISEASE 2019 PANDEMIC

In addition to the direct health effects of COVID-19, the pandemic has had adverse collateral health impacts on children due to the impacts of COVID-19 in adults, community-wide mitigation efforts, and school closures. Early in the pandemic, the number of primary care preventive and acute care visits decreased.[237] Changes in health-care–seeking behavior have led to decreased routine screening tests, such as blood lead level testing[238] and a decrease in childhood vaccination rates.[239] Delays in care have exacerbated health-related outcomes, including appendicitis,[240] asthma

Table 6
MIS-C workup and treatment

Pediatric Organization	American College of Rheumatology[220]	American Academy of Pediatrics[222]	PIMS-TS National Consensus Management Study Group[221]
	Children presenting with unremitting high fever, an epidemiologic link to SARS-CoV-2 and suggestive clinical symptoms of MIS-C	Persistent fever (≥3 d) without a clear clinical source accompanied by symptoms concerning in their severity or coincident with recent exposure to a person with COVID-19	Children presenting to the hospital with fever, abdominal pain, gastrointestinal, respiratory or neurologic symptoms who are stable
Laboratory studies	Tier 1: Complete blood cell count with differential, complete metabolic panel, ESR, CRP, and testing for SARS-CoV-2 (by PCR or serology); If ESR or CRP are elevated and at least 1 other laboratory feature: lymphopenia, neutrophilia, thrombocytopenia, hyponatremia, or hypoalbuminemia, then proceed to tier 2; Tier 2: includes cardiac assessment and markers of systemic inflammation, which may include D-dimer, ferritin, procalcitonin, LDH, cytokine panels (including IL-6, tumor necrosis factor, or IL-10), and Cardiac laboratory values: troponin, B-type natriuretic peptide; a peripheral blood smear for assessment of microangiopathic changes can be considered	Initial: Complete blood cell count with differential, urine analysis, ESR, and CRP Subsequent studies based on initial clinical suspicion or evidence of inflammation: Ferritin, LDH, comprehensive metabolic panel, proBNP, troponin, and fibrinogen In addition to the above, hospitalized children should also obtain triglycerides, creatinine kinase, amylase, blood and urine culture, D-dimer, prothrombin time/partial thromboplastin time, INR, SARS-CoV-2 PCR and SARS-CoV-2 serology (before the administration of IVIG) In severely ill-appearing or hemodynamically fragile patients, laboratory testing should be obtained regardless of duration of fever	Initial: Full blood count, CRP, urea, creatinine, electrolytes, and liver function Second line (done within 12 h of admission): blood gas and lactate, fibrinogen, ferritin, D-dimer, troponin, NT-proBNP, LDH, SARS-CoV-2 RT-PCR test, and SARS-CoV-2 serology, septic and viral screen (lumbar puncture only if specifically indicated)
Imaging	Echocardiogram; cardiac computed tomography should be considered in patients with suspected distal	Chest radiograph, consider echocardiogram and/or cardiac MRI	Done within 12 h of admission: chest radiograph; echocardiogram (daily in those who are physiologically

Other studies	coronary artery aneurysms not well visualized on echocardiogram	under consultation with pediatric cardiology	unstable)
	ECG every 48 h; telemetry in those with conduction abnormalities	ECG	Abdominal ultrasound to rule out alternative diagnoses
			ECG
Treatment	Depending on the severity of symptoms, in addition to supportive care, the following therapies are recommended: First tier: IVIG (2 g/kg) should be given to patients with MIS-C who are hospitalized and/or fulfill KD criteria; Adjunctive: low to moderate dose steroids can be considered in children with milder forms of MIS-C who are persistently febrile and symptomatic despite IVIG; low to moderate dose glucocorticoids should be used with IVIG in those with severe or refractory disease; high and pulse dose glucocorticoids can be considered in those who do not respond to IVIG and low to moderate dose glucocorticoids Refractory disease: Anakinra (>4 mg/kg per d) can be considered in those refractory to IVIG and glucocorticoids. Low-dose aspirin (3–5 mg/kg per d) should be used until normalization of platelet count and normal coronary arteries at ≥4 wk after	IVIG (2 g/kg with max of 100 g) In patients who do not improve either clinically or by laboratory values, additional treatment can include steroid therapy (2–30 mg/kg per d of methylprednisolone depending on illness severity) and biologics (anakinra, 2–10 mg/kg per d, subcutaneously or intravenously, divided every 6–12 h) All patients with MIS-C should be started on low-dose aspirin (except for those with platelets < 100,000 or active bleeding)	Continue treatment for presumed sepsis until microbiological cultures are available and preferred enrollment in a clinical trial for additional therapies; in the absence of a clinical trial, then the following was recommended: Children with KD-like phenotype (fulfills complete or incomplete KD criteria): First line: IVIG (2 g/kg single or divided dose) is recommended and a second dose can be considered for children who partially responded or have not responded at all to the first dose; Second line: methylprednisolone is recommended (10–30 mg/kg per d for 3 d) 24 h after IVIG if child remains unwell; given at the same time as IVIG in high-risk children (eg, age <12 mo and those with coronary artery changes) Third line: biological therapy is recommended with infliximab as biological therapy of choice for KD-like phenotype Children with nonspecific

(continued on next page)

Table 6
(continued)

Pediatric Organization	American College of Rheumatology[220]	American Academy of Pediatrics[222]	PIMS-TS National Consensus Management Study Group[221]
	diagnosis (except in those with active bleeding, risk of bleeding, or platelet count ≤80,000/µL) Patients with MIS-C with coronary artery aneurysm with z-score ≥10 should be treated with low-dose aspirin and therapeutic anticoagulation with enoxaparin or warfarin		presentation and evidence of coronary artery abnormality, meeting criteria for toxic shock syndrome, evidence of progressive disease or extended duration of fever >5 d: First line: IVIG (2 g/kg single or divided dose) is recommended and a second dose can be considered for children who partially responded or have not responded at all to the first dose; Second line: methylprednisolone is recommended (10–30 mg/kg per d for 3 d) Third line: biological therapy is recommended (may include anakinra, infliximab, and tocilizumab) All children <12 y should wear compression stockings Follow local KD guidelines for aspirin dosing and continued for a minimum of 6 wk Follow local protocols for children with a thrombotic event Discuss with hematologist regarding long-term antiplatelet and anticoagulation therapy in children with abnormal coronary arteries

| Follow-up | Echocardiogram: 7–14 d then 4–6 wk after presentation; consider 1 y echocardiogram in those with cardiac abnormalities
Cardiac MRI at 2–6 mo in those with moderate to severe left ventricular dysfunction
ECG: at each follow-up; consider a Holter monitor in those with conduction abnormalities | Close follow-up 1–2 wk after discharge with pediatric cardiology and, if steroids or biologics were used, pediatric rheumatology | Recommended follow-up at 1–2 wk and 6 wk after discharge with echocardiography; multidisciplinary follow-up with pediatric infectious disease, immunology, and cardiology in those with coronary artery abnormalities or who have required organ support |

Abbreviations: CRP, C-reactive protein; ECG, electrocardiogram; ESR, erythrocyte sedimentation rate; IL, interleukin; INR, international normalized ratio; IVIG, intravenous immunoglobulin; KD, Kawasaki disease; LDH, lactate dehydrogenase; MIS-C, multisystem inflammatory syndrome in children; NT-proBNP, N-terminal pro brain natriuretic peptide; PCR, polymerase chain reaction; PIMS-TS, pediatric inflammatory multisystem syndrome temporally associated with SARS-CoV-2; RT-PCR, reverse-transcriptase polymerase chain reaction; SARS-CoV-2, severe acute respiratory distress syndrome coronavirus 2.

exacerbation,[241] and cancer treatment.[242] The global prevalence of depression and anxiety in children highlight the persistent exacerbation of mental health illnesses.[243] In addition to these acute medical issues, the pandemic has altered the daily habits of families, resulting in decreases in physical activity[244] and increase in hours of screen time in children.[245] These and other social disruptions have had substantial adverse effects on mental health[246,247] and behavior.[248] Family units have also been disrupted because of the deaths of parents and caregivers as a result of COVID-19,[249] exacerbating income inequalities[250] and food insecurity.[251,252] Early studies during the pandemic suggested increases in cases of child abuse and neglect[253,254]; however, there is some evidence to suggest that the increase in family time and strengthening of family support systems helped mitigate instances of physical abuse of children.[255] With school closures, learning was adapted to minimize face-to-face contact.[256] Although schools have resumed in-person learning for the most part, the full impact of changes in childhood education during the pandemic has yet to be fully quantified.

SUMMARY

The SARS-CoV-2 pandemic has led to unprecedented worldwide morbidity and mortality impacting children of all ages. Pediatric acute COVID-19 has likely been underestimated given the milder presentation of disease and testing paradigms, although severe outcomes have been experienced by all age groups. The post-acute sequelae of acute COVID-19, including MIS-C and chronic persistent symptoms, experienced by children who recovered from acute COVID-19 emphasize the importance of infection mitigation. Safe and effective SARS-CoV-2 vaccines are available to most pediatric age groups and are becoming more available worldwide, with booster doses available in some settings. There is a dearth of clinical trial data to determine the ideal treatment in children; future studies must include children to help guide therapy. In addition to direct impacts of infection, children have suffered disproportionately given the closure of schools, loss of adult caregivers, and disruption to household stability. Further changes in the pandemic are likely as SARS-CoV-2 variants arise and public health measures are loosened, but community-wide public health interventions aimed at curbing the pandemic will have important consequences for children's health.

CLINICS CARE POINTS

- SARS-CoV-2 infections are more commonly asymptomatic, with milder disease presentations of COVID-19 in children, although children of all ages are at risk for severe outcomes; SARS-CoV-2 vaccines remain a mainstay of COVID-19 prevention in children.

- MIS-C and persistent symptoms after SARS-CoV-2 infection are important post-acute COVID-19 sequelae in children and emphasize the need for preventing pediatric infections.

- The management of acute COVID-19 and MIS-C requires clinical and laboratory investigations to rule out alternative etiologies for which treatment is available, and follow-up may be required.

- Optimal therapy for acute COVID-19 and MIS-C is unknown and is guided by expert panels; consultation with subspecialists is advised when therapy is considered in children.

- Maintaining regular preventive care and ensuring high rates of childhood vaccine uptake are vital to prevent long-term consequences of non–COVID-19 disease and other infectious disease outbreaks.

- Indirect impacts of the SARS-CoV-2 pandemic threaten the health and well-being of children worldwide.

DISCLOSURE

E.J. Chow has no conflicts of interest to disclose. J.A. Englund reports research support from AstraZeneca, Merck, and Pfizer, and has been a consultant for Sanofi Pasteur, Meissa Vaccines, Teva Pharmaceuticals, AstraZeneca.

REFERENCES

1. Dong Y, Mo X, Hu Y, et al. Epidemiology of COVID-19 among children in China. Pediatrics 2020;145(6). https://doi.org/10.1542/peds.2020-0702.
2. Leidman E, Duca LM, Omura JD, et al. COVID-19 trends among persons aged 0-24 years - United States, March 1-December 12, 2020. MMWR Morb Mortal Wkly Rep 2021;70(3):88–94.
3. Centers for Disease Control and Prevention. COVID Data Tracker: Demographic Trends of COVID-19 Cases and Deaths in the US Reported to CDC. Available at: https://covid.cdc.gov/covid-data-tracker/#demographics. Accessed January 12, 2022.
4. Team CC-R. Coronavirus disease 2019 in children - United States, February 12-April 2, 2020. MMWR Morb Mortal Wkly Rep 2020;69(14):422–6.
5. Kim L, Whitaker M, O'Halloran A, et al. Hospitalization rates and characteristics of children aged <18 years hospitalized with laboratory-confirmed COVID-19 - COVID-NET, 14 States, March 1-July 25, 2020. MMWR Morb Mortal Wkly Rep 2020;69(32):1081–8.
6. Lu X, Zhang L, Du H, et al. SARS-CoV-2 infection in children. N Engl J Med 2020; 382(17):1663–5.
7. Davies NG, Klepac P, Liu Y, et al. Age-dependent effects in the transmission and control of COVID-19 epidemics. Nat Med 2020;26(8):1205–11.
8. Yousaf AR, Duca LM, Chu V, et al. A prospective cohort study in nonhospitalized household contacts with severe acute respiratory syndrome coronavirus 2 infection: symptom profiles and symptom change over time. Clin Infect Dis 2021; 73(7):e1841–9.
9. Stokes EK, Zambrano LD, Anderson KN, et al. Coronavirus disease 2019 case surveillance - United States, January 22-May 30, 2020. MMWR Morb Mortal Wkly Rep 2020;69(24):759–65.
10. UNICEF: Child Mortality and COVID-19. Available at: https://data.unicef.org/topic/child-survival/covid-19/. Accessed January 12, 2022.
11. Rodriguez Velasquez S, Jacques L, Dalal J, et al. The toll of COVID-19 on African children: a descriptive analysis on COVID-19-related morbidity and mortality among the pediatric population in Sub-Saharan Africa. Int J Infect Dis 2021; 110:457–65.
12. Indenbaum V, Lustig Y, Mendelson E, et al. Under-diagnosis of SARS-CoV-2 infections among children aged 0-15 years, a nationwide seroprevalence study, Israel, January 2020 to March 2021. Euro Surveill 2021;26(48). https://doi.org/10.2807/1560-7917.ES.2021.26.48.2101040.
13. Jeewandara C, Guruge D, Abyrathna IS, et al. Seroprevalence of SARS-CoV-2 infection in the Colombo Municipality Region, Sri Lanka. Front Public Health 2021;9. https://doi.org/10.3389/fpubh.2021.724398. 724398.

14. Zinszer K, McKinnon B, Bourque N, et al. Seroprevalence of SARS-CoV-2 antibodies among children in school and day care in Montreal, Canada. JAMA Netw Open 2021;4(11):e2135975.
15. Pollan M, Perez-Gomez B, Pastor-Barriuso R, et al. Prevalence of SARS-CoV-2 in Spain (ENE-COVID): a nationwide, population-based seroepidemiological study. Lancet 2020;396(10250):535–44.
16. Stringhini S, Wisniak A, Piumatti G, et al. Seroprevalence of anti-SARS-CoV-2 IgG antibodies in Geneva, Switzerland (SEROCoV-POP): a population-based study. Lancet 2020;396(10247):313–9.
17. Tonshoff B, Muller B, Elling R, et al. Prevalence of SARS-CoV-2 infection in children and their parents in Southwest Germany. JAMA Pediatr 2021;175(6): 586–93.
18. Rostami A, Sepidarkish M, Leeflang MMG, et al. SARS-CoV-2 seroprevalence worldwide: a systematic review and meta-analysis. Clin Microbiol Infect 2021; 27(3):331–40.
19. Stringhini S, Zaballa ME, Pullen N, et al. Seroprevalence of anti-SARS-CoV-2 antibodies 6 months into the vaccination campaign in Geneva, Switzerland, 1 June to 7 July 2021. Euro Surveill 2021;26(43). https://doi.org/10.2807/1560-7917.ES. 2021.26.43.2100830.
20. Maltezou HC, Krumbholz B, Mavrouli M, et al. A study of the evolution of the third COVID-19 pandemic wave in the Athens metropolitan area, Greece, through two cross-sectional seroepidemiological surveys: March, June 2021. J Med Virol 2021. https://doi.org/10.1002/jmv.27465.
21. United States Census Bureau Quick Facts. Available at: https://www.census. gov/quickfacts/fact/table/US/AGE295219#AGE295219. Accessed January 12, 2022.
22. Centers for Disease Control and Prevention. Estimated COVID-19 Burden. Available at: https://www.cdc.gov/coronavirus/2019-ncov/cases-updates/burden. html. Accessed January 12, 2022.
23. Dhar MS, Marwal R, Vs R, et al. Genomic characterization and epidemiology of an emerging SARS-CoV-2 variant in Delhi, India. Science 2021;374(6570): 995–9.
24. Delahoy MJ, Ujamaa D, Whitaker M, et al. Hospitalizations associated with COVID-19 among children and adolescents - COVID-NET, 14 States, March 1, 2020-August 14, 2021. MMWR Morb Mortal Wkly Rep 2021;70(36):1255–60.
25. Siegel DA, Reses HE, Cool AJ, et al. Trends in COVID-19 cases, emergency department visits, and hospital admissions among children and adolescents aged 0-17 years - United States, August 2020-August 2021. MMWR Morb Mortal Wkly Rep 2021;70(36):1249–54.
26. Oeser C, Whitaker H, Linley E, et al. Large increases in SARS-CoV-2 seropositivity in children in England: effects of the delta wave and vaccination. J Infect 2021. https://doi.org/10.1016/j.jinf.2021.11.019.
27. Ito K, Piantham C, Nishiura H. Relative instantaneous reproduction number of Omicron SARS-CoV-2 variant with respect to the Delta variant in Denmark. J Med Virol 2021. https://doi.org/10.1002/jmv.27560.
28. World Health Organization. Classification of Omicron (B.1.1.529): SARS-CoV-2 Variant of Concern. Available at: https://www.who.int/news/item/26-11-2021-classification-of-omicron-(b.1.1.529)-sars-cov-2-variant-of-concern. Accessed January 12, 2022.
29. Team CC-R. SARS-CoV-2 B.1.1.529 (Omicron) Variant - United States, December 1-8, 2021. MMWR Morb Mortal Wkly Rep 2021;70(50):1731–4.

30. Centers for Disease Control and Prevention. New admissions of patients with confirmed COVID-19 per 100,000 population by age group, United States. Available at: https://covid.cdc.gov/covid-data-tracker/#new-hospital-admissions. Accessed January 12, 2022.

31. Chowkwanyun M, Reed AL Jr. Racial health disparities and Covid-19 - caution and context. N Engl J Med 2020;383(3):201–3.

32. Gold JAW, Wong KK, Szablewski CM, et al. Characteristics and clinical outcomes of adult patients hospitalized with COVID-19 - Georgia, March 2020. MMWR Morb Mortal Wkly Rep 2020;69(18):545–50.

33. Webb Hooper M, Napoles AM, Perez-Stable EJ. COVID-19 and racial/ethnic disparities. JAMA 2020;323(24):2466–7.

34. Bhala N, Curry G, Martineau AR, et al. Sharpening the global focus on ethnicity and race in the time of COVID-19. Lancet 2020;395(10238):1673–6.

35. Chamie G, Marquez C, Crawford E, et al. Community transmission of severe acute respiratory syndrome Coronavirus 2 disproportionately affects the Latinx population during shelter-in-place in San Francisco. Clin Infect Dis 2021; 73(Suppl 2):S127–35.

36. Bandi S, Nevid MZ, Mahdavinia M. African American children are at higher risk of COVID-19 infection. Pediatr Allergy Immunol 2020;31(7):861–4.

37. McCormick DW, Richardson LC, Young PR, et al. Deaths in children and adolescents associated with COVID-19 and MIS-C in the United States. Pediatrics 2021;148(5). https://doi.org/10.1542/peds.2021-052273.

38. Hatcher SM, Agnew-Brune C, Anderson M, et al. COVID-19 among American Indian and Alaska Native persons - 23 states, January 31-July 3, 2020. MMWR Morb Mortal Wkly Rep 2020;69(34):1166–9.

39. Martinez DA, Hinson JS, Klein EY, et al. SARS-CoV-2 positivity rate for Latinos in the Baltimore-Washington, DC Region. JAMA 2020;324(4):392–5.

40. Goyal MK, Simpson JN, Boyle MD, et al. Racial and/or ethnic and socioeconomic disparities of SARS-CoV-2 infection among children. Pediatrics 2020; 146(4). https://doi.org/10.1542/peds.2020-009951.

41. Tan TQ, Kullar R, Swartz TH, et al. Location matters: geographic disparities and impact of coronavirus disease 2019. J Infect Dis 2020;222(12):1951–4.

42. Kong STJ, Lee RY, Rodriguez F, et al. Racial and ethnic disparities in household contact with individuals at higher risk of exposure to COVID-19. J Gen Intern Med 2021;36(5):1470–2.

43. Rane MS, Robertson MM, Westmoreland DA, et al. Intention to vaccinate children against COVID-19 among vaccinated and unvaccinated US parents. JAMA Pediatr 2021. https://doi.org/10.1001/jamapediatrics.2021.5153.

44. Honein MA, Christie A, Rose DA, et al. Summary of guidance for public health strategies to address high levels of community transmission of SARS-CoV-2 and related deaths, December 2020. MMWR Morb Mortal Wkly Rep 2020; 69(49):1860–7.

45. Haston JC, Pickering LK. Non-household transmission of SARS-CoV-2 underscores importance of stay-at-home orders. Available at: https://www.aappublications.org/news/2020/05/21/mmwr052120?utm_source=TrendMD&utm_medium=TrendMD&utm_campaign=AAPNews_TrendMD_1. Accessed January 12, 2022.

46. Ghinai I, Woods S, Ritger KA, et al. Community transmission of SARS-CoV-2 at two family gatherings - Chicago, Illinois, February-March 2020. MMWR Morb Mortal Wkly Rep 2020;69(15):446–50.

47. Rajmil L. Role of children in the transmission of the COVID-19 pandemic: a rapid scoping review. BMJ Paediatr Open 2020;4(1):e000722.
48. Kelvin AA, Halperin S. COVID-19 in children: the link in the transmission chain. Lancet Infect Dis 2020;20(6):633–4.
49. Coffin SE, Rubin D. Yes, children can transmit COVID, but we need not fear. JAMA Pediatr 2021;175(11):1110–2.
50. Wu JT, Cowling BJ, Lau EH, et al. School closure and mitigation of pandemic (H1N1) 2009, Hong Kong. Emerg Infect Dis 2010;16(3):538–41.
51. Weycker D, Edelsberg J, Halloran ME, et al. Population-wide benefits of routine vaccination of children against influenza. Vaccine 2005;23(10):1284–93.
52. Anderson EJ, Daugherty MA, Pickering LK, et al. Protecting the community through child vaccination. Clin Infect Dis 2018;67(3):464–71.
53. Cohen SA, Chui KK, Naumova EN. Influenza vaccination in young children reduces influenza-associated hospitalizations in older adults, 2002-2006. J Am Geriatr Soc 2011;59(2):327–32.
54. Centers for Disease Control and Prevention. Scientific brief: SARS-CoV-2 transmission. Available at: https://www.cdc.gov/coronavirus/2019-ncov/science/science-briefs/sars-cov-2-transmission.html. Accessed January 12, 2022.
55. Yehya N, Venkataramani A, Harhay MO. Statewide interventions and coronavirus disease 2019 mortality in the United States: An Observational Study. Clin Infect Dis 2021;73(7):e1863–9.
56. Courtemanche C, Garuccio J, Le A, et al. Strong social distancing measures in the United States reduced the COVID-19 growth rate. Health Aff (Millwood) 2020;39(7):1237–46.
57. Zhou L, Ayeh SK, Chidambaram V, et al. Modes of transmission of SARS-CoV-2 and evidence for preventive behavioral interventions. BMC Infect Dis 2021; 21(1):496.
58. Paul LA, Daneman N, Schwartz KL, et al. Association of age and pediatric household transmission of SARS-CoV-2 infection. JAMA Pediatr 2021;175(11): 1151–8.
59. Park YJ, Choe YJ, Park O, et al. Contact tracing during coronavirus disease outbreak, South Korea, 2020. Emerg Infect Dis 2020;26(10):2465–8.
60. Rostad CA, Kamidani S, Anderson EJ. Implications of SARS-CoV-2 viral load in children: getting back to school and normal. JAMA Pediatr 2021;175(10): e212022.
61. Su L, Ma X, Yu H, et al. The different clinical characteristics of corona virus disease cases between children and their families in China - the character of children with COVID-19. Emerg Microbes Infect 2020;9(1):707–13.
62. Kam KQ, Yung CF, Cui L, et al. A well infant with coronavirus disease 2019 with high viral load. Clin Infect Dis 2020;71(15):847–9.
63. Chan JF, Yuan S, Kok KH, et al. A familial cluster of pneumonia associated with the 2019 novel coronavirus indicating person-to-person transmission: a study of a family cluster. Lancet 2020;395(10223):514–23.
64. Posfay-Barbe KM, Wagner N, Gauthey M, et al. COVID-19 in children and the dynamics of infection in families. Pediatrics 2020;146(2). https://doi.org/10.1542/peds.2020-1576.
65. Maltezou HC, Vorou R, Papadima K, et al. Transmission dynamics of SARS-CoV-2 within families with children in Greece: A study of 23 clusters. J Med Virol 2021;93(3):1414–20.

66. Li F, Li YY, Liu MJ, et al. Household transmission of SARS-CoV-2 and risk factors for susceptibility and infectivity in Wuhan: a retrospective observational study. Lancet Infect Dis 2021;21(5):617–28.
67. Hall CB, Douglas RG Jr. Modes of transmission of respiratory syncytial virus. J Pediatr 1981;99(1):100–3.
68. Madewell ZJ, Yang Y, Longini IM Jr, et al. Factors associated with household transmission of SARS-CoV-2: an updated systematic review and meta-analysis. JAMA Netw Open 2021;4(8):e2122240.
69. Grijalva CG, Rolfes MA, Zhu Y, et al. Transmission of SARS-COV-2 infections in households - Tennessee and Wisconsin, April-September 2020. MMWR Morb Mortal Wkly Rep 2020;69(44):1631–4.
70. Kawasuji H, Takegoshi Y, Kaneda M, et al. Transmissibility of COVID-19 depends on the viral load around onset in adult and symptomatic patients. PLoS One 2020;15(12):e0243597.
71. Goyal A, Reeves DB, Cardozo-Ojeda EF, et al. Viral load and contact heterogeneity predict SARS-CoV-2 transmission and super-spreading events. Elife 2021;10. https://doi.org/10.7554/eLife.63537.
72. Marks M, Millat-Martinez P, Ouchi D, et al. Transmission of COVID-19 in 282 clusters in Catalonia, Spain: a cohort study. Lancet Infect Dis 2021;21(5): 629–36.
73. Chung E, Chow EJ, Wilcox NC, et al. Comparison of symptoms and RNA levels in children and adults with SARS-CoV-2 infection in the community setting. JAMA Pediatr 2021;175(10):e212025.
74. Xiao F, Sun J, Xu Y, et al. Infectious SARS-CoV-2 in feces of patient with severe COVID-19. Emerg Infect Dis 2020;26(8):1920–2.
75. Hua CZ, Miao ZP, Zheng JS, et al. Epidemiological features and viral shedding in children with SARS-CoV-2 infection. J Med Virol 2020;92(11):2804–12.
76. Han MS, Seong MW, Kim N, et al. Viral RNA load in mildly symptomatic and asymptomatic children with COVID-19, Seoul, South Korea. Emerg Infect Dis 2020;26(10):2497–9.
77. Buddingh EP, Vossen A, Lamb HJ, et al. Reinfection with severe acute respiratory syndrome coronavirus 2 without recurrence of multisystem inflammatory syndrome in children. Pediatr Infect Dis J 2021;40(12):e491–2.
78. Viner R, Waddington C, Mytton O, et al. Transmission of SARS-CoV-2 by children and young people in households and schools: a meta-analysis of population-based and contact-tracing studies. J Infect 2021. https://doi.org/10.1016/j.jinf.2021.12.026.
79. Heavey L, Casey G, Kelly C, et al. No evidence of secondary transmission of COVID-19 from children attending school in Ireland, 2020. Euro Surveill 2020;(21):25. https://doi.org/10.2807/1560-7917.ES.2020.25.21.2000903.
80. Kim C, McGee S, Khuntia S, et al. Characteristics of COVID-19 cases and outbreaks at child care facilities - District of Columbia, July-December 2020. MMWR Morb Mortal Wkly Rep 2021;70(20):744–8.
81. Lam-Hine T, McCurdy SA, Santora L, et al. Outbreak associated with SARS-CoV-2 B.1.617.2 (Delta) variant in an elementary school - Marin County, California, May-June 2021. MMWR Morb Mortal Wkly Rep 2021;70(35):1214–9.
82. Yin S, Barnes K, Fisher R, et al. COVID-19 case rates in transitional kindergarten through grade 12 schools and in the community - Los Angeles County, California, September 2020-March 2021. MMWR Morb Mortal Wkly Rep 2021;70(35): 1220–2.

83. Jehn M, McCullough JM, Dale AP, et al. Association between K-12 school mask policies and school-associated COVID-19 outbreaks - Maricopa and Pima Counties, Arizona, July-August 2021. MMWR Morb Mortal Wkly Rep 2021; 70(39):1372–3.

84. Budzyn SE, Panaggio MJ, Parks SE, et al. Pediatric COVID-19 cases in counties with and without school mask requirements - United States, July 1-September 4, 2021. MMWR Morb Mortal Wkly Rep 2021;70(39):1377–8.

85. Nemoto N, Dhillon S, Fink S, et al. Evaluation of test to stay strategy on secondary and tertiary transmission of SARS-CoV-2 in K-12 schools - Lake County, Illinois, August 9-October 29, 2021. MMWR Morb Mortal Wkly Rep 2021;70(5152): 1778–81.

86. Harris-McCoy K, Lee VC, Munna C, et al. Evaluation of a test to stay strategy in transitional kindergarten through grade 12 schools - Los Angeles County, California, August 16-October 31, 2021. MMWR Morb Mortal Wkly Rep 2021; 70(5152):1773–7.

87. World Health Organization. COVID-19 vaccines WHO EUL issued. Available at: https://extranet.who.int/pqweb/vaccines/vaccinescovid-19-vaccine-eul-issued. Accessed January 12, 2022.

88. World Health Organization. COVID-19 advice for the public: getting vaccinated. Available at: https://www.who.int/emergencies/diseases/novel-coronavirus-2019/covid-19-vaccines/advice. Accessed January 12, 2022.

89. Oliver SE, Gargano JW, Marin M, et al. The Advisory Committee on Immunization Practices' Interim Recommendation for Use of Pfizer-BioNTech COVID-19 Vaccine - United States, December 2020. MMWR Morb Mortal Wkly Rep 2020; 69(50):1922–4.

90. Wallace M, Woodworth KR, Gargano JW, et al. The Advisory Committee on Immunization Practices' Interim Recommendation for Use of Pfizer-BioNTech COVID-19 Vaccine in Adolescents Aged 12-15 Years - United States, May 2021. MMWR Morb Mortal Wkly Rep 2021;70(20):749–52.

91. Woodworth KR, Moulia D, Collins JP, et al. The Advisory Committee on Immunization Practices' Interim Recommendation for Use of Pfizer-BioNTech COVID-19 Vaccine in Children Aged 5-11 Years - United States, November 2021. MMWR Morb Mortal Wkly Rep 2021;70(45):1579–83.

92. U.S. Food and Drug Administration: FDA Takes Key Action in Fight Against COVID-19 By Issuing Emergency Use Authorization for First COVID-19 Vaccine. Available at: https://www.fda.gov/news-events/press-announcements/fda-takes-key-action-fight-against-covid-19-issuing-emergency-use-authorization-first-covid-19. Accessed January 12, 2022.

93. U.S. Food and Drug Administration: FDA Approves First COVID-19 Vaccine. Available at: https://www.fda.gov/news-events/press-announcements/fda-approves-first-covid-19-vaccine. Accessed January 12, 2022.

94. U.S. Food and Drug Administration: Coronavirus (COVID-19) Update: FDA Authorizes Pfizer-BioNTech COVID-19 Vaccine for Emergency Use in Adolescents in Another Important Action in Fight Against Pandemic. Available at: https://www.fda.gov/news-events/press-announcements/coronavirus-covid-19-update-fda-authorizes-pfizer-biontech-covid-19-vaccine-emergency-use. Accessed January 12, 2022.

95. U.S. Food and Drug Administration. FDA Authorizes Pfizer-BioNTech COVID-19 Vaccine for Emergency Use in Children 5 through 11 Years of Age. Available at: https://www.fda.gov/news-events/press-announcements/fda-authorizes-pfizer-

biontech-covid-19-vaccine-emergency-use-children-5-through-11-years-age. Accessed January 12, 2022.

96. U.S. Food and Drug Administration. Coronavirus (COVID-19) Update: FDA Expands Eligibility to Pfizer-BioNTech COVID-19 Booster Dose to 16- and 17-Year-Olds. Available at: https://www.fda.gov/news-events/press-announcements/coronavirus-covid-19-update-fda-expands-eligibility-pfizer-biontech-covid-19-booster-dose-16-and-17. Accessed January 12, 2022.

97. U.S. Food and Drug Administration. Coronavirus (COVID-19) Update: FDA Takes Multiple Actions to Expand Use of Pfizer-BioNTech COVID-19 Vaccine. Available at: https://www.fda.gov/news-events/press-announcements/coronavirus-covid-19-update-fda-takes-multiple-actions-expand-use-pfizer-biontech-covid-19-vaccine. Accessed January 12, 2022.

98. Cameroni E, Bowen JE, Rosen LE, et al. Broadly neutralizing antibodies overcome SARS-CoV-2 Omicron antigenic shift. Nature 2021. https://doi.org/10.1038/s41586-021-04386-2.

99. U.S. Food and Drug Administration. Coronavirus (COVID-19) Update: FDA Authorizes New Long-Acting Monoclonal Antibodies for Pre-exposure Prevention of COVID-19 in Certain Individuals. Available at: https://www.fda.gov/news-events/press-announcements/coronavirus-covid-19-update-fda-authorizes-new-long-acting-monoclonal-antibodies-pre-exposure. Accessed January 12, 2022.

100. Polack FP, Thomas SJ, Kitchin N, et al. Safety and efficacy of the BNT162b2 mRNA Covid-19 vaccine. N Engl J Med 2020;383(27):2603–15.

101. Frenck RW Jr, Klein NP, Kitchin N, et al. Safety, immunogenicity, and efficacy of the BNT162b2 Covid-19 vaccine in adolescents. N Engl J Med 2021;385(3):239–50.

102. Walter EB, Talaat KR, Sabharwal C, et al. Evaluation of the BNT162b2 Covid-19 vaccine in children 5 to 11 years of age. N Engl J Med 2022;386(1):35–46.

103. Ali K, Berman G, Zhou H, et al. Evaluation of mRNA-1273 SARS-CoV-2 vaccine in adolescents. N Engl J Med 2021;385(24):2241–51.

104. Bar-On YM, Goldberg Y, Mandel M, et al. Protection against Covid-19 by BNT162b2 booster across age groups. N Engl J Med 2021;385(26):2421–30.

105. Olson SM, Newhams MM, Halasa NB, et al. Effectiveness of Pfizer-BioNTech mRNA vaccination against COVID-19 hospitalization among persons aged 12-18 years - United States, June-September 2021. MMWR Morb Mortal Wkly Rep 2021;70(42):1483–8.

106. Lutrick K, Rivers P, Yoo YM, et al. Interim estimate of vaccine effectiveness of BNT162b2 (Pfizer-BioNTech) vaccine in preventing SARS-CoV-2 infection among adolescents aged 12-17 years - Arizona, July-December 2021. MMWR Morb Mortal Wkly Rep 2021;70(5152):1761–5.

107. Naleway AL, Groom HC, Crawford PM, et al. Incidence of SARS-CoV-2 infection, emergency department visits, and hospitalizations because of COVID-19 among persons aged >/=12 years, by COVID-19 vaccination status - Oregon and Washington, July 4-September 25, 2021. MMWR Morb Mortal Wkly Rep 2021;70(46):1608–12.

108. Levy M, Recher M, Hubert H, et al. Multisystem inflammatory syndrome in children by COVID-19 vaccination status of adolescents in France. JAMA 2021. https://doi.org/10.1001/jama.2021.23262.

109. Zambrano LD, Newhams MM, Olson SM, et al. Effectiveness of BNT162b2 (Pfizer-BioNTech) mRNA vaccination against multisystem inflammatory

syndrome in children among persons aged 12–18 years — United States, July–December 2021. MMWR Morbidity Mortality Weekly Rep 2022;71(2):52–8.

110. Centers for Disease Control and Prevention. Demographic Trends of People Receiving COVID-19 Vaccinations in the United States. Available at: https://covid.cdc.gov/covid-data-tracker/#vaccination-demographics-trends. Accessed January 12, 2022.

111. Morgan L, Schwartz JL, Sisti DA. COVID-19 vaccination of minors without parental consent: respecting emerging autonomy and advancing public health. JAMA Pediatr 2021;175(10):995–6.

112. Hause AM, Baggs J, Marquez P, et al. COVID-19 vaccine safety in children aged 5-11 years - United States, November 3-December 19, 2021. MMWR Morb Mortal Wkly Rep 2021;70(5152):1755–60.

113. Hause AM, Gee J, Baggs J, et al. COVID-19 vaccine safety in adolescents aged 12-17 years - United States, December 14, 2020-July 16, 2021. MMWR Morb Mortal Wkly Rep 2021;70(31):1053–8.

114. Truong DT, Dionne A, Muniz JC, et al. Clinically suspected myocarditis temporally related to COVID-19 vaccination in adolescents and young adults. Circulation 2021. https://doi.org/10.1161/CIRCULATIONAHA.121.056583.

115. Barda N, Dagan N, Ben-Shlomo Y, et al. Safety of the BNT162b2 mRNA Covid-19 vaccine in a nationwide setting. N Engl J Med 2021;385(12):1078–90.

116. Diaz GA, Parsons GT, Gering SK, et al. Myocarditis and Pericarditis After Vaccination for COVID-19. JAMA 2021;326(12):1210–2.

117. Dionne A, Sperotto F, Chamberlain S, et al. Association of myocarditis with BNT162b2 messenger RNA COVID-19 vaccine in a case series of children. JAMA Cardiol 2021;6(12):1446–50.

118. Gargano JW, Wallace M, Hadler SC, et al. Use of mRNA COVID-19 vaccine after reports of myocarditis among vaccine recipients: update from the Advisory Committee on Immunization Practices - United States, June 2021. MMWR Morb Mortal Wkly Rep 2021;70(27):977–82.

119. Boehmer TK, Kompaniyets L, Lavery AM, et al. Association between COVID-19 and myocarditis using hospital-based administrative data - United States, March 2020-January 2021. MMWR Morb Mortal Wkly Rep 2021;70(35):1228–32.

120. Li B, Zhang S, Zhang R, et al. Epidemiological and clinical characteristics of COVID-19 in children: a systematic review and meta-analysis. Front Pediatr 2020;8. https://doi.org/10.3389/fped.2020.591132. 591132.

121. Liguoro I, Pilotto C, Bonanni M, et al. SARS-COV-2 infection in children and newborns: a systematic review. Eur J Pediatr 2020;179(7):1029–46.

122. Centers for Disease Control and Prevention. COVID-19: Information for Pediatric Healthcare Providers. Available at: https://www.cdc.gov/coronavirus/2019-ncov/hcp/pediatric-hcp.html. Accessed January 12, 2022.

123. Lauer SA, Grantz KH, Bi Q, et al. The incubation period of coronavirus disease 2019 (COVID-19) from publicly reported confirmed cases: estimation and application. Ann Intern Med 2020;172(9):577–82.

124. Molteni E, Sudre CH, Canas LS, et al. Illness duration and symptom profile in symptomatic UK school-aged children tested for SARS-CoV-2. Lancet Child Adolesc Health 2021;5(10):708–18.

125. Ng KF, Bandi S, Bird PW, et al. COVID-19 in neonates and infants: progression and recovery. Pediatr Infect Dis J 2020;39(7):e140–2.

126. National Institutes of Health. COVID-19 Treatment Guidelines: Clinical Spectrum of SARS-CoV-2 infection. Available at: https://www.covid19treatmentguidelines.nih.gov/overview/clinical-spectrum/. Accessed January 12, 2022.

127. Gandhi RT, Lynch JB, Del Rio C. Mild or moderate Covid-19. N Engl J Med 2020; 383(18):1757–66.
128. Shekerdemian LS, Mahmood NR, Wolfe KK, et al. Characteristics and outcomes of children with coronavirus disease 2019 (COVID-19) infection admitted to US and Canadian pediatric intensive care units. JAMA Pediatr 2020. https://doi.org/ 10.1001/jamapediatrics.2020.1948doi:10.1001/jamapediatrics.2020.1948.
129. Bixler D, Miller AD, Mattison CP, et al. SARS-CoV-2-associated deaths among persons aged <21 years - United States, February 12-July 31, 2020. MMWR Morb Mortal Wkly Rep 2020;69(37):1324–9.
130. Bailey LC, Razzaghi H, Burrows EK, et al. Assessment of 135794 pediatric patients tested for severe acute respiratory syndrome coronavirus 2 across the United States. JAMA Pediatr 2021;175(2):176–84.
131. Ouldali N, Yang DD, Madhi F, et al. Factors associated with severe SARS-CoV-2 infection. Pediatrics 2021;147(3). https://doi.org/10.1542/peds.2020-023432.
132. Gotzinger F, Santiago-Garcia B, Noguera-Julian A, et al. COVID-19 in children and adolescents in Europe: a multinational, multicentre cohort study. Lancet Child Adolesc Health 2020;4(9):653–61.
133. Wanga V, Gerdes ME, Shi DS, et al. Characteristics and clinical outcomes of children and adolescents aged <18 years hospitalized with COVID-19 - six hospitals, United States, July-August 2021. MMWR Morb Mortal Wkly Rep 2021; 70(5152):1766–72.
134. Tsabouri S, Makis A, Kosmeri C, et al. Risk factors for severity in children with coronavirus disease 2019: a comprehensive literature review. Pediatr Clin North Am 2021;68(1):321–38.
135. Kompaniyets L, Agathis NT, Nelson JM, et al. Underlying medical conditions associated with severe COVID-19 illness among children. JAMA Netw Open 2021;4(6):e2111182.
136. Newman AM, Jhaveri R, Patel AB, et al. Trisomy 21 and coronavirus disease 2019 in pediatric patients. J Pediatr 2021;228:294–6.
137. Arlet JB, de Luna G, Khimoud D, et al. Prognosis of patients with sickle cell disease and COVID-19: a French experience. Lancet Haematol 2020;7(9):e632–4.
138. Sanna G, Serrau G, Bassareo PP, et al. Children's heart and COVID-19: up-to-date evidence in the form of a systematic review. Eur J Pediatr 2020;179(7): 1079–87.
139. DeBiasi RL, Song X, Delaney M, et al. Severe coronavirus disease-2019 in children and young adults in the Washington, DC, Metropolitan Region. J Pediatr 2020;223:199–203.e1.
140. Kosmeri C, Koumpis E, Tsabouri S, et al. Hematological manifestations of SARS-CoV-2 in children. Pediatr Blood Cancer 2020;67(12):e28745.
141. Centers for Disease Control and Prevention. Underlying medical conditions associated with higher risk for severe COVID-19: information for healthcare providers. Available at: https://www.cdc.gov/coronavirus/2019-ncov/hcp/clinical-care/underlyingconditions.html. Accessed January 12, 2022.
142. Walker KF, O'Donoghue K, Grace N, et al. Maternal transmission of SARS-COV-2 to the neonate, and possible routes for such transmission: a systematic review and critical analysis. BJOG 2020;127(11):1324–36.
143. American Academy of Pediatrics. FAQs: management of infants born to mothers with suspected or confirmed COVID-19. Available at: https://www.aap.org/en/ pages/2019-novel-coronavirus-covid-19-infections/clinical-guidance/faqs-management-of-infants-born-to-covid-19-mothers/. Accessed January 12, 2022.

144. Ray STJ, Abdel-Mannan O, Sa M, et al. Neurological manifestations of SARS-CoV-2 infection in hospitalised children and adolescents in the UK: a prospective national cohort study. Lancet Child Adolesc Health 2021;5(9):631–41.
145. Trogen B, Gonzalez FJ, Shust GF. COVID-19-associated myocarditis in an adolescent. Pediatr Infect Dis J 2020;39(8):e204–5.
146. Lara D, Young T, Del Toro K, et al. Acute fulminant myocarditis in a pediatric patient with COVID-19 infection. Pediatrics 2020;146(2). https://doi.org/10.1542/peds.2020-1509.
147. Raymond TT, Das A, Manzuri S, et al. Pediatric COVID-19 and pericarditis presenting with acute pericardial tamponade. World J Pediatr Congenit Heart Surg 2020;11(6):802–4.
148. Dimopoulou D, Spyridis N, Dasoula F, et al. Pericarditis as the main clinical manifestation of COVID-19 in adolescents. Pediatr Infect Dis J 2021;40(5): e197–9.
149. Panjabi AL, Foster RC, McCarthy AM, et al. Pulmonary embolism as the initial presentation of coronavirus disease 2019 in adolescents. Pediatr Infect Dis J 2021;40(5):e200–2.
150. Samuel S, Friedman RA, Sharma C, et al. Incidence of arrhythmias and electrocardiographic abnormalities in symptomatic pediatric patients with PCR-positive SARS-CoV-2 infection, including drug-induced changes in the corrected QT interval. Heart Rhythm 2020;17(11):1960–6.
151. Persson J, Shorofsky M, Leahy R, et al. ST-elevation myocardial infarction due to acute thrombosis in an adolescent with COVID-19. Pediatrics 2021;148(2). https://doi.org/10.1542/peds.2020-049793.
152. Andina D, Belloni-Fortina A, Bodemer C, et al. Skin manifestations of COVID-19 in children: Part 1. Clin Exp Dermatol 2021;46(3):444–50.
153. Andina D, Belloni-Fortina A, Bodemer C, et al. Skin manifestations of COVID-19 in children: Part 2. Clin Exp Dermatol 2021;46(3):451–61.
154. Paz L, Eslava E, Ribes M, et al. Acute pancreatitis in a teenager with SARS-CoV-2 infection. Pediatr Infect Dis J 2021;40(4):e161–2.
155. Brisca G, Mallamaci M, Tardini G, et al. SARS-CoV-2 infection may present as acute hepatitis in children. Pediatr Infect Dis J 2021;40(5):e214–5.
156. Perez A, Kogan-Liberman D, Sheflin-Findling S, et al. Presentation of severe acute respiratory syndrome-coronavirus 2 infection as cholestatic jaundice in two healthy adolescents. J Pediatr 2020;226:278–80.
157. Stewart DJ, Hartley JC, Johnson M, et al. Renal dysfunction in hospitalised children with COVID-19. Lancet Child Adolesc Health 2020;4(8):e28–9.
158. Marr KA, Platt A, Tornheim JA, et al. Aspergillosis complicating severe coronavirus disease. Emerg Infect Dis 2021;27(1). https://doi.org/10.3201/eid2701. 202896.
159. Dulski TM, DeLong M, Garner K, et al. Notes from the field: COVID-19-associated mucormycosis - Arkansas, July-September 2021. MMWR Morb Mortal Wkly Rep 2021;70(50):1750–1.
160. Samprathi M, Jayashree M. Biomarkers in COVID-19: an up-to-date review. Front Pediatr 2020;8. https://doi.org/10.3389/fped.2020.607647. 607647.
161. Henry BM, Benoit SW, de Oliveira MHS, et al. Laboratory abnormalities in children with mild and severe coronavirus disease 2019 (COVID-19): A pooled analysis and review. Clin Biochem 2020;81:1–8.
162. Irfan O, Muttalib F, Tang K, et al. Clinical characteristics, treatment and outcomes of paediatric COVID-19: a systematic review and meta-analysis. Arch Dis Child 2021. https://doi.org/10.1136/archdischild-2020-321385.

163. Wang Y, Zhu F, Wang C, et al. Children hospitalized with severe COVID-19 in Wuhan. Pediatr Infect Dis J 2020;39(7):e91–4.

164. Qiu H, Wu J, Hong L, et al. Clinical and epidemiological features of 36 children with coronavirus disease 2019 (COVID-19) in Zhejiang, China: an observational cohort study. Lancet Infect Dis 2020;20(6):689–96.

165. Shelmerdine SC, Lovrenski J, Caro-Dominguez P, et al. Collaborators of the European Society of Paediatric Radiology Cardiothoracic Imaging T. Coronavirus disease 2019 (COVID-19) in children: a systematic review of imaging findings. Pediatr Radiol 2020;50(9):1217–30.

166. Cameroni E, Saliba C, Bowen JE, et al. Broadly neutralizing antibodies overcome SARS-CoV-2 Omicron antigenic shift. bioRxiv 2021. https://doi.org/10.1101/2021.12.12.472269.

167. Langford BJ, So M, Raybardhan S, et al. Antibiotic prescribing in patients with COVID-19: rapid review and meta-analysis. Clin Microbiol Infect 2021;27(4):520–31.

168. U.S. Food and Drug Administration. Fact Sheet for Health Care Providers Emergency Use Authorization (EUA) of Bamlanivimab and Etesevimab. Available at: https://www.fda.gov/media/145802/download. Accessed January 12, 2022.

169. National Institutes of Health. COVID-19 Treatment Guidelines. Available at: https://files.covid19treatmentguidelines.nih.gov/guidelines/covid19treatmentguidelines.pdf. Accessed January 12, 2022.

170. Wolf J, Abzug MJ, Wattier RL, et al. Initial guidance on use of monoclonal antibody therapy for treatment of coronavirus disease 2019 in children and adolescents. J Pediatr Infect Dis Soc 2021;10(5):629–34.

171. U.S. Food and Drug Administration: Veklury (remdesivir) EUA Letter of Approval, reissued 10/22/2020. Available at: https://www.fda.gov/media/137564/download. Accessed January 12, 2022.

172. Beigel JH, Tomashek KM, Dodd LE, et al. Remdesivir for the treatment of Covid-19 - final report. N Engl J Med 2020;383(19):1813–26.

173. Goldman JD, Lye DCB, Hui DS, et al. Remdesivir for 5 or 10 days in patients with severe Covid-19. N Engl J Med 2020;383(19):1827–37.

174. Spinner CD, Gottlieb RL, Criner GJ, et al. Effect of remdesivir vs standard care on clinical status at 11 days in patients with moderate COVID-19: a randomized clinical trial. JAMA 2020;324(11):1048–57.

175. National Institutes of Health. The COVID-19 treatment guidelines panel's statement of therapies for high-risk, nonhospitalized patients with mild to moderate COVID-19. Available at: https://www.covid19treatmentguidelines.nih.gov/therapies/statement-on-therapies-for-high-risk-nonhospitalized-patients/. Accessed January 12, 2022.

176. Gottlieb RL, Vaca CE, Paredes R, et al. Early remdesivir to prevent progression to severe Covid-19 in outpatients. N Engl J Med 2021. https://doi.org/10.1056/NEJMoa2116846.

177. Chiotos K, Hayes M, Kimberlin DW, et al. Multicenter interim guidance on use of antivirals for children with coronavirus disease 2019/severe acute respiratory syndrome coronavirus 2. J Pediatr Infect Dis Soc 2021;10(1):34–48.

178. World Health Organization: Therapeutics and COVID-19: Living Guidelines. Available at: https://www.who.int/publications/i/item/WHO-2019-nCoV-therapeutics-2021.3. Accessed January 12, 2022.

179. Chow EJ, Maust B, Kazmier KM, et al. Sinus bradycardia in a pediatric patient treated with remdesivir for acute coronavirus disease 2019: a case report and a review of the literature. J Pediatr Infect Dis Soc 2021;10(9):926–9.

180. U.S. Food and Drug Administration. Coronavirus (COVID-19) update: FDA authorizes additional oral antiviral treatment of COVID-19 in certain adults. Available at: https://www.fda.gov/news-events/press-announcements/coronavirus-covid-19-update-fda-authorizes-additional-oral-antiviral-treatment-covid-19-certain. Accessed January 12, 2022.

181. U.S. Food and Drug Administration. Coronavirus (COVID-19) update: FDA authorizes first oral antiviral for treatment of COVID-19. Available at: https://www.fda.gov/news-events/press-announcements/coronavirus-covid-19-update-fda-authorizes-first-oral-antiviral-treatment-covid-19. Accessed January 12, 2022.

182. Villar J, Ferrando C, Martinez D, et al. Dexamethasone treatment for the acute respiratory distress syndrome: a multicentre, randomised controlled trial. Lancet Respir Med 2020;8(3):267–76.

183. Group RC, Horby P, Lim WS, et al. Dexamethasone in hospitalized patients with Covid-19. N Engl J Med 2021;384(8):693–704.

184. Tomazini BM, Maia IS, Cavalcanti AB, et al. Effect of dexamethasone on days alive and ventilator-free in patients with moderate or severe acute respiratory distress syndrome and COVID-19: the CoDEX randomized clinical trial. JAMA 2020;324(13):1307–16.

185. World Health Organization: Corticosteroids for COVID-19. Available at: https://www.who.int/publications/i/item/WHO-2019-nCoV-Corticosteroids-2020.1. Accessed January 12, 2022.

186. Dulek DE, Fuhlbrigge RC, Tribble AC, et al. Multidisciplinary guidance regarding the use of immunomodulatory therapies for acute coronavirus disease 2019 in pediatric patients. J Pediatr Infect Dis Soc 2020;9(6):716–37.

187. Whittaker E, Bamford A, Kenny J, et al. Clinical characteristics of 58 children with a pediatric inflammatory multisystem syndrome temporally associated with SARS-CoV-2. JAMA 2020;324(3):259–69.

188. Paediatric Intensive Care Society Statement: increased number of reported cases of novel presentation of multisystem inflammatory disease. Available at: https://pccsociety.uk/wp-content/uploads/2020/04/PICS-statement-re-novel-KD-C19-presentation-v2-27042020.pdf. Accessed January 12, 2022.

189. Verdoni L, Mazza A, Gervasoni A, et al. An outbreak of severe Kawasaki-like disease at the Italian epicentre of the SARS-CoV-2 epidemic: an observational cohort study. Lancet 2020;395(10239):1771–8.

190. Riphagen S, Gomez X, Gonzalez-Martinez C, et al. Hyperinflammatory shock in children during COVID-19 pandemic. Lancet 2020;395(10237):1607–8.

191. Grimaud M, Starck J, Levy M, et al. Acute myocarditis and multisystem inflammatory emerging disease following SARS-CoV-2 infection in critically ill children. Ann Intensive Care 2020;10(1):69.

192. Dufort EM, Koumans EH, Chow EJ, et al. Multisystem inflammatory syndrome in children in New York State. N Engl J Med 2020;383(4):347–58.

193. Feldstein LR, Rose EB, Horwitz SM, et al. Multisystem inflammatory syndrome in U.S. children and adolescents. N Engl J Med 2020;383(4):334–46.

194. Royal College of Paediatrics and Child Health. Guidance: paediatric multisystem inflammatory syndrome temporally associated with COVID-19. Available at: https://www.rcpch.ac.uk/sites/default/files/2020-05/COVID-19-Paediatric-multisystem-%20inflammatory%20syndrome-20200501.pdf. Accessed January 12, 2022.

195. Levin M. Childhood Multisystem Inflammatory Syndrome - A New Challenge in the Pandemic. N Engl J Med 2020;383(4):393–5.

196. Centers for Disease Control and Prevention. Multisystem inflammatory syndrome in children (MIS-C) associated with coronavirus disease 2019 (COVID-19). Available at: https://emergency.cdc.gov/han/2020/han00432.asp. Accessed October 28, 2021.

197. Morris SB, Schwartz NG, Patel P, et al. Case series of multisystem inflammatory syndrome in adults associated with SARS-CoV-2 infection - United Kingdom and United States, March-August 2020. MMWR Morb Mortal Wkly Rep 2020;69(40): 1450–6.

198. Hekimian G, Kerneis M, Zeitouni M, et al. Coronavirus disease 2019 acute myocarditis and multisystem inflammatory syndrome in adult intensive and cardiac care units. Chest 2021;159(2):657–62.

199. Davogustto G, Clark DE, Hardison E, et al. Characteristics associated with multisystem inflammatory syndrome among adults with SARS-CoV-2 infection. JAMA Netw Open 2021;4(5):e2110323.

200. Chow EJ. The multisystem inflammatory syndrome in adults with SARS-CoV-2 infection-another piece of an expanding puzzle. JAMA Netw Open 2021;4(5): e2110344.

201. World Health Organization. Multisystem inflammatory syndrome in children and adolescents temporally related to COVID-19. Available at: https://www.who.int/news-room/commentaries/detail/multisystem-inflammatory-syndrome-in-children-and-adolescents-with-covid-19. Accessed January 12, 2022.

202. Payne AB, Gilani Z, Godfred-Cato S, et al. Incidence of multisystem inflammatory syndrome in children among US persons infected with SARS-CoV-2. JAMA Netw Open 2021;4(6):e2116420.

203. Rowley AH. Understanding SARS-CoV-2-related multisystem inflammatory syndrome in children. Nat Rev Immunol 2020;20(8):453–4.

204. Consiglio CR, Cotugno N, Sardh F, et al. The immunology of multisystem inflammatory syndrome in children with COVID-19. Cell 2020;183(4):968–81.e7.

205. Godfred-Cato S, Bryant B, Leung J, et al. COVID-19-associated multisystem inflammatory syndrome in children - United States, March-July 2020. MMWR Morb Mortal Wkly Rep 2020;69(32):1074–80.

206. Sharma C, Ganigara M, Galeotti C, et al. Multisystem inflammatory syndrome in children and Kawasaki disease: a critical comparison. Nat Rev Rheumatol 2021; 17(12):731–48.

207. Feldstein LR, Tenforde MW, Friedman KG, et al. Characteristics and outcomes of US children and adolescents with multisystem inflammatory syndrome in children (MIS-C) compared with severe acute COVID-19. JAMA 2021;325(11): 1074–87.

208. Lee EH, Kepler KL, Geevarughese A, et al. Race/ethnicity among children with COVID-19-associated multisystem inflammatory syndrome. JAMA Netw Open 2020;3(11):e2030280.

209. Abrams JY, Godfred-Cato SE, Oster ME, et al. Multisystem inflammatory syndrome in children associated with severe acute respiratory syndrome coronavirus 2: a systematic review. J Pediatr 2020;226:45–54.e1.

210. Stierman B, Abrams JY, Godfred-Cato SE, et al. Racial and ethnic disparities in multisystem inflammatory syndrome in children in the United States, March 2020 to February 2021. Pediatr Infect Dis J 2021;40(11):e400–6.

211. Javalkar K, Robson VK, Gaffney L, et al. Socioeconomic and racial and/or ethnic disparities in multisystem inflammatory syndrome. Pediatrics 2021;147(5). https://doi.org/10.1542/peds.2020-039933.

212. Ahmed M, Advani S, Moreira A, et al. Multisystem inflammatory syndrome in children: a systematic review. EClinicalMedicine 2020;26. https://doi.org/10.1016/j.eclinm.2020.100527. 100527.

213. Lo Vecchio A, Garazzino S, Smarrazzo A, et al. Factors associated with severe gastrointestinal diagnoses in children with SARS-CoV-2 infection or multisystem inflammatory syndrome. JAMA Netw Open 2021;4(12):e2139974.

214. Young TK, Shaw KS, Shah JK, et al. Mucocutaneous manifestations of multisystem inflammatory syndrome in children during the COVID-19 pandemic. JAMA Dermatol 2021;157(2):207–12.

215. Carlin RF, Fischer AM, Pitkowsky Z, et al. Discriminating multisystem inflammatory syndrome in children requiring treatment from common febrile conditions in outpatient settings. J Pediatr 2021;229:26–32.e2.

216. Sperotto F, Friedman KG, Son MBF, et al. Cardiac manifestations in SARS-CoV-2-associated multisystem inflammatory syndrome in children: a comprehensive review and proposed clinical approach. Eur J Pediatr 2021;180(2):307–22.

217. Kaushik A, Gupta S, Sood M, et al. A systematic review of multisystem inflammatory syndrome in children associated with SARS-CoV-2 infection. Pediatr Infect Dis J 2020;39(11):e340–6.

218. Penner J, Abdel-Mannan O, Grant K, et al. 6-month multidisciplinary follow-up and outcomes of patients with paediatric inflammatory multisystem syndrome (PIMS-TS) at a UK tertiary paediatric hospital: a retrospective cohort study. Lancet Child Adolesc Health 2021;5(7):473–82.

219. Davies P, du Pre P, Lillie J, et al. One-year outcomes of critical care patients post-COVID-19 multisystem inflammatory syndrome in children. JAMA Pediatr 2021;175(12):1281–3.

220. Henderson LA, Canna SW, Friedman KG, et al. American College of Rheumatology clinical guidance for multisystem inflammatory syndrome in children associated with SARS-CoV-2 and hyperinflammation in pediatric COVID-19: version 2. Arthritis Rheumatol 2021;73(4):e13–29.

221. Harwood R, Allin B, Jones CE, et al. A national consensus management pathway for paediatric inflammatory multisystem syndrome temporally associated with COVID-19 (PIMS-TS): results of a national Delphi process. Lancet Child Adolesc Health 2021;5(2):133–41.

222. American Academy of Pediatrics: multisystem inflammatory syndrome in children (MIS-C) interim guidance. Available at: https://www.aap.org/en/pages/2019-novel-coronavirus-covid-19-infections/clinical-guidance/multisystem-inflammatory-syndrome-in-children-mis-c-interim-guidance/. Accessed January 12, 2022.

223. Ouldali N, Toubiana J, Antona D, et al. Association of intravenous immunoglobulins plus methylprednisolone vs immunoglobulins alone with course of fever in multisystem inflammatory syndrome in children. JAMA 2021;325(9):855–64.

224. Son MBF, Murray N, Friedman K, et al. Multisystem inflammatory syndrome in children - initial therapy and outcomes. N Engl J Med 2021;385(1):23–34.

225. Nalbandian A, Sehgal K, Gupta A, et al. Post-acute COVID-19 syndrome. Nat Med 2021;27(4):601–15.

226. Ashkenazi-Hoffnung L, Shmueli E, Ehrlich S, et al. Long COVID in children: observations from a designated pediatric clinic. Pediatr Infect Dis J 2021;40(12):e509–11.

227. Zimmermann P, Pittet LF, Curtis N. How common is long COVID in children and adolescents? Pediatr Infect Dis J 2021;40(12):e482–7.

228. Ludvigsson JF. Case report and systematic review suggest that children may experience similar long-term effects to adults after clinical COVID-19. Acta Paediatr 2021;110(3):914–21.
229. Buonsenso D, Munblit D, De Rose C, et al. Preliminary evidence on long COVID in children. Acta Paediatr 2021;110(7):2208–11.
230. Brackel CLH, Lap CR, Buddingh EP, et al. Pediatric long-COVID: an overlooked phenomenon? Pediatr Pulmonol 2021;56(8):2495–502.
231. Radtke T, Ulyte A, Puhan MA, et al. Long-term symptoms after SARS-CoV-2 infection in children and adolescents. JAMA 2021. https://doi.org/10.1001/jama.2021.11880.
232. Say D, Crawford N, McNab S, et al. Post-acute COVID-19 outcomes in children with mild and asymptomatic disease. Lancet Child Adolesc Health 2021;5(6):e22–3.
233. Kumar S, Veldhuis A, Malhotra T. Neuropsychiatric and cognitive sequelae of COVID-19. Front Psychol 2021;12:577529. https://doi.org/10.3389/fpsyg.2021.577529.
234. Morrow AK, Ng R, Vargas G, et al. Postacute/Long COVID in pediatrics: development of a multidisciplinary rehabilitation clinic and preliminary case series. Am J Phys Med Rehabil 2021;100(12):1140–7.
235. Stephenson T, Shafran R, De Stavola B, et al. Long COVID and the mental and physical health of children and young people: national matched cohort study protocol (the CLoCk study). BMJ Open 2021;11(8):e052838.
236. National Institutes of Health. RECOVER: research COVID to enhance recovery. Available at: https://recovercovid.org/. Accessed January 12, 2022.
237. Schweiberger K, Patel SY, Mehrotra A, et al. Trends in pediatric primary care visits during the coronavirus disease of 2019 pandemic. Acad Pediatr 2021;21(8):1426–33.
238. Courtney JG, Chuke SO, Dyke K, et al. Decreases in young children who received blood lead level testing during COVID-19 - 34 jurisdictions, January-May 2020. MMWR Morb Mortal Wkly Rep 2021;70(5):155–61.
239. DeSilva MB, Haapala J, Vazquez-Benitez G, et al. Association of the COVID-19 pandemic with routine childhood vaccination rates and proportion up to date with vaccinations across 8 US health systems in the Vaccine Safety Datalink. JAMA Pediatr 2022;176(1):68–77.
240. Gerall CD, DeFazio JR, Kahan AM, et al. Delayed presentation and sub-optimal outcomes of pediatric patients with acute appendicitis during the COVID-19 pandemic. J Pediatr Surg 2021;56(5):905–10.
241. Levene R, Fein DM, Silver EJ, et al. The ongoing impact of COVID-19 on asthma and pediatric emergency health-seeking behavior in the Bronx, an epicenter. Am J Emerg Med 2021;43:109–14.
242. Graetz D, Agulnik A, Ranadive R, et al. Global effect of the COVID-19 pandemic on paediatric cancer care: a cross-sectional study. Lancet Child Adolesc Health 2021;5(5):332–40.
243. Racine N, McArthur BA, Cooke JE, et al. Global prevalence of depressive and anxiety symptoms in children and adolescents during COVID-19: a meta-analysis. JAMA Pediatr 2021;175(11):1142–50.
244. Chaffee BW, Cheng J, Couch ET, et al. Adolescents' substance use and physical activity before and during the COVID-19 pandemic. JAMA Pediatr 2021;175(7):715–22.

245. Tandon PS, Zhou C, Johnson AM, et al. Association of children's physical activity and screen time with mental health during the COVID-19 pandemic. JAMA Netw Open 2021;4(10):e2127892.

246. Gassman-Pines A, Ananat EO, Fitz-Henley J 2nd. COVID-19 and parent-child psychological well-being. Pediatrics 2020;146(4). https://doi.org/10.1542/peds.2020-007294.

247. Raffagnato A, Iannattone S, Tascini B, et al. The COVID-19 pandemic: a longitudinal study on the emotional-behavioral sequelae for children and adolescents with neuropsychiatric disorders and their families. Int J Environ Res Public Health 2021;18(18). https://doi.org/10.3390/ijerph18189880.

248. Hanno EC, Fritz LS, Jones SM, et al. School learning format and children's behavioral health during the COVID-19 pandemic. JAMA Pediatr 2022. https://doi.org/10.1001/jamapediatrics.2021.5698.

249. Hillis SD, Unwin HJT, Chen Y, et al. Global minimum estimates of children affected by COVID-19-associated orphanhood and deaths of caregivers: a modelling study. Lancet 2021;398(10298):391–402.

250. Dooley DG, Bandealy A, Tschudy MM. Low-income children and coronavirus disease 2019 (COVID-19) in the US. JAMA Pediatr 2020;174(10):922–3.

251. Parekh N, Ali SH, O'Connor J, et al. Food insecurity among households with children during the COVID-19 pandemic: results from a study among social media users across the United States. Nutr J 2021;20(1):73.

252. Adams EL, Caccavale LJ, Smith D, et al. Food insecurity, the home food environment, and parent feeding practices in the era of COVID-19. Obesity (Silver Spring) 2020;28(11):2056–63.

253. Swedo E, Idaikkadar N, Leemis R, et al. Trends in U.S. emergency department visits related to suspected or confirmed child abuse and neglect among children and adolescents aged <18 years before and during the COVID-19 pandemic - United States, January 2019-September 2020. MMWR Morb Mortal Wkly Rep 2020;69(49):1841–7.

254. Ortiz R, Kishton R, Sinko L, et al. Assessing child abuse hotline inquiries in the wake of COVID-19: answering the call. JAMA Pediatr 2021;175(8):859–61.

255. Sege R, Stephens A. Child physical abuse did not increase during the pandemic. JAMA Pediatr 2021. https://doi.org/10.1001/jamapediatrics.2021.5476.

256. Parks SE, Zviedrite N, Budzyn SE, et al. COVID-19-related school closures and learning modality changes - United States, August 1-September 17, 2021. MMWR Morb Mortal Wkly Rep 2021;70(39):1374–6.

257. U.S. Food and Drug Administration. Coronavirus (COVID-19) update: FDA authorizes additional vaccine dose for certain immunocompromised individuals. Available at: https://www.fda.gov/news-events/press-announcements/fda-authorizes-booster-dose-pfizer-biontech-covid-19-vaccine-certain-populations. Accessed January 12, 2022.

258. U.S. Food and Drug Administration. FDA authorizes booster dose of Pfizer-BioNTech COVID-19 vaccine for certain populations. Available at: https://www.fda.gov/news-events/press-announcements/fda-authorizes-booster-dose-pfizer-biontech-covid-19-vaccine-certain-populations. Accessed January 12, 2022.

259. U.S. Food and Drug Administration. Coronavirus (COVID-19) update: FDA expands eligibility for COVID-19 vaccine boosters. Available at: https://www.fda.gov/news-events/press-announcements/coronavirus-covid-19-update-fda-expands-eligibility-covid-19-vaccine-boosters. Accessed January 12, 2022.

260. U.S. Food and Drug Administration. Moderna COVID-19 Vaccine. Available at: https://www.fda.gov/emergency-preparedness-and-response/coronavirus-disease-2019-covid-19/moderna-covid-19-vaccine. Accessed January 12, 2022.
261. U.S. Food and Drug Administration. Coronavirus (COVID-19) update: FDA shortens interval for booster dose of Moderna COVID-19 vaccine to five months. Available at: https://www.fda.gov/news-events/press-announcements/coronavirus-covid-19-update-fda-shortens-interval-booster-dose-moderna-covid-19-vaccine-five-months. Accessed January 12, 2022.
262. U.S. Food and Drug Administration. Janssen. COVID-19 vaccine. Available at: https://www.fda.gov/emergency-preparedness-and-response/coronavirus-disease-2019-covid-19/janssen-covid-19-vaccine. Accessed January 12, 2022.
263. Centers for Disease Control and Prevention. CDC endorses ACIP's updated COVID-19 vaccine recommendations. Available at: https://www.cdc.gov/media/releases/2021/s1216-covid-19-vaccines.html. Accessed January 12, 2022.
264. A manual for pediatric house officers: the Harriet Lane handbook, 21st edition., 2018, Elsevier, https://www.lebpedsoc.org/doc/HIGHLIGHTS%20FROM%20THE%20LITERATURE/Harriet%20Lane%20Handbook%20%202021st%20ed%20%20%202018.pdf.

COVID-19 Vaccines

William O. Hahn, MD[a],[*], Zanthia Wiley, MD[b]

KEYWORDS

- COVID-19 • Janssen (Ad.26.CoV2) • SARS-CoV-2 • Vaccine • mRNA vaccine
- vaccine efficacy trials • post-marketing vaccine surveillance

KEY POINTS

- The degree of clinical protection against COVID-19 provided by vaccination remains an incredible triumph of modern science.
- Analysis of data generated from "real-world" vaccination cohorts have recapitulated the striking degree of efficacy of vaccination against clinical disease, especially severe disease, observed in randomized controlled trials.
- Although there may be subtle differences with respect to the duration of protection against mild illness conferred by various vaccine products, these differences pale in comparison to the difference between the unvaccinated and those with only immunity following natural infection.

INTRODUCTION

Within 1 year of the first identification of severe acute respiratory syndrome coronavirus 2 (SARS-CoV-2), a series of landmark clinical trials involving a variety of vaccine approaches unequivocally demonstrated that coronavirus disease 2019 (COVID-19) was a vaccine-preventable illness.[1–7] Since the initial demonstration of clinical efficacy in the fall of 2020, several products have achieved authorization or licensure and billions of persons have been vaccinated worldwide. All vaccine candidates to date have demonstrated a high degree of efficacy against hospitalization and severe disease. However, there has been wide variation in the reported efficacy against infection and mildly symptomatic disease, and questions remain whether there are significant differences in the durability of the clinical protection elicited by various vaccine platforms. This review is an attempt to briefly summarize a fast-moving field, with an emphasis on clinical efficacy established in both randomized trials and postmarketing surveillance. Important efforts to address concerns regarding vaccine equity, including the racial and ethnic disparities associated with vaccine access, are addressed elsewhere in Chapter 4.

[a] Division of Infectious Diseases, Department of Medicine, University of Washington, Seattle, WA, USA; [b] Division of Infectious Diseases, Department of Medicine, Emory University, Infectious Diseases Clinic, 550 Peachtree Street NE, 7th Floor - Medical Office Tower, Atlanta, GA 30308, USA
* Corresponding author:
E-mail address: willhahn@uw.edu

Infect Dis Clin N Am 36 (2022) 481–494
https://doi.org/10.1016/j.idc.2022.01.008
0891-5520/22/© 2022 Elsevier Inc. All rights reserved.

Overview of Vaccine Efficacy Trials: Rapid Design and Implementation

Approximately 6 months after the initial description of a respiratory virus syndrome associated with SARS-CoV-2 infection, efficacy trials were initiated in several countries. Within 10 months several products were clinically available, which have now been administered to billions of persons worldwide. The incredible pace of the development schedule has prompted questions from the public regarding whether safety or data quality were compromised in the pursuit of speed. For reference, the shortest development cycle under modern approval mechanisms was approximately 5 years for an Ebola vaccine, and a typical vaccine approval cycle takes 10 to 15 years[8]; the old paradigm for vaccine development timelines has been shattered.

The time savings during the development of COVID-19 vaccines was achieved via unparalleled degrees of public financial support and a higher tolerance for at-risk investment into the technology and process, when compared with previous vaccine development cycles. Some of the key efficiency gains were achieved by immediately initiating efficacy trials after establishing that vaccines were safe and immunogenic rather than waiting for information regarding the durability of the immune response (as would be typical). To further increase the pace of the COVID-19 vaccine trials, a large population was enrolled with a "time-to-event" trial design, whereby prespecified efficacy analysis was based on a specific number of observed infections rather than a predefined observation period. From the implementation side, large amounts of vaccines were manufactured before the establishment of clinical efficacy, meaning that there was substantial risk that resources devoted to manufacturing a vaccine with unknown efficacy could have been wasted if the vaccine failed to provide clinical protection. By manufacturing a large amount of candidate vaccines before demonstrating these vaccines are effective, national health authorities were able to rapidly roll out massive vaccination campaigns immediately after the vaccines were shown to be clinically efficacious. It is important to note that whereas private industry developed and sponsored many of the trials, public dollars supported the trials, substantially decreasing the risk to a particular company from both the clinical trial and manufacturing perspectives.

Currently Approved Vaccines: Overview

The current regulatory landscape is rapidly evolving, but 3 vaccines have achieved emergency use authorization (EUA) in the United States as of 2021: BNT162b2 from Pfizer-BioNTech, mRNA-1273 from Moderna, and the Ad26.COV2.S product from Janssen Pharmaceuticals. The Pfizer (BNT162b2) vaccine has since achieved biologic license application approval from the US Food and Drug Administration (FDA). All 3 have seen widespread implementation, with mRNA vaccines comprising most vaccinations in the United States. Both the Pfizer (BNT162b2) and Moderna (mRNA-1273) vaccines comprise 2 doses, whereas the Janssen vaccine (Ad26.COV2.S) is approved as a one-dose regimen. Advanced candidate vaccines that have undergone (or are undergoing) phase 3 trials to support licensure in the United States include products from Sanofi, Novavax, and AstraZeneca (AZ); these products are undergoing FDA regulatory review, but the approval timeline for these products has not been established as of early 2022. Other vaccines have achieved international licensure but are not, to date, conducting trials to support licensure in the United States.

All vaccines to date target the spike protein of the SARS-CoV-2 virus using a variety of platforms to deliver the spike antigen, including mRNA encapsulated in lipid nanoparticles (LNP) (Pfizer and Moderna), replication-incompetent viruses (AZ/University of Oxford, Janssen, Gameleya), or recombinant proteins (Novavax). Except for the AZ product, all other vaccines in advanced stages in the United States use a modified spike protein designed to be more stable in the prefusion state; the AZ product uses a native sequence. There are more than 50 candidate vaccines in various stages of clinical testing using a variety of approaches; the specific details of these products are beyond the scope of this review.

All phase 3 efficacy trials have been randomized, placebo-controlled trials with laboratory confirmed SARS-CoV-2 infection in combination with symptomatic COVID-19 disease considered the primary end points. The prespecified statistical analysis plan of each trial to date conducted in the United States included a minimum number of clinical end points that triggered an interim analysis (typically around 100–150 cases). In general, the protocols were designed assuming a much lower rate of community transmission than was observed (an assumption of ~1% of placebo recipients per year becoming infected vs an observed rate of ~5%–10% per year); the high rate of community transmission was an underappreciated contributor to the rapid pace of determining that a given vaccine was effective. All the landmark trials reported in the following discussion were conducted before the emergence of the Delta or Omicron variants. Sanofi is currently testing their product and likely will have data from the period coinciding with the emergence of the Delta and Omicron variants.

Safety Data from Phase 3 Efficacy Trials

Although it is somewhat counterintuitive given the rapid pace of vaccine approval, the COVID-19 vaccine trials generated substantially more short-term safety data than would be available during a typical vaccine approval process. For example, each of the efficacy trials intended for licensure in the United States have enrolled (or plan to enroll) approximately 30,000 participants, with between 15,000 and 20,000 administered study product. For comparison, the RESOLVE trial, which was intended to support licensure of a vaccine against lower respiratory tract infection caused by respiratory syncytial virus in older adults only enrolled 11,856 participants with 1:1 randomization, meaning only 5921 participants were administered the study product (https://clinicaltrials.gov/ct2/show/NCT02608502).

Despite the large number of trial participants leading to abundant safety data, important safety signals for these vaccines were only determined with postmarketing surveillance after widespread implementation (see later discussion).

The generally consistent vaccination strategy between products (with 5 of the 6 major vaccine platforms produced in the United States including the same inserts of the spike protein of SARS-CoV-2) offers an unprecedented capacity for comparing the safety profile and performance across various platforms. An important technical note is the conceptual differentiation in safety outcomes between reactogenicity (eg, transient symptoms such as malaise or arm pain) and serious adverse events attributable to the vaccine (eg, Guillain-Barré syndrome [GBS]). The former are quite common with all vaccines, whereas the latter are extremely rare. The Centers for Disease Control and Prevention (CDC) is actively monitoring vaccines implemented using an EUA with several postmarketing surveillance programs.

All vaccines in which trial data have been reported were found to be safe and effective against both mild and severe disease (the Sanofi trial has not reported outcomes as of this writing). All vaccines used the same insert, a SARS-CoV-2 full-length spike, modified with 2 prolines that lock the protein into a form similar to the form the protein has before fusion with the target host cell. Both the Moderna (mRNA 1273) and the

Pfizer (BNT162b2) vaccines require an established cold chain capable of storage at −20°C to 70°C depending on the product, whereas the Janssen adenovirus vector vaccine (Ad26.COV2.S) can be stored for months in a refrigerator (4°C).

Although it is now incontrovertible that clinical COVID-19 can be prevented by vaccination, there are major outstanding questions about how SARS-CoV-2 will evolve in response to immune pressure from both natural immunity and immunity induced by the current generation of SARS-CoV-2 vaccines. In addition, as new variants, such as Delta and Omicron spread, the efficacy of current vaccines against asymptomatic and mild infection, and therefore also in interrupting transmission, is less clear, even while vaccines designed against the ancestral strain retain strong effectiveness against severe disease and death.

Moderna (mRNA-1273)

The Moderna vaccine (mRNA-1273) product is a 100 µg dose of the SARS-CoV-2 spike protein encoded by mRNA and LNP, developed by Moderna and the Vaccine Research Center within the National Institutes of Health. The regimen tested was a 2-dose regimen, administered with a 4-week interval between doses.

Phase 3 clinical trial ("COVE" trial) (**Table 1**) gave the following results:

- Results from a phase 3 randomized, observer-blinded, placebo-controlled trial of the Moderna SARS-CoV-2 vaccine candidate (mRNA-1273) indicated that the vaccine showed 94.1% efficacy at preventing COVID-19 (ancestral and alpha variants), including severe disease. A total of 30,420 volunteers were enrolled (15,210 placebo, 15,210 vaccine).
- Efficacy was similar across key secondary analyses, including in participants who had evidence of SARS-CoV-2 infection at baseline and analyses in participants aged 65 years or older.
- Serious adverse events were rare, and the incidence was similar to placebo.
- Reactogenicity after 1 dose was generally mild to moderate with pain reported as the most common injection site symptom. For systemic reactogenicity symptoms, 54.9% of participants reported solicited adverse events after the first dose (compared with 42.2% of placebo), and this increased to 79.4% with the second dose (compared with 36.5% with placebo). To place this rate in context with other vaccines, the rate of systemic reactogenicity after the first dose is less than that observed for the recombinant adjuvanted zoster vaccine and after the second mRNA-1273 dose is similar.[9] The Shingrix vaccine is a licensed vaccine generally considered to have a "moderate" degree of reactogenicity.

PFIZER (BNT162b2)

The Pfizer product (BNT162b2) is a 30 µg dose of the SARS-CoV-2 spike protein encoded by mRNA and encapsulated with LNP, developed by BioNTech and Pfizer.

Table 1 Phase 3 clinical trial ("COVE" trial)		
	Cases that Meet Primary End Point	Severe Cases
Vaccine	11	0
Placebo	185	30

Data from Baden LR, El Sahly HM, Essink B, et al. Efficacy and safety of the mRNA-1273 SARS-CoV-2 vaccine. N Engl J Med. 2021;384(5):403–16.

The regimen tested was a 2-dose regimen, administered with a 3-week interval between doses.

Results of the phase 3 double-blind, randomized, placebo-controlled trial for the BioNTech and Pfizer mRNA vaccine (BNT162b2) (n = 21,720 in vaccine group, and 21,728 in placebo group) showed a vaccine efficacy of 95% (95% confidence interval [CI], 90.3–97.6) against ancestral strain and Alpha variant, with 8 cases of COVID-19 (1 severe case) in the vaccine group and 162 cases (9 severe cases) in the placebo group (Table 2).

Efficacy was similar across subgroups defined by age, sex, race, ethnicity, body mass index, and presence of coexisting conditions.

Mild to moderate reactogenicity was commonly observed and more frequent with the second dose. Severe fatigue was observed in approximately 4% of Pfizer (BNT162b2) vaccine recipients.

Few participants in either group had severe or serious adverse events, and the 6 deaths (2 in vaccine group, 4 in placebo group) were determined by investigators not to be related to the vaccine or placebo.

JANSSEN (Ad26.COV2.S)

The Janssen (pharmaceutical division of Johnson and Johnson) vaccine product was tested as single-dose regimen in the ENSEMBLE trial (Table 3). The vaccine includes the same insert as the Pfizer (BNT162b2) and Moderna (mRNA-1273) products but uses a well-established replication-incompetent adenovirus (Ad26) as a delivery package. The trial was conducted internationally, with 44% of participants enrolled in the United States, 41% of participants enrolled in South America, and 15% in South Africa. Of note, unlike either the Moderna (mRNA-1273) or Pfizer (BNT162b2) trial, the timing of the ENSEMBLE trial coincided with the emergence of the beta variant (B1.351) in South Africa.[3] As the vaccine was administered as a 1-dose regimen, data regarding protection at both 14 and 28 days (more analogous to the mRNA trials) after administration are presented.

The level of protection against moderate to severe COVID-19 infection was 72% in the United States, 66% in Latin America, and 57% in South Africa 28 days postvaccination. Molecular sequencing of the breakthrough cases suggests a much higher presence of the beta variant in breakthrough cases, in line with the reported epidemiology of the pandemic in South Africa.

VACCINE SAFETY GATHERED FROM POSTMARKETING SURVEILLANCE STUDIES
Allergic Reactions

Anaphylaxis has been rarely observed following vaccination with the mRNA vaccines. In one postmarketing study, 21 cases of anaphylaxis were determined to be related to vaccination (a rate of 11.1 per million doses administered), including 17 in people with prior documented history of allergies/allergic reactions, 7 of whom had a prior history of anaphylaxis. The median interval from vaccine receipt to symptom onset was

Table 2
Pfizer-BioNtech (BNT162b2)

	Cases that Meet Primary End Point	Severe Cases
Vaccine	8	1
Placebo	162	9

Table 3 Janssen (Ad26.COV2.S) ENSEMBLE trial			
	Cases that Meet Primary End Point at D14	Cases that Meet Primary End Point at Day 28	Severe Cases at Day 14	Severe Cases at Day 28
Vaccine	114	65	14	5
Placebo	365	193	60	34

13 minutes.[10] The incidence of acute allergic reactions in health care workers (HCW) who received mRNA COVID-10 vaccines from December 16, 2020, to February 12, 2021, was assessed in a prospective observational cohort study conducted in Boston, Massachusetts. Of the HCW who received an mRNA COVID-19 vaccine and completed a symptom survey, 98% had no symptoms of an allergic reaction (different from true anaphylaxis). Acute allergic reactions were slightly more frequent with the Moderna vaccine (mRNA-1273) (2.20%) compared with Pfizer (BNT162b2) (1.95%), and anaphylaxis occurred at a rate of 2.47 cases per 100,000 vaccinations (similar rates between the Moderna [mRNA-1273] and Pfizer [BNT162b2]). Anaphylaxis was confirmed in 16 HCW, of whom 63% (n = 10) reported prior allergic reaction and 31% (n = 5) reported prior anaphylaxis.[11,12]

Another study performed analysis of safety surveillance data from Vaccine Safety Datalink of 10,162,227 vaccine-eligible members of 8 participating US health plans from December 14, 2020, through June 26, 2021. A total of 11,845,128 doses of mRNA vaccines (57% Pfizer [BNT162b2]: 6,175,813 first doses and 5,669,315 second doses) were administered to 6.2 million individuals (mean age, 49 years; 54% female individuals). Incidence of confirmed anaphylaxis was 4.8 (95% CI, 3.2–6.9) per million doses of Pfizer (BNT162b2) and 5.1 (95% CI, 3.3–7.6) per million doses of Moderna (mRNA-1273).

The current hypothesis is that the reaction is to polyethylene glycol, a preservative used in the vaccines. Persons with a history of hypersensitivity to polyethylene glycol or anaphylaxis to the first dose of an mRNA series should be vaccinated with an alternate product, such as the Janssen (Ad26.COV2.S) vaccine. Similarly, rare persons are known to have severe allergies to polysorbate—present in the Janssen adenovirus vaccine—and these individuals should be vaccinated with an mRNA vaccine.

In addition, there are a wide range of rashes and other skin findings associated with mRNA vaccine administration. None of these are life threatening. One notable finding with the mRNA vaccine is a delayed, local reaction where substantial erythema/induration is observed at the injection site on or around day 8 postvaccine administration; these do not represent true allergy, and patients have safely received repeat vaccinations.

KEY POINTS [TEXT BOX]

- Allergic reactions occur a median of ~15 minutes after product administration
- No cross-reactivity between mRNA and adenoviral vectors, so even a person with documented allergy should be eligible for continuing the series or boosting with an alternative product.
- Delayed injection site reactions (onset on or after day 8) have been reported in ~0.5% to 1% of participants after the first dose; subsequent doses are well tolerated, and therefore delayed injection site reactions are not a contraindication to booster doses.

Myocarditis

Several studies have reported the rare diagnoses of myocarditis following the COVID-19 mRNA vaccines, typically in young men and adolescent boys. In one population-based cohort study of 2,292,924 individuals (median age 49 year old) who received at least 1 dose of COVID-19 mRNA vaccines, acute myocarditis was rare, at an incidence of 5.8 cases per 1 million individuals after the second dose (1 case per 172,414 fully vaccinated individuals).[13] Another study noted that during a 3-month period between February 1, 2021, and April 30, 2021, 7 patients with acute myocarditis were identified, of which 4 occurred within 5 days of COVID-19 vaccination. Three were younger men (age, 23–36 years), and 1 was a 70-year-old woman. All 4 had received the second dose of an mRNA vaccine (2 received Moderna [mRNA-1273], and 2 received Pfizer [BNT162b2]).[14] A retrospective case series of patients within the US Military Health System who experienced myocarditis after COVID-19 vaccination between January and April 2021 identified 23 men (median [range] age, 25 [20–51] years); during this time period more than 2.8 million doses of mRNA COVID-19 vaccine were administered.[15] Data from the largest health care organization in Israel to evaluate the safety of the Pfizer vaccine (BNT162b2) also noted an excess risk of myocarditis in the vaccinated. The control and vaccinated groups each included a mean of 884,828 persons, and vaccination was most strongly associated with an elevated risk of myocarditis (risk ratio, 3.24; 95% CI, 1.55–12.44).

SARS-CoV-2 infection itself is much more strongly associated with increased risk of myocarditis (risk ratio 18.28; 95% CI, 3.95–25.12) with an excess risk of myocarditis (1–5 events per 100,000 persons).[16] In another study of more than 2.5 million vaccinated persons (who were $\geq$16 years old) in this same large health care system, 54 cases met the criteria for myocarditis. Of those who received at least one dose of the Pfizer (BNT162b2) vaccine, the estimated incidence of myocarditis was 2.13 cases per 100,000 persons; the highest incidence was among male patients between the ages of 16 and 29 years (10.69 cases per 100,000 persons). Most cases of myocarditis were mild or moderate in severity.[17] Although the rare risk of myocarditis with mRNA vaccines has been reported, the known risk of morbidity, including cardiac injury and myocarditis, following COVID-19 infection should be taken into consideration.[15]

KEY POINTS

- Risk of myocarditis with COVID-19 infection is higher than with COVID-19 vaccination.
- Myocarditis risk is highest in the first week after a second dose of mRNA vaccine.
- The risk is highest in adolescent boys and young men

Vaccine-Induced Thrombosis and Thrombocytopenia

Cerebral venous sinus thrombosis (CVST) associated with severe thrombocytopenia and disseminated intravascular coagulation that resembles autoimmune heparin-induced thrombocytopenia has been reported in recipients of the Janssen (Ad26.COV2.S) vaccine and recipients of the AZ vaccine (AZD1222 (ChAdOx1-S nCCoV-19). By April 12, 2021, approximately 7 million Janssen (Ad26.COV2.S) vaccine doses were administered in the United States and 6 cases of CVST with thrombocytopenia were diagnosed among recipients, resulting in a temporary pause in vaccination on April 13, 2021. A case series of 12 US patients with CVST and thrombocytopenia following use of the Janssen (Ad26.COV2.S) vaccine was reported to the Vaccine Adverse Event Reporting System (VAERS) from March 2 to April 21, 2021 (with follow-up reported through April 21, 2021). Patient ages ranged from 18 to less than 60 years; all were white women. The time from vaccination to symptom onset ranged from 6 to 15 days. Of the 12 patients with CVST, 7 also had intracerebral bleed; 8 had non-CVST thromboses.[18] On April 23, 2021, the CDC and the FDA recommended that the use of Janssen (Ad26.COV2.S) vaccines resume in the United States, noting that the potential benefits of the vaccine outweigh the potential and known risks.[19] The CDC and FDA also noted that women younger than 50 years should be made aware of alternative COVID-19 vaccine options for which this risk has not been seen and should be made aware of the rare, but increased, risk for CVST. For these reasons, the CDC generally recommends use of mRNA vaccines over the Janssen (Ad26.COV2.S) product in most situations.

KEY POINTS

- Even with extremely low risk of vaccine-induced thrombosis and thrombocytopenia due to adenovirus-vectored vaccines, women younger than 50 years should be made aware of mRNA vaccines if available.
- The CDC currently recommends mRNA vaccines over Janssen (Ad26.COV2.S) based on the differences in safety profile

Guillain-Barré Syndrome

The US FDA also identified a potential safety concern for GBS following Janssen (Ad26.COV2.S) vaccination.[20] Presumptive GBS reports were noted via VAERS between February and July 2021, and as of July 24, 2021, 130 reports of presumptive GBS were identified following Janssen (Ad26.COV2.S) vaccination (median age, 56 years; 111 persons [86.0%] were < 65 years; 77 men [59.7%]). Most reports (93.1%, n = 121) were serious, including 1 death. The estimated crude reporting rate was 1 case of GBS per 100,000 doses administered. The overall estimated observed to expected rate ratio was 4.18 (95% CI, 3.47–4.98) for the 42-day window following immunization, and in the worst-case scenario analysis for adults 18 years or older, corresponded to an estimated absolute rate increase of 6.36 per 100,000 person-years compared with a background rate of approximately 2 cases per 100,000 person-years. For both risk windows, the observed to expected rate ratio was elevated in all age groups except persons aged 18 through 29 years. These findings suggest a small but statistically significant safety concern for GBS following receipt of the Janssen (Ad26.COV2.S) vaccine.[20] Notably, this increase in risk is less than the increased risk of GBS observed following natural SARS-CoV-2 infection.[21]

KEY POINTS

- Risk of GBS is higher with natural SARS-CoV-2 infection than with vaccination with adenovirus-vectored vaccines.

POSTMARKETING STUDIES OF REAL-WORLD EFFICACY
mRNA Vaccines

Adults older than 50 years

High mRNA vaccine effectiveness among older adults has been reported. A common approach to establishing efficacy in a real-world setting is a "test-negative" design. In this approach, patients tested clinically for SARS-CoV-2 infection are compared with those who tested negative. These analyses are relatively easy to conduct, but one potential criticism is that the underlying indication for testing can change based on the population (eg, asymptomatic screening vs patients presenting with upper respiratory tract symptoms). A study of adults (>50 years old) with COVID-19-like illness who underwent SARS-CoV-2 molecular testing evaluated 41,552 hospital admissions and 21,522 visits to emergency department or urgent care clinics in multiple states from January 1 through June 22, 2021. The effectiveness of full mRNA vaccination (>14 days after the second dose) was 89% against laboratory-confirmed SARS-CoV-2 infection leading to hospitalization, 90% against infection leading to an intensive care unit admission, and 91% against infection leading to an emergency department or urgent care clinic visit (against ancestral or Alpha strains). The effectiveness of full vaccination with respect to a COVID-19-associated hospitalization or emergency department or urgent care clinic visit was similar with the Pfizer (BNT162b2) and Moderna (mRNA-1273) vaccines and ranged from 81% to 95% among adults aged 85 year or older, those with chronic medical conditions, and black or Hispanic adults.[22] Another study found that among adults aged 65 to 74 years, effectiveness of full vaccination for preventing hospitalization was 96% for Pfizer (BNT162b2) and 96% for Moderna (mRNA-1273) and among adults aged 75 years or older, effectiveness of full vaccination for preventing hospitalizations was 91% for Pfizer (BNT162b2) and 96% for Moderna (mRNA-1273).[23]

All adult populations

One early study was conducted during a nationwide mass vaccination in Israel's largest health care organization of persons newly vaccinated with Pfizer (BNT162b2) between December 20, 2020, and February 1, 2021. Each study group (vaccinated and unvaccinated controls) included 596,618 persons. Estimated vaccine effectiveness at days 14 through 20 after the first dose and at 7 days or more after the second dose was as follows: for documented infection, 46% and 92%; for symptomatic COVID-19, 57% and 94%; for hospitalization, 74% and 87%; and for severe disease, 62% and 92%, respectively (ancestral strain and Alpha variant). Estimated effectiveness in preventing death from COVID-19 was 72% for days 14 through 20 after the first dose. The effectiveness in specific subgroups evaluated for documented infection and symptomatic COVID-19 was consistent across age groups, with potentially slightly lower effectiveness in persons with multiple coexisting conditions.[24] Another early study during December 14, 2020, to April 10, 2021, with data from the HEROES-RECOVER Cohorts, a network of prospective cohorts among frontline workers, found that both the Pfizer (BNT162b2) and Moderna (mRNA-1273) mRNA COVID-19 vaccines were approximately 90% effective in preventing symptomatic and asymptomatic COVID-19 infections.[25]

US studies noted high mRNA vaccine effectiveness as well. The effectiveness of mRNA vaccines against COVID-19-associated hospitalization among 1175 US veterans aged 18 years or older at 5 Veterans Affairs Medical Centers (VAMCs) during February 1 to August 6, 2021 (when the B.1.617.2 [Delta] variant was dominant) was measured. The overall adjusted vaccine effectiveness against COVID-19-associated hospitalization was 86.8% and was similar before (February 1 to June 30) and during

(July 1 to August 6) SARS-CoV-2 Delta variant predominance (84.1% vs 89.3%, respectively). Vaccine effectiveness was 79.8% among adults aged 65 years or older and 95.1% among veterans aged 18 to 64 years.[26] A test-negative, case-control analysis of 3689 US adults aged 18 years or older hospitalized at 21 US hospitals across 18 states during March 11 to August 15, 2021, was performed, and among adults without immunocompromising conditions, vaccine effectiveness against COVID-19 hospitalization was 93% for the Moderna (mRNA-1273) vaccine and 88% for the Pfizer (BNT162b2) vaccine.[27]

Studies of mRNA vaccine effectiveness that extended over longer periods and further into the Delta variant surge continued to note high vaccine effectiveness, although declines in effectiveness from earlier studies were reported. A matched test-negative, case-control study designed to estimate vaccine effectiveness against any SARS-CoV-2 infection and against any severe, critical, or fatal case of COVID-19, from January 1 to September 5, 2021, was performed, and the estimated Pfizer (BNT162b2) vaccine effectiveness against any SARS-CoV-2 infection reached its peak at 77.5% in the first month after the second dose. Thereafter, the effectiveness gradually declined, with the decline accelerating (after the fourth month) to approximately 20% in months 5 through 7 after the second dose. Variant-specific effectiveness waned in the same pattern. This contrasted with the pattern seen for severe disease where following vaccination, effectiveness against any severe, critical, or fatal case of COVID-19 was 66.1% by the third week after the first dose and reached 96% or higher in the first 2 months after the second dose; effectiveness persisted at approximately this level for 6 months.[28] Another large US health care system study assessed Pfizer (BNT162b2) vaccine effectiveness against SARS-CoV-2 infections and COVID-19-related hospital admissions among more than 3.4 million individuals between December 14, 2020, and August 8, 2021. For the fully vaccinated, effectiveness against SARS-CoV-2 infections was 73%, and against COVID-19-related hospital admissions it was 90%. Effectiveness against infections declined from 88% during the first month after full vaccination to 47% after 5 months. For those who received 2 doses, effectiveness against SARS-CoV-2 infections was 73%, and against COVID-19-related hospital admissions it was 90%. Effectiveness against infections declined from 88% during the first month after full vaccination to 47% after 5 months.[29]

Janssen (Ad26.COV2.S) Vaccine

Adults older than 50 years
A study of adults (>50 years of age) with COVID-19-like illness who underwent molecular testing for SARS-CoV-2) assessed 41,552 hospital admissions and 21,522 visits to emergency department or urgent care clinics between January 1 and June 22, 2021, in multiple states. The effectiveness of the Janssen vaccine (Ad26.COV2.S) was 68% against laboratory-confirmed SARS-CoV-2 infection leading to an emergency department or urgent care clinic visit.[22] Among adults aged 65 to 74 years, effectiveness of full vaccination for preventing hospitalization was 84%, and among adults aged 75 years or older effectiveness of full vaccination for preventing hospitalizations was 85%.[23]

All adults
A case-control analysis among 3689 adults aged 18 years or older who were hospitalized at 21 US hospitals across 18 states during March 11 to August 15, 2021, among adults without immunocompromising conditions, vaccine effectiveness against COVID-19 hospitalization was 71%.[27] A comparative effectiveness US study across

multistate Mayo Clinic Health System between February 27 and July 22, 2021, of 8889 vaccinated persons and 88,898 unvaccinated persons (mean age, 52.4 years and 51.7, respectively) found a vaccine effectiveness of 73.6% (95% CI, 65.9%–79.9%) and a 3.73-fold reduction in SARS-CoV-2 infections.[30]

NEED FOR ADDITIONAL DOSES BEYOND PRIMARY SERIES ("BOOSTER DOSES")

The initial large-scale vaccinations against COVID-19 occurred less than 1 year before the drafting of this publication. Data regarding the long-term durability of clinical protection are rapidly emerging. Nevertheless, it has been repeatedly observed that neutralizing antibody titers wane, albeit with some variation by product. Titers induced by the Janssen (Ad26.COV2.S) vaccine seem lower but more stable over time, whereas neutralizing titers induced by the mRNA vaccines are initially higher but seem to decline with a steeper slope.[31] There seem to be subtle differences in the durability of clinical protection, with the Moderna (mRNA-1273) vaccine appearing to provide a slightly longer period of protection when compared with the Pfizer (BNT162b2) or Janssen (Ad26.COV2.S) vaccines.[32] Neutralizing antibody titers were a clear surrogate of protection observed in the initial randomized trial of the Moderna (mRNA-1273) product.[33] In combination with the observation that there are emerging data suggesting a waning of clinical immunity[32] and the observation that boosting with any product leads to an increase in antibody titers,[34] a mass-scale booster program was initiated in the United States toward the end of 2021.

The FDA authorized a booster dose for all persons regardless of primary series. In addition, the CDC does not differentiate their recommendations for a booster based on the initial product or platform. Finally, it is important to note that the approved dose of the booster is different from the dose approved for the primary series with respect to the Moderna (mRNA-1273) vaccine, where the dose is half of the initial dose. The Pfizer (BNT162b2) dose is the same as the primary series, and the Janssen booster dose (Ad26.COV2.S) is the same dose as the initial series. The reduced dose of the mRNA was selected to relieve pressure on manufacturing capacity and also to potentially reduce reactogenicity.

SUMMARY

The degree of clinical protection against COVID-19 provided by vaccination remains an incredible triumph of modern science. Analysis of data generated from "real-world" vaccination cohorts have recapitulated the striking degree of efficacy of vaccination against clinical disease, especially severe disease, observed in randomized controlled trials. Extremely rare severe adverse events, such as myocarditis, are much more likely to occur with clinical COVID-19 than after vaccination. Even for persons with documented anaphylaxis to a vaccine component, alternative vaccination strategies exist. Although there may be subtle differences with respect to the duration of protection against mild illness conferred by various vaccine products, these differences pale in comparison to the difference between the unvaccinated and those with only immunity following natural infection. The emergence of the Omicron variant has been associated with substantial immune escape, and the full degree of loss of protection against clinical disease is not yet clear at the time this article was prepared. It is clear, however, that substantial protection against severe disease has been maintained with vaccination, and it is clear that vaccination remains the best method for preventing severe disease.

CLINICS CARE POINTS

- Even for persons with documented anaphylaxis to a vaccine component, alternative vaccination strategies exist.

- There may be subtle differences with respect to the duration of protection against mild illness conferred by various vaccine products, these differences pale in comparison to the difference between the unvaccinated and those with only immunity following natural infection.

- The degree of clinical protection against COVID-19 provided by vaccination remains an incredible triumph of modern science.

REFERENCES

1. Polack FP, Thomas SJ, Kitchin N, et al. Safety and efficacy of the BNT162b2 mRNA Covid-19 vaccine. N Engl J Med 2020;383(27):2603–15.
2. Baden LR, El Sahly HM, Essink B, et al. Efficacy and safety of the mRNA-1273 SARS-CoV-2 vaccine. N Engl J Med 2021;384(5):403–16.
3. Sadoff J, Gray G, Vandebosch A, et al. Safety and efficacy of single-dose Ad26.-COV2.S vaccine against Covid-19. N Engl J Med 2021;384(23):2187–201.
4. Falsey AR, Sobieszczyk ME, Hirsch I, et al. Phase 3 safety and efficacy of AZD1222 (ChAdOx1 nCoV-19) Covid-19 vaccine. N Engl J Med 2021. https://doi.org/10.1056/NEJMoa2105290.
5. Heath PT, Galiza EP, Baxter DN, et al. Safety and efficacy of NVX-CoV2373 Covid-19 vaccine. N Engl J Med 2021;385(13):1172–83.
6. Jara A, Undurraga EA, González C, et al. Effectiveness of an inactivated SARS-CoV-2 vaccine in Chile. N Engl J Med 2021;385(10):875–84.
7. Logunov DY, Dolzhikova IV, Shcheblyakov DV, et al. Safety and efficacy of an rAd26 and rAd5 vector-based heterologous prime-boost COVID-19 vaccine: an interim analysis of a randomised controlled phase 3 trial in Russia. Lancet 2021;397(10275):671–81.
8. Wolf J, Bruno S, Eichberg M, et al. Applying lessons from the Ebola vaccine experience for SARS-CoV-2 and other epidemic pathogens. NPJ Vaccines 2020;5(1):51.
9. Cunningham AL, Lal H, Kovac M, et al. Efficacy of the herpes zoster subunit vaccine in adults 70 years of age or older. N Engl J Med 2016;375(11):1019–32.
10. CDC COVID-19 Response Team, Food and Drug Administration. Allergic Reactions Including Anaphylaxis After Receipt of the First Dose of Pfizer-BioNTech COVID-19 Vaccine - United States, December 14-23, 2020. MMWR Morb Mortal Wkly Rep 2021;70(2):46–51.
11. Blumenthal KG, Robinson LB, Camargo CA, et al. Acute allergic reactions to mRNA COVID-19 vaccines. JAMA 2021;325(15):1562–5.
12. Klein NP, Lewis N, Goddard K, et al. Surveillance for adverse events After COVID-19 mRNA vaccination. JAMA 2021;326(14):1390–9.
13. Simone A, Herald J, Chen A, et al. Acute myocarditis following COVID-19 mRNA vaccination in adults aged 18 years or older. JAMA Intern Med 2021;181(12):1668–70.
14. Kim JH, Levine BD, Phelan D, et al. Coronavirus disease 2019 and the athletic heart: emerging perspectives on pathology, risks, and return to play. JAMA Cardiol 2021;6(2):219–27.

15. Montgomery J, Ryan M, Engler R, et al. Myocarditis following immunization with mRNA COVID-19 vaccines in members of the US military. JAMA Cardiol 2021; 6(10):1202–6.

16. Barda N, Dagan N, Ben-Shlomo Y, et al. Safety of the BNT162b2 mRNA Covid-19 vaccine in a nationwide setting. N Engl J Med 2021;385(12):1078–90.

17. Witberg G, Barda N, Hoss S, et al. Myocarditis after Covid-19 vaccination in a large health care organization. N Engl J Med 2021;385(23):2132–9.

18. See I, Su JR, Lale A, et al. US case reports of cerebral venous sinus thrombosis with thrombocytopenia after Ad26.COV2.S vaccination, March 2 to April 21, 2021. JAMA 2021;325(24):2448–56.

19. CDC. CDC recommends use of johnson & johnson's janssen COVID-19 Vaccine Resume. 2021. Accessed. https://www.cdc.gov/coronavirus/2019-ncov/vaccines/safety/JJUpdate.html. [Accessed 12 November 2021]. Available at.

20. Woo EJ, Mba-Jonas A, Dimova RB, et al. Association of receipt of the Ad26.-COV2.S COVID-19 vaccine with presumptive guillain-barré syndrome, February-July 2021. JAMA 2021;326(16):1606–13.

21. Fragiel M, Miró Ò, Llorens P, et al. Incidence, clinical, risk factors and outcomes of Guillain-Barré in Covid-19. Ann Neurol 2021;89(3):598–603.

22. Thompson MG, Burgess JL, Naleway AL, et al. Prevention and ATtenuation of Covid-19 with the BNT162b2 and mRNA-1273 vaccines. N Engl J Med 2021; 385(4):320–9.

23. Moline HL, Whitaker M, Deng L, et al. Effectiveness of COVID-19 vaccines in preventing hospitalization among adults Aged ≥65 Years - COVID-NET, 13 States, February-April 2021. MMWR Morb Mortal Wkly Rep 2021;70(32):1088–93.

24. Dagan N, Barda N, Kepten E, et al. BNT162b2 mRNA Covid-19 vaccine in a nationwide mass vaccination setting. N Engl J Med 2021;384(15):1412–23.

25. Thompson MG, Burgess JL, Naleway AL, et al. Interim estimates of vaccine effectiveness of BNT162b2 and mRNA-1273 COVID-19 vaccines in preventing SARS-CoV-2 Infection among health care personnel, first responders, and other essential and frontline workers - Eight U.S. Locations, December 2020-March 2021. MMWR Morb Mortal Wkly Rep 2021;70(13):495–500.

26. Bajema KL, Dahl RM, Prill MM, et al. Effectiveness of COVID-19 mRNA vaccines against COVID-19-associated hospitalization - five veterans affairs medical centers, United States, February 1-August 6, 2021. MMWR Morb Mortal Wkly Rep 2021;70(37):1294–9.

27. Self WH, Tenforde MW, Rhoads JP, et al. Comparative effectiveness of moderna, Pfizer-BioNTech, and janssen (johnson & johnson) vaccines in preventing COVID-19 hospitalizations among adults without immunocompromising conditions - United States, March-August 2021. MMWR Morb Mortal Wkly Rep 2021;70(38): 1337–43.

28. Chemaitelly H, Tang P, Hasan MR, et al. Waning of BNT162b2 vaccine protection against SARS-CoV-2 Infection in Qatar. N Engl J Med 2021. https://doi.org/10.1056/NEJMoa2114114.

29. Tartof SY, Slezak JM, Fischer H, et al. Effectiveness of mRNA BNT162b2 COVID-19 vaccine up to 6 months in a large integrated health system in the USA: a retrospective cohort study. Lancet 2021;398(10309):1407–16.

30. Corchado-Garcia J, Zemmour D, Hughes T, et al. Analysis of the effectiveness of the Ad26.COV2.S adenoviral vector vaccine for preventing COVID-19. JAMA Netw Open 2021;4(11):e2132540.

31. Collier A-RY, Yu J, McMahan K, et al. Differential Kinetics of Immune Responses Elicited by Covid-19 Vaccines. N Engl J Med 2021. https://doi.org/10.1056/NEJMc2115596.
32. Uschner D, Bott M, Santacatterina M, et al. Breakthrough SARS-CoV-2 infections after vaccination in North Carolina. bioRxiv 2021. https://doi.org/10.1101/2021.10.10.21264812.
33. Gilbert PB, Montefiori DC, McDermott A, et al. Immune correlates analysis of the mRNA-1273 COVID-19 vaccine efficacy trial. medRxiv 2021. https://doi.org/10.1101/2021.08.09.21261290.
34. Atmar RL, Lyke KE, Deming ME, et al. Heterologous SARS-CoV-2 booster vaccinations - preliminary report. medRxiv 2021. https://doi.org/10.1101/2021.10.10.21264827.

9780323919791